State of Immunity

CALIFORNIA/MILBANK BOOKS ON HEALTH AND THE PUBLIC

State of Immunity

*The Politics of Vaccination
in Twentieth-Century America*

James Colgrove

UNIVERSITY OF CALIFORNIA PRESS
Berkeley · Los Angeles · London

MILBANK MEMORIAL FUND
New York

University of California Press
Berkeley and Los Angeles, California

University of California Press, Ltd.
London, England

Library of Congress Cataloging-in-Publication Data

Colgrove, James Keith.
    State of immunity : the politics of vaccination
in twentieth-century America / James Colgrove.
        p. ; cm. — (California/Milbank books on health
and the public ; 16)
    Includes bibliographical references and index.
    ISBN-13, 978-0-520-24749-3 (cloth : alk. paper),
ISBN-10, 0-520-24749-3 (cloth : alk. paper)
    1. Vaccination—United States—History—20th century.
    2. Medical policy—United States—History—20th
century. I. Title. II. Series. [DNLM: 1. Vaccination—
history—United States. 2. Attitude to Health—United
States. 3. Health Policy—history—United States.
4. History, 20th Century—United States. QW 806
C695s 2006]
    RA638.C64 2006
    614.4'7—dc22   2006002049

Manufactured in the United States of America

15   14   13   12   11   10   09   08   07   06
10   9   8   7   6   5   4   3   2   1

This book is printed on New Leaf EcoBook 50, a 100%
recycled fiber of which 50% is de-inked post-consumer
waste, processed chlorine-free. EcoBook 50 is acid-free and
meets the minimum requirements of ANSI/ASTM D 5634–01
(*Permanence of Paper*). ∞

Contents

Illustrations

Foreword

The Milbank Memorial Fund is an endowed operating foundation that works to improve health by helping decision makers in the public and private sectors acquire and use the best available evidence to inform policy for health care and population health. The Fund has engaged in nonpartisan analysis and research on and communication about significant issues in health policy since its inception in 1905.

State of Immunity: The Politics of Vaccination in Twentieth-Century America is the sixteenth of the California/Milbank Books on Health and the Public. The publishing partnership between the Fund and University of California Press seeks to encourage the synthesis and communication of findings from research that could contribute to more effective health policy.

James Colgrove argues that the history of vaccination policy "is one of politics as much as of science." He describes how "vaccination policy evolved through a series of confrontations" between decision makers in local, state, and national government and both individuals and interest groups. The courts and popular media were central to most of these confrontations. Each of these events in the history of vaccination policy, Colgrove writes, can only be understood by studying the political effects of "differing values, beliefs, and standards of proof."

The history Colgrove presents has implications for contemporary policy. An important current dispute, for example, is about how many children can be exempted from vaccination at the request of their parents before the size of the unvaccinated population could threaten the health of the community. Scientists can calculate when this threat could arise, but elected officials must be willing to apply their findings in policy and public education.

Daniel M. Fox
President

Samuel L. Milbank
Chairman

Acknowledgments

Many people contributed both directly and indirectly to the writing of this book, and I am pleased to have the opportunity to thank them.

The patient and diligent help of numerous archivists and librarians made this research possible. I am grateful for the assistance of Kenneth Cobb, Gabriel Gervais, and Leonora Gidlund at the New York City Municipal Archives; Jim Folts and his staff at the New York State Archives; Marjorie Ciarlante at the National Archives and Records Administration, College Park, Maryland; Charles Reeves and Richard Rayburn at the National Archives and Records Administration, East Point, Georgia; David Rose at the March of Dimes archives; Jack Termine at the Medical Research Library of Brooklyn, State University of New York; Stephen Novak at the Hammer Health Sciences Library, Columbia University; Elisabeth Wittman and Joel Thoreson at the archives of the Evangelical Lutheran Church in America; Stephen Greenberg and the reference staff of the History of Medicine Division at the National Library of Medicine; and the librarians at the New York Academy of Medicine. I give a special thanks to Walter Orenstein, former director of the National Immunization Program at the Centers for Disease Control and Prevention, for providing me with a complete set of the proceedings of the national immunization conferences.

This book began as a dissertation in the Department of Sociomedical Sciences at Columbia University's Mailman School of Public Health. I owe an incalculable debt to the five members of my dissertation committee, whose critiques of draft chapters greatly improved the final work. Most of all I thank Ronald Bayer, who has been an extraordinary mentor and friend throughout the years I worked on this manuscript. Ron's insight, rigor, and ability to ask the right questions were guiding forces behind this research from its inception to its completion. Amy Fairchild offered astute editing and assistance at every stage. David Rosner gave me many helpful comments and suggestions. Elizabeth Blackmar, in addition to providing thoughtful advice on the final manuscript, challenged me at an early stage of my research to shape my arguments more carefully. Allan Brandt's incisive feedback helped me think about my findings in new ways. I was fortunate to conduct my research in the Center for the History and Ethics of Public Health, which is as collegial and intellectually stimulating an environment as any scholar could wish for. I thank Richard Parker, my department chair, for his support of my work and that of my colleagues in the center. My fellow doctoral students at the Mailman School of Public Health have provided encouragement and empathy. I especially thank Dina Feivelson, Beth Filiano, Marian Jones, Paola Mejía-Rodríguez, Sheena Morrison, Elizabeth Robilotti, Nick Turse, and Daniel Wolfe.

Many colleagues have helped me think through ideas and provided valuable insights. I have benefited from conversations with John Ballard, Virginia Berridge, Héctor Carrillo, Cynthia Connolly, Nadav Davidovitch, Steve Epstein, Kenneth Jackson, Constance Nathanson, Gerald Oppenheimer, Naomi Rogers, and Charles Rosenberg. I thank Alison Bateman-House for carefully proofreading the manuscript.

The editorial staff of the University of California Press has been unfailingly helpful. I am grateful for the guidance of Stan Holwitz, Randy Heyman, Dore Brown, and Lynne Withey, and for the thorough copyediting of Peter Dreyer. I also thank Daniel Fox of the Milbank Memorial Fund for his support of the manuscript as part of the California/Milbank series on health and the public.

A portion of chapter 1 originally appeared in the *Bulletin of the History of Medicine* and is reprinted here by permission of Johns Hopkins University Press. A shorter version of chapter 2 originally appeared in *Isis*, © 2005 by the History of Science Society, and is reprinted by permission. A portion of chapter 3 originally appeared in *Public Health Reports* and is reprinted by permission.

I would have been unable to complete this book without a devoted family of friends. David Dunbar's daily messages and regular visits were wonderful sources of support. Naomi Schegloff's humor and empathy helped me through many difficult spots. My work would have been much more challenging without the friendship of Carole Cooper, James Holmes, Martina Lynch, Anthony Myers, Cookie Neil, Julie Potts, Catherine Rohweder, Silja Talvi, Nancy Worthington, and Vanessa Vichit-Vadakan. The generous spirit of the late Tom Lindsay remained an inspiration to me after Tom's death in 2003.

Finally, I express my love and gratitude to Robert Sember for the many things he has taught me.

Introduction

Vaccination Politics and Law
in American History

In January 1931, Charles Hoppe, a Brooklyn theosophist, vegetarian, and self-described "conscientious objector to vaccination," appealed to New York City's health commissioner for help. Hoppe's eight-year-old son Robert faced exclusion from school because he lacked the legally required protection against smallpox. "It is revolting to say the least," the elder Hoppe wrote to the commissioner, "to think I must have diseased animal matter injected into the blood of my child before he can receive an education."[1] In addition to philosophical scruples against the procedure, Hoppe's resistance was rooted in a past tragedy: one of his other sons had died several years earlier after being immunized against diphtheria, and Hoppe was convinced the injection was responsible. The commissioner was a strong proponent of immunization, having spearheaded one of the largest advertising campaigns ever seen in the city to persuade parents to protect their children against diphtheria, but he was moved by the persistence of Hoppe's pleas and the sincerity of his beliefs. He was also sensitive to the dangers of antagonizing a local anti-vaccination society that was engaged in a vigorous effort to overturn the state law requiring the procedure for students. Against the advice of the health department's legal counsel—New York state law provided no exemption from vaccination based on religious or philosophical beliefs—the commissioner arranged for a special certificate of admission so that Robert Hoppe could attend school.[2]

One of the most fundamental and enduring tensions in the enterprise of public health is the balance between the rights of the individual and the claims of the collective, and nowhere is this dynamic more salient than in policies and practices surrounding immunization. For two centuries, vaccines, first against smallpox and then a host of other contagions, have protected communities from diseases that in previous eras were responsible for the majority of the world's illness and death. Like any medical intervention, vaccination carries the small risk of sometimes severe adverse reactions. But unlike other procedures, vaccination is performed on healthy people. It has also been mandated by law, most commonly for children attending school, because of its unique social benefit. It has been one of the most highly lauded public health activities, but it has also been vilified by a small minority because of disbelief in its efficacy and safety, religious or philosophical objections, opposition to state coercion, or some combination of these factors.

A century ago, just a handful of vaccines had been developed, and only one, for smallpox, was commonly used in the United States. A loose patchwork of widely varying local and state laws governed the practice, some requiring it only during epidemics and others for students in public schools. Enforcement was often haphazard, and large segments of the population, both adults and children, remained unimmunized. In 2006, there are more than two dozen vaccines in use, fourteen of which are universally recommended for children. Levels of coverage among youth have topped 90 percent for most vaccines, and as a result, almost all of the conditions they protect against have declined to the vanishing point in the United States. To achieve this state of immunity, vaccine proponents have used a variety of strategies to secure the trust, cooperation, and compliance of the public; their efforts have provoked a wide range of reactions, including enthusiasm, indifference, skepticism, and hostility. They have trodden carefully between respect for individual liberty in medical matters and the need to protect the community against disease. As the case of Charles Hoppe illustrates, pragmatism and political acuity, rather than doctrinaire adherence to epidemiological theory or ethical principles, typically guided their decision making.

Seventy-five years after Hoppe pled his case, many of the fundamental policy issues surrounding vaccination remain the same. Mistrust of the safety of vaccines has waxed and waned since then, but it has experienced a dramatic resurgence in the past two decades, in the course of which a diverse and loosely organized social movement opposed to vaccination has challenged the judgment and integrity of the scientific and medical establishment. In response to pressure from parent activists who believed their children had been harmed by vaccines, a U.S. House of Representatives committee held repeated hearings on vaccine safety beginning in 1999, at which public health officials and scientists were often cast in an adversarial role against groups and individuals questioning whether the risks of vaccines outweighed their benefits. The Institute of Medicine, a branch of the National Academies that advises the government on health issues, has published eight reports in the past five years examining—and generally rejecting—the hypothesized connections between vaccinations and a variety of disorders, including autism. Not coincidentally, state laws requiring vaccinations before children may enroll in school have continued to generate controversy, and the question of which children, if any, may be exempt from these laws remains highly contentious.

This book tells the story of how vaccination became a widely accepted component of the American health care system over the course of the twentieth century and analyzes the social context that has shaped this evolution. I examine the motivations and actions of a range of stakeholders—public health officials, physicians, charitable organizations, pharmaceutical manufacturers, parents, school administrators, and lawmakers—and the most significant points of consensus, discord, and controversy among them. Because it enters into the lives of the vast majority of Americans and has exerted such a powerful, if often unseen, influence on patterns of illness and death, vaccination serves as a lens through which we may view some of the most important issues in twentieth-century social history: the changing role of the state and its duties to maintain the health of citizens; popular attitudes toward scientific expertise and authority; the acceptance of unorthodox and alternative views of health, illness, and medicine; the limits of parental autonomy when child-rearing practices conflict with socially accepted norms; and shifting views of the legal and ethical responsibility for risks both naturally occurring and human-made.

RISK, COERCION, AND THE ETHICS OF VACCINATION

The epidemiologic foundation for vaccination is the phenomenon, first formally described in the 1920s, of herd immunity, by which an entire community will be protected against a contagion if a sufficiently large percentage of the group is immune. The optimal situation for the community occurs when each member assumes the small risk of undergoing vaccination in order to protect both himself or herself and the group as a whole; a successful vaccination program thus depends at least in part on individuals making an altruistic decision. But as one analysis noted, "an individual's ideal strategy would be to encourage everyone else to be vaccinated, [except] himself or herself (or his or her child)."[3] Thus a paradox exists: the decision of any one individual to refuse vaccination will not affect the group's protection, but if too many people make that choice, those decisions in the aggregate will undermine herd immunity. Those who are fit to undergo vaccination but do not do so have been termed "free riders" since they enjoy the benefit of herd immunity that results from other members of the community having assumed the small risk of vaccination.[4]

One of the most eloquent explorations of the failure of altruism was provided by the environmentalist Garrett Hardin in a 1968 essay in the journal *Science*. Hardin described the "tragedy of the commons," in which each individual, placing self-interest first, acts in ways that are contrary to the good of the collective and, ultimately, his own good. Hardin's trenchant critique of libertarian philosophy was directed at the issue of environmental degradation, but it was also highly applicable to immunization policy, because it suggested an ethical foundation for the acceptability of coercive measures to ensure the common welfare. "To many, the word *coercion* implies arbitrary decisions of distant and irresponsible bureaucrats; but this is not a necessary part of its meaning," Hardin wrote. "The only kind of coercion I recommend is mutual coercion, mutually agreed upon by the majority of the people affected."[5]

The acceptability of coercion in the United States has been shaped by a strong cultural ethos antagonistic to paternalism. In what has become known as the "harm principle," the nineteenth-century utilitarian philosopher John Stuart Mill famously contended that the only justification for coercive action against an individual was the presence of imminent harm to other members of society: a person's own good, Mill wrote, "is not sufficient warrant."[6] Opponents of mandatory vaccination have often cited Mill's dictum, arguing that the individual who declines the procedure places only himself at risk. But even the most effective vaccines do not provide 100 percent protection; a small number of people who undergo vaccination will fail to develop the intended immunity (cases known as "vaccine failures"). Furthermore, some vaccines are medically contraindicated for people with certain biological susceptibilities such as weakened immune systems. Thus some members of the community who, though willing to assume the risk, are unable to benefit may be placed in danger by vaccine refusers. Because the decision not to be vaccinated does have "other-regarding" consequences, to use Mill's phrase, some philosophers have advanced the harm principle as the key ethical justification for compulsory vaccination.[7]

As these analyses make clear, the use of vaccination has required that society confront two closely interrelated issues that must frequently be resolved in policy and law: risk and coercion. Risk—the possibility that a negative event will occur—is a complex phenomenon with cultural, political, and legal dimensions. As a large body of social science literature has shown, the risks that both individuals and society deem significant serve as a revealing barometer of their attitudes and values.[8] Several types of risk figure in decisions to be vaccinated: the risk of contracting the disease a vaccine is designed to prevent; the risk of suffering an adverse event caused by the vaccination; and the risk an individual may impose on others by remaining without protection.

Vaccines today are very safe. The vast majority of side effects are transient and superficial, including pain and swelling at the injection site or moderately elevated fever. But rare severe events have been well documented, such as paralytic polio caused by one in several million doses of the oral polio vaccine, or dangerous encephalitis resulting from one in several thousand doses of the smallpox vaccine (neither product is routinely used any longer in the United States). Determining the true incidence of vaccine adverse events—disentangling correlation from causation—has often pitted epidemiologists against grieving parents, statistical significance against the "truth" of personal experience. "The death rate from all causes during the first few months of life is comparatively high," cautioned one physician in the 1940s as new vaccines were becoming more widely used, "thus widespread use of any vaccine during the first few months of life requires caution lest some of the deaths due to usual causes may be wrongly attributed to the vaccine."[9] While the proposition that risk is an inevitable part of modern medicine is self-evident to many, it has nevertheless been controversial. "The public (and even much of the medical profession) has not been sufficiently educated to realize that there is some measurable risk in every medical intervention," one analysis asserted in the 1970s, "and when that risk is spread over thousands or millions of persons subject to the intervention, it results in countable numbers of individuals paying the whole price for the benefit provided to the larger population."[10]

Coercion, like risk, can take many forms. It is invoked in varied contexts to protect the community overall from harms that affect members, although when such force is ethically acceptable remains a matter of dispute in political and moral philosophy.[11] In the field of bioethics, where respect for patient autonomy is the polestar, coercion is anathema. But in the still-developing field of public health ethics, which is concerned with population-level interventions rather than the clinical encounter, it is less clear whether or when compulsory measures are appropriate.[12] In vaccination programs, coercion has involved the threat of the deprivation of liberty; the imposition of monetary or other penalties; and the denial of social goods to which one may otherwise be entitled, such as free education for children or welfare benefits. It has been exercised through the formal mechanisms of law, as well as by "softer" or informal means, including pressure from authority figures such as physicians and the figurative and metaphorical forms found in health promotion messages that attempt to stigmatize the failure to vaccinate.

Those skeptical of vaccination, especially parents, have forcefully rejected the use of coercion. Their stance is succinctly captured by an anti-vaccination Internet site called Vaccination News, which declares itself to be "against a parent, any parent, being forced to do something that has even a remote chance of harming their child."[13] This attitude exemplifies an important psychological phenomenon relevant to vaccination and risk: the preference for errors of *omission* over errors of *commission*.[14] The counterargument that the *failure* to immunize has a far greater chance of harming the child has generally gained little traction in the face of parental anxiety.

In addition to being embodied in philosophy and law, risk and coercion are, of course, historical constructs that have taken on different meanings over successive eras: what constitutes, or is perceived as, a risk or a coercive measure is always the product of a particular set of circumstances. Conceptions of risk and coercion have shaped the discourse and practices around vaccination since its earliest use in this country.

Vaccination was introduced in the United States in 1801, just a few years after being discovered by the British physician Edward Jenner, who fortuitously observed that milkmaids who contracted cowpox from cattle seemed to be immune to smallpox. Vaccination replaced inoculation, an older method of immunization in which smallpox material was transferred from the arm of a sick person to that of a healthy one in order to artificially induce a milder form of the illness. Inoculation occasionally produced a full-blown case of smallpox, however, and could inadvertently spread the disease instead of preventing it.[15] Vaccination, in contrast, involved the use of cowpox, a related disease of cattle, which produced only mild illness in humans and provided cross-protection against its more dangerous cousin.

While the use of cowpox was an improvement, because it eliminated the possibility of unintentionally spreading smallpox, the process of arm-to-arm transfer of pustular material retained the older procedure's other major drawback, the possibility of also transferring blood-borne illnesses such as syphilis. In the 1860s, a few "vaccine farms," usually run by doctors, began to produce vaccine matter made from the lymph of infected cows, thus eliminating the need to immunize directly from person to person. The forerunners of commercial medical laboratories, the farms sold their preparations to health departments and private practitioners.[16] While the use of calf's lymph made the practice considerably safer than the older arm-to-arm method, the care and skill with which practitioners administered the procedure varied widely, and sloppy vaccination sometimes resulted in other infections or inadequate protection against the disease. Moreover, the operation provided relatively short-term immunity; experts disagreed on precisely how often people needed to be revaccinated, since the duration of protection could in general only be estimated.[17]

Empirical evidence suggested that vaccination was highly effective at protecting a community from smallpox, and nineteenth-century medical and scientific journals featured numerous articles discussing its efficacy, as demonstrated by the experience of places where the practice was widespread, compared with those where it was not. Proponents of vaccination noted, for example, that Germany, which had made vaccination compulsory in 1874, enjoyed far greater immunity from the disease than any of its neighbors without such a law.[18] Comparisons in U.S. cities of the incidence and death rates among protected and unprotected populations offered similar support for its efficacy.[19] In calculating statistics such as standardized mortality rates, which enabled the comparison of countries and cities with different population sizes, such investigations articulated in an inchoate form some of the epidemiological parameters that would become cornerstones of public health practice in the next century. The idea that vaccination's protective value could be empirically proved by comparative statistics also gained currency in the popular press when newspaper editorials cited these studies approvingly.[20]

The numerical demonstration of vaccination's efficacy both drew on and contributed to the rise of quantification during the nineteenth century, when the counting of things—people, births, deaths, livestock, commercial goods—became an increasingly important way in which

Americans ordered their reality.[21] Quantification has been central to
notions of risk in general, and vaccination in particular, with both supporters and opponents of the practice invoking the certainty of numbers
to buttress their positions. "There is only one chance in twenty-four of
catching smallpox," declared an anti-vaccination activist in the late
nineteenth century. "Why should the twenty-four be poisoned to save
one?"[22] A physician in that era seeking to reassure the public about the
low risk of vaccine-related harm offered another type of calculation:

> When one rides in a railroad or street car, on a ferryboat or ocean liner,
> drives in a pleasure vehicle, visits the theater or promenades upon the side-
> walk, he takes a definite risk which may be mathematically calculated. We
> read almost daily of deaths from accidents under such circumstances. While
> in the aggregate the number of accidents and deaths throughout the world
> from each of these causes may be considerable, yet the individual risk is so
> small as to be generally disregarded.
>
> The case is the same with respect to vaccination. When we consider the
> thousands upon thousands of vaccinations performed throughout the world,
> and note how rare it is for any death or serious complication to result, we
> are justified in concluding that the risk attending vaccination in any individ-
> ual case is practically a negligible quantity.[23]

Since the 1970s, health economists have justified vaccination through
cost-benefit analysis, a technique for quantifying and measuring the value
of an intervention by weighing the likely costs—including the consequences of adverse events—against the positive outcomes. Cost-benefit
analysis rose to prominence in the mid-twentieth century on the grounds
that it offered a better, more "objective" basis for public policy formation
than the potentially biased judgments of experts.[24] Of all public health
interventions, vaccination has one of the best cost-benefit profiles, reducing enormous expenditures on medical care and adding years of produc-
tive life to society's members for a small per-person cost.[25] But the failure
of such statistical justifications to reassure those with philosophical objections has recently led to calls to explicitly incorporate moral and ethical
values, such as respect for liberty and autonomy, into this traditionally
quantitative process.[26]

Because the benefit vaccination offers—the absence of disease—is a
"negative" or unapparent one, its risks, though rare, seem more salient.
This property has had a significant effect on perceptions of risks and
benefits: the invocation of a certain number of illnesses or deaths that
did not occur has much less rhetorical force when placed against numbers of vaccine adverse events, even if the latter are very few. As early as

the nineteenth century, when smallpox had declined dramatically due to the wide application of vaccination, this phenomenon drew a lament from New York City Health Commissioner Cyrus Edson. "It is easy to be bold against an absent danger," Edson said of his fellow citizens' scorn of vaccination, "to despise the antidote while one has no experience with the bane!"[27] The more infectious diseases declined, the worse this problem became. "[E]ffective vaccines are self-defeating in that success itself is a deterrent to program maintenance," noted one analysis in the 1970s. "In proportion to the suppression of overt disease and visible threat, urgency for immunization lessens, acceptance of negative side effects diminishes, and criticism increases."[28]

The emergence of organized resistance to vaccination has historically been in reaction to the dual elements of risk and coercion. The first anti-vaccinationists arose in the nineteenth century in England, which made the procedure compulsory as part of a series of health laws that were bitterly resisted by both middle-class and poor citizens. The British laws, aimed broadly at controlling infectious disease, expanded the purview of the state over previously private spheres such as child-rearing and sexual behavior; the imposition of fines on those refusing vaccination drew the wrath of libertarians opposed in principle to government intervention and aroused more concrete fears about the physical violation of the body.[29] The British movement spawned several energetic pamphleteers and political rabble-rousers, at least one of whom, William Tebb, was so devoted to the cause that he traveled abroad in order to convince Americans of the evils of the practice. Tebb was instrumental in founding several organizations in major U.S. cities, including the Anti-Vaccination Society of America, established in New York in 1879.[30] In addition to portraying the practice as dangerous and ineffective, such groups asserted that any effort to compel it through legal means was a tyrannical violation of individual liberty.

In the United States, the efficacy of vaccination in protecting communities from smallpox prompted laws to compel the practice, in spite of its recognized risks. In 1809, Massachusetts was the first state to make it compulsory for the general population, requiring that all infants undergo the procedure before their second birthday and again before entering a public school; during epidemics, local public health officers could also require revaccination for all citizens in their area who had not undergone the procedure within the previous five years.[31] State laws imposed a variety of penalties on those refusing, ranging from fines to imprisonment.[32]

As public education became widespread, cities quickly realized that the schoolhouse, as a natural site for the spread of contagion, could also serve as a locus for prevention, and they began to pass laws requiring protection from smallpox before children could attend school.[33] Such regulations provoked numerous legal challenges and legislative battles, especially in the second half of the nineteenth century, when many states repealed or modified their laws in response to activist pressure.[34] Although controversy over public health regulations was not uncommon during this period, vaccination provoked an especially vociferous response. Other regulations that limited individual liberty in order to protect the common good generally required that people *refrain from* an action or behavior. Vaccination, in contrast, required people to *submit to* a procedure, one that involved discomfort and whose safety and efficacy remained uncertain in the minds of many.[35]

Court disputes over the practice arose as early as 1820, when the constable of North Hero, Vermont, confiscated Dan Hazen's cow after he refused to contribute to a municipal fund to pay a doctor to vaccinate all the town's residents.[36] Although the legal question in that case hinged not on vaccination per se but rather on the authority of town governments to levy taxes, the tension between the individual and the collective would be a recurring element in court challenges to compulsory vaccination programs. By the end of the nineteenth century, courts around the country had handed down dozens of decisions on the subject.[37] In one of the most significant pieces of public health jurisprudence in U.S. history, the 1905 Supreme Court case of *Jacobson v. Massachusetts*, the justices ruled that compulsory vaccination falls within the category of "police powers," the constitutional authority of state governments to guard the health, welfare, safety, and morals of their citizens.[38] The acceptability of compulsion was subsequently affirmed in the context of school attendance in the 1922 case of *Zucht v. King*. In spite of these rulings, the courtroom has been, and remains, a site of contention over vaccination, and judicial rulings have had an important effect on shaping policy.

The *Jacobson* decision did not, ironically, exert a determinative influence on the ways in which new vaccinations were deployed in the community over the next several decades. Perhaps the most counterintuitive aspect of the history of vaccination in the United States, given the early use of legal enforcement to protect against smallpox and the extensive network of laws currently in place, is that throughout the middle of the twentieth century, health officials relied very little on coercion.

The preference for persuasion was rooted partly in respect for the principles of liberty and autonomy that have occupied such a central position in American civic and political life. Equally important were pragmatic reasons. Laws enforced through schools would distract from efforts to protect infants, health officials believed, while attempts to force adults would provoke potentially violent resistance. Above all, persuasion was felt to be a surer source of behavior change. "Persuasion is a slow process," wrote New York State Health Commissioner Matthias Nicoll in 1927. "Its results are seldom spectacular but they are certain and durable, accomplishing far more among average human beings than attempts at legal compulsion."[39]

But persuasion, for all its virtues, had limits—a fact that Nicoll, with years of experience as a public health administrator, was keenly aware of when he wrote that "it is far less difficult to induce the first thousand of a population to cooperate in a public health movement than the last stubborn indifferent hundred."[40] How to convince those least likely to be vaccinated—the group that in midcentury became widely labeled the "hard to reach"—was a source of ongoing frustration. Explanations of why people did not seek vaccination for themselves or their children varied over successive eras. In the first half of the century, their inaction was largely viewed as an individual failing; "ignorance and apathy" was the standard gloss on the behavior of the unwilling. Beginning in the late 1950s, critiques of the health care system began to partially supplant behavioral explanations. In this view, suboptimal vaccination rates were not the fault of the individual but of society and its inadequate structures for providing preventive services.

The most notable feature of the persuasive efforts has been the adoption of the tools of advertising and public relations. Beginning with the emergence of modern marketing techniques in the 1920s, health officials have sought to "sell" the public on the importance of immunization. Like advertisements for consumer goods, these appeals have attempted to play on a range of emotions—including guilt, fear, and the desire to conform to a publicly approved norm—to motivate their target audiences. Many of the campaigns overtly sought to characterize the failure to immunize a child as morally culpable neglect. A 1978 radio spot featuring Marion Ross, the actress who played the mother on the popular television sitcom *Happy Days,* made this charge: "If your child comes down with polio, measles, diphtheria or mumps, it's probably your fault, because your child was not properly immunized."[41] Along with inducing parental guilt, a prominent rhetorical tactic in persuasive efforts has been to create a sense of urgency by emphasizing—or magnifying—the risk of illness. A 1963 guide published by the federal Communicable Disease Center to help local health officials plan their anti-polio programs contended that "the full use of the word *epidemic* itself in public statements is the most effective single means of stimulating the public to action."[42] But as infectious disease became an increasingly insignificant, even vestigial, source of illness and death in this country, this strategy grew more untenable.

While persuasion rather than coercion dominated vaccination policy through the middle of the century, the landscape changed in the late 1960s. In the context of a nationwide anti-measles campaign, an ideological commitment to the eradication of infectious disease sparked a national push to enact laws requiring vaccination before children could attend school. The belief that parents were basically willing, but needed special stimulus to help them act responsibly, provided a justification for the recourse to coercion. These laws have been challenged both on their foundations and in their particulars, but for the most part have been remarkably well accepted by the public and successful at increasing coverage rates among school-aged youth. The use of persuasion remained a cornerstone of vaccination programs, with school laws serving in the eyes of health officials as a kind of societal safety net to catch the children of the "hard to reach."

Because infants and children have been the primary focus of immunization campaigns in the twentieth century, the issue of parental control over children has been overlaid on the tension between the individual and the collective. To what extent should the wishes of parents who may have philosophical or religious reasons for not wishing their children to be vaccinated prevail over society's interest in protecting children from preventable illness and building herd immunity through high levels of vaccination? The questions of whether society has a right—or a duty—to override parental choice has sparked controversy in both medical and nonmedical contexts, with debates centering on groups such as Christian Scientists, Jehovah's Witnesses, and the Amish, and issues such as compliance with mandatory education laws, prohibitions on child labor, and consent for life-saving blood transfusions.[43] American culture and politics generally place a high premium on parental autonomy in matters of conscience, and health officials have sought to provide reasonable exemptions to vaccination laws based on religious or philosophical objections. But the scope of these provisions has been challenged on constitutional grounds. If too narrow, they may represent an unacceptable establishment of religion by the state; on the other hand, their very existence may violate the equal protection of the nonexempt majority.[44]

The question of exemption is not simply an ethical or legal one, but has epidemiological consequences, since a large number of exemptions will ultimately undermine herd immunity. Those sympathetic to greater parental control over children's health care have argued that reasonable accommodations can be made without threatening the safety of the community. "If a small minority of parents decide not to have their children vaccinated, it is unlikely to alter significantly the level of population immunity and the chance of susceptible individuals contracting infectious disease," argued one commentator in favor of more expansive exemptions.[45] But such an analysis sidesteps the difficult question of how large the exempt minority should be allowed to become, and whether the recourse to coercion becomes more acceptable if a sufficiently large number of parents decide against vaccinating their children. Epidemiological studies of the effects of unvaccinated clusters of children on the spread of illness suggest that, especially in the case of highly contagious conditions such as measles, even small numbers of susceptible youth can endanger the community's health.[46]

As with most other aspects of health care in the United States, a strong socioeconomic gradient has characterized vaccination uptake; people of lower income and less formal education, and their children, have been much less likely to be vaccinated than those of higher income and more formal education. This phenomenon was observed as early as the 1920s in the first nationwide surveys of vaccination status, and was rediscovered in the 1950s in the wake of the introduction of the Salk vaccine, when national surveillance of vaccination coverage became routinized. As infectious disease became increasingly limited to poverty areas, the issue of immunization was the subject of extensive social science research, and it was recast as a problem of inequality and social justice in the 1960s. This conceptualization informed efforts in the last decades of the century, when the primary focus of reformers was on improving the health care delivery system to make it more equitable and accessible.

THE EVOLUTION OF VACCINATION POLICY AND LAW

This narrative opens in the years leading up to the landmark case of *Jacobson v. Massachusetts* in 1905. The book's chapters map the trajectory of twentieth-century vaccination policy, as decision making evolved gradually from being local to being national in scope. In the first decades of the century, decisions about who should be targeted and how they should be reached were made largely by city, county, or state health officials. The first three chapters of this book focus primarily on New York City and State. The city, a national leader in organized public health since the early days of the sanitary revolution, was at the forefront of setting vaccination policies.

In chapter 1, I describe events that set the stage for the decision in *Jacobson*. Epidemics of smallpox in Brooklyn and New York around the turn of the century led to a series of protracted court cases and legislative battles over the issue of whether those who resisted vaccination could be compelled, through the threat of quarantine, civil or criminal penalties, or other forms of censure, to undergo vaccination. Chapter 2 examines the surprising aftermath of *Jacobson* during the Progressive Era and the 1920s, a period of intensified anti-vaccination agitation in New York and around the country. As smallpox declined in incidence and receded from the public eye, adverse events arising from vaccination assumed new salience. A variety of individuals and organizations, espousing diverse philosophies ranging from libertarian politics to visions of natural and alternative healing practices, were able, through agitation and passive resistance, to frustrate the efforts of health officials to achieve high coverage levels. The dramatic rise of new techniques of advertising and public relations forms the backdrop for the events of chapter 3, which considers the introduction of toxin-antitoxin injections against diphtheria, the second immunization to become widespread. A new public health ethos took hold during this period, as persuasive measures replaced—in theory, if not always in fact—the coercive tactics of the nineteenth century. As the medical profession became increasingly homogeneous in its use of allopathic medicine and established itself as the authoritative arbiter in matters of health, illness, and the body, tensions arose about the "ownership" of vaccination, which straddled the boundaries of a medical procedure and a public health intervention.

In chapters 4 through 7, my focus expands to events nationally, with examples drawn selectively from New York and other cities and states to illustrate local and regional variation. Beginning in the 1950s, in the wake of the licensing of the polio vaccine, the federal government took the first tentative steps toward a substantive role in vaccination; this involvement expanded in the 1960s, as an immunization-focused bureaucracy within the U.S. Public Health Service became a strong force in programming around the country. Chapter 4 describes the introduction of the polio vaccine, a pivotal event in the history of vaccination policy in America. The arrival of Jonas Salk's vaccine was a media sensation and marked the first time that meeting public demand for a vaccination was a greater challenge than persuading the reluctant. This initial dynamic proved ephemeral, however, and health officials once again turned to the advertising techniques that had been used with mixed success during the anti-diphtheria campaigns two decades earlier. Social science research and new epidemiological surveillance methods also assumed a prominent role in policymaking. In chapter 5, I examine the efforts to control infectious diseases during a period when their decline led to unprecedented hope that vaccination could free society of ancient scourges. The almost complete disappearance of polio from the United States, the planning of a global smallpox eradication campaign, and the widespread use of antibiotics and other medical advances fueled the development of a philosophy of "eradicationism" that became a dominant feature of vaccination policy. It was in the context of a national campaign to eradicate measles that the most significant policy transformation of the century occurred: the enactment and vigorous enforcement of laws requiring a wide range of vaccinations prior to entry into public schools.

Controversies over vaccine safety and the ethical and strategic complexities of compulsory policies are the subject of chapter 6. As the doctrine of informed consent became the norm in clinical and research settings, health officials were increasingly under pressure to ensure that vaccine recipients had full knowledge and appreciation of risks and benefits, but struggled to reconcile consent with the use of legal mandates. The widespread recognition that a small number of people are inevitably harmed by vaccine adverse events led to debates over who should be accountable for this risk and what forms this responsibility should take. These debates culminated in the enactment in 1986 of landmark federal legislation that created a financial compensation system for vaccine injuries. Finally, chapter 7 looks at vaccination policy, politics, and law at the turn of the twenty-first century. The major initiative to boost coverage rates in the 1990s, a federal program to provide free vaccine to children of low-income families, lifted levels of coverage to their highest ever. At the same time, however, new concerns about safety sparked a dramatic resurgence of anti-vaccination activism, facilitated by the democratizing effects of the Internet. The potential reemergence of smallpox as a weapon of bioterrorism, and the specter of coercive measures on a potentially wide scale, gave sudden new relevance to the century-old ruling on compulsory powers in *Jacobson v. Massachusetts*.

Over the course of the twentieth century, advances in scientific medicine produced an impressive armamentarium of vaccines that dramatically transformed the public health landscape. But the story of vaccination is one of politics as much as of science. Vaccination policy evolved through a series of confrontations with political, ethical, and legal questions concerning risks and benefits, individual rights and communal duties, and the balance between persuasion and compulsion. These issues have been contested not just in meetings of public health and medical advisory bodies, but also in legislatures, courtrooms, the popular media, and, most recently, on the Internet. In all of these forums, differing values, beliefs, and standards of proof hold sway.

CHAPTER I

Between Persuasion and Compulsion

Vaccination at the Turn of the Twentieth Century

"Carelessness in the matter of vaccination is sure to tell against the health of a community, sooner or later," the *New York Daily Tribune* editorialized in the winter of 1902, as a smallpox epidemic was raging in the city.[1] In urging those who had not undergone the procedure recently to update their protection, the newspaper gave public voice to the private frustration of many municipal health officials. They should have been eminently capable of controlling smallpox, since a reliable preventive had existed for over a century, yet the very success of widespread vaccination had caused many people to take their freedom from the disease for granted. How best to overcome this civic complacency—how to persuade people to protect themselves, for their own good and that of the community—was a recurring problem in a city where a huge population and the constant influx of immigrants meant an ongoing struggle with infectious threats.

At the turn of the twentieth century, the power of health officials to control smallpox through vaccination was argued in numerous legal actions and debated in state legislatures, in the popular and medical press, and in city neighborhoods. At issue was the question of whether those who did not wish to undergo the procedure should or could be compelled, legally or practically, to do so. When an epidemic loomed, many people waited voluntarily in long lines to receive their protection. For reluctant citizens, the Brooklyn and New York health departments sent teams of vaccinators door to door in affected neighborhoods and on-site

to large employers. Although these programs were ostensibly voluntary—
New York State never placed a law on its books making vaccination compulsory for adults—the manner in which they were conducted was at
least arguably coercive, and gave many people the impression that they
had no choice but to submit.

This chapter analyzes the conflicts and tensions in vaccination policy
during a transitional era in which health officials expanded their influence
but negotiated an ambiguous relationship with both legal authority and
public opinion. During two major outbreaks of smallpox, the health commissioners in Brooklyn and New York exercised de facto compulsion but
portrayed their practices in the language of voluntarism, because they
lacked a clear legal mandate and believed this strategy was the most effective way to accomplish their goals and reduce the likelihood of organized
resistance. The inconsistent and sometimes conflicting rulings that
emerged from the court battles over vaccination reveal how mutable were
ideas about the proper role of the government in guarding the community's health during this period. These rulings set the stage for the landmark U.S. Supreme Court opinion in *Jacobson v. Massachusetts* in 1905,
which explicitly addressed the question of how far individual liberty could
be constrained in order to prevent the spread of disease. Both the court
cases and the public reactions to vaccination reflected persistent doubts
about the competence of the medical profession to prevent and treat illness, even as scientific advances were increasing doctors' diagnostic and
therapeutic capacities. The events of this period—a crucial turning point in
the history of vaccination in America—illustrate the growth and the
limitations of the power wielded by municipal health departments and
their difficult task as they sought to assert both their authority and their
ability to ensure the welfare of the city's residents.

THE EPIDEMIC OF 1893–1894

At the turn of the twentieth century, public attitudes about smallpox were
a mixture of complacency and dread. Although it had once been one of
the most devastating diseases, it had long ceased to be a major source of
either sickness or death in the United States and elsewhere in the Western
world; other contagions, such as measles, scarlet fever, and diphtheria,
exacted a far greater toll. Years of relative freedom from smallpox—due,
many argued, to the success of vaccination—had engendered complacency among the public, and many physicians could no longer accurately
diagnose it in its early stages, often mistaking it for measles or chicken pox.[2]

At the same time, the disease's gruesome symptoms, high fatality rate, and rapid spread made it greatly feared among any who had had personal experience with it. So it was that a Brooklyn Health Department report noted that when outbreaks occurred, "the proximity of the contagion act[ed] as an efficient aid to the efforts of the vaccinators."[3]

The safety of vaccination had improved considerably by the end of the nineteenth century as the use of calf's lymph gradually replaced the old arm-to-arm transfer of pustular material, but many people remained reluctant to undergo the procedure because of its checkered history of unpleasant and occasionally life-threatening side effects. Fears lingered about accidental infections, especially lockjaw, and vaccination was well known to cause soreness that lasted for several days. Physicians who championed vaccination saw its proper administration as crucial to assuaging public qualms. The arm was scraped several times with a sharpened "point," usually of ivory, to break the skin, and a preparation of glycerinated lymph from a calf infected with cowpox was then applied to the incision. Discussions of the safest and most efficacious ways of vaccinating—how deeply to scratch the arm, how best to disinfect the site—featured prominently in the medical literature and at meetings of professional organizations.[4] A physician writing in a medical journal scolded his colleagues for too often being slipshod, charging that "this perfunctoriness on the physician's part teaches parents to wish their children to have as little vaccination as possible, and encourages in them an active opposition."[5] The use by some colleagues of impure or improperly prepared lymph from disreputable drug firms was a source of continuing consternation for doctors; every swollen, infected, or abscessed arm that resulted was a black eye to the profession and its efforts to gain respectability with an often skeptical public.

When smallpox reappeared in Brooklyn in 1893 after an absence of several years, many health officials were frustrated that they had no legal authority to compel the vaccination of reluctant citizens. To control the disease, vaccinators were dispatched to a site where a case had been diagnosed, and they then fanned out to the houses on either side, offering protection to the neighbors—"surrounding each case by an impenetrable wall of vaccination," as one health department report described the process.[6] In the face of resistance, city doctors complained, "we can only persuade; arguments are our only resource."[7] The limited legal authority to enforce vaccination reflected broader debates about the rights and responsibilities of the government in guarding the public welfare. State and local health departments had begun to be created in the

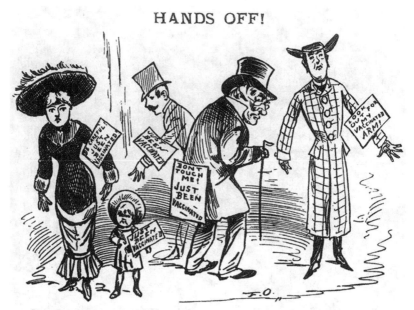

The Only Way to Avoid Unpleasant Collisions During a Small-pox Scare.

Figure 1. This 1882 cartoon in the popular magazine *Puck*, illustrating the pain and discomfort that vaccination caused, signified both acceptance of the procedure and the uneasiness many people felt about undergoing it.

1860s, and, in general, health officials' authority had expanded over the next decades. Spurred by the initial success of sanitary reforms in limiting the spread of cholera, they later used dramatic advances in bacteriology following Robert Koch's 1882 identification of the tubercle bacillus to bring more and more areas of city life under their purview. A new class of professionals trained in the latest techniques of chemistry, engineering, and medicine established regulations governing the production and distribution of meat and milk, tenement construction, garbage collection, private and public privies, and water supplies.[8] Enforcement in all of these areas remained patchy, however, and officials often encountered opposition from private citizens who resented government intrusion into their lives, as well as from businessmen who viewed health regulations as interference with commerce.[9]

The Brooklyn Health Department began taking a more aggressive stance toward smallpox when, at the height of the epidemic, a new commissioner took office. (Brooklyn at this time was independent of

New York City and had its own well-established department of health.)
Z. Taylor Emery, a physician and former president of the county medical
society who had been practicing in the city for almost twenty years,
started work on February 1, 1894, newly appointed by Brooklyn's popular Republican mayor Charles Schieren. Confronted with an alarming
increase in the number of smallpox cases, Emery moved aggressively,
expanding the number of vaccinators, the scope of their activities, and
the forcefulness with which they conducted their rounds.

In one of his first actions, he dispatched teams of doctors to the
twenty-seventh ward, which had a predominately German population. The city's German immigrants were well known not just for
opposing vaccination but for their more general suspicion of health
officials. "Case after case occurred and was concealed, meanwhile
the inmates were going about their usual work, many taking in tai-
loring and the children going to school," according to a report by the
city's chief of contagious diseases. "There seemed to have been a
mutual understanding among them to keep the cases from the Health
Department."[10]

The immigrants' resistance to state authority in this matter may have
been influenced by their sentiments about Germany's compulsory vaccination law, which imposed a fine or three days' detention for refusal to
be vaccinated. The law, enacted two decades earlier, had provoked widespread opposition, based both on skepticism about the efficacy of the
procedure and on ideological objections to state interference with private
matters such as parents' decisions about how to protect their children
from illness.[11] A health officer in Buffalo who encountered similar resistance among that city's German immigrants saw their refusal to be vaccinated as a repudiation of their native country's unpopular law: "The
moment they land on our free soil, they imbibe the spirit of freedom,
especially as regards vaccination."[12]

Resistance to vaccination was also strong among Brooklyn's Italian
immigrants. As one health department physician recalled,

> The Italians are in great fear of vaccination, and resort to all sorts of
> means to hide themselves and their children. If the child is small enough
> they will put it in the bureau drawer. I have found dozens of babies
> there, and my experience has taught me never to overlook the smallest
> nook or cranny in searching for persons in the tenement houses. One
> woman whom we vaccinated admitted that she had escaped inoculation
> on four previous visits of the Health Department's vaccinators by
> crawling under the bed, and she bewailed her luck in at last getting
> caught.[13]

Under Emery's direction, the department established free vaccination clinics at more than two dozen locations around the city, and doctors visited more than 200 factories and other places of business over the next several weeks to vaccinate the employees.[14] They also continued house-to-house sweeps in areas adjacent to cases that were discovered. The official "Rules for Vaccinators" issued by Emery to his teams gave the following guidance on dealing with public reluctance: "In case persons are found who have never been vaccinated, every effort should be made to induce them to accept it, and, if necessary, they should be visited a second or third time to bring about this result.... When the inmates of infected houses refuse to be vaccinated, the vaccinator may, at his discretion, direct the Sanitary Police to maintain a quarantine until all are vaccinated."[15] As the policy was implemented, however, it was not only those in "infected houses" who became subject to quarantine.

An example of the department's tactics and public resistance to them was the case of the McCauley family, a 65-year-old couple and their 27-year-old son, who were placed under quarantine after refusing vaccination. Smallpox had been diagnosed a block away, on Atlantic Avenue, and Emery ordered all the neighborhood's residents to bare their arms. The McCauleys alone refused, fearing dire health consequences from the procedure, and after the elder McCauley threatened the city's doctors with a rifle, two policemen were stationed at their doors.[16] "They were forbidden to leave their apartment, and the other tenants were warned, under penalty of arrest, not to deliver any messages for them," the *New York Times* reported. "The grocers, butchers, and bakers in the vicinity were also forbidden to deliver provisions."[17] The next day, shocked police discovered a two-foot-square hole in a closet wall, through which the family had crawled into an adjacent apartment that was unoccupied; a neighbor reported that the three had fled to New Jersey. Three days later, after being convinced by family members with whom they had taken refuge in Hoboken that they had nothing to fear from the procedure, the three surrendered themselves at the Atlantic Avenue police station and consented to be vaccinated.[18] In applying quarantine in this way, Emery was testing the elasticity of a state law that empowered local boards of health to "guard against the introduction of contagious and infectious disease" and to "require the isolation of all persons infected with and exposed to such disease."[19] How broad a net could be cast over those "exposed to" disease was unclear.

By the middle of March, the aggressive tactics of Emery's staff of vaccinators had begun to attract some public opposition. The *Brooklyn*

Daily Eagle criticized the department's "loose methods of quarantining," citing complaints that "families are shut up in tenement and apartment houses without any reason."[20] One Brooklynite wrote to the *Eagle* charging that the system of paying health department vaccinators 30 cents for each operation they performed created an incentive for them to "terrorize or intimidate healthy people to be revaccinated by them under penalty of quarantine for refusal."[21]

Well aware of the influence of the press, Emery used the *Eagle* throughout the epidemic to advance his case, issuing regular statements and giving interviews to the newspaper, in which he attempted to enlist public support for his actions. The day after the McCauleys' return, for example, Emery gave an interview to the *Eagle* in which he addressed himself to those who accused the department of overstepping its bounds in the name of public health. "The law clothes the department with ample authority to do all which it deems necessary, and it is pursuing a systematic course of vaccinating, disinfecting and quarantining," he said. "For the most part the citizens have shown a patriotic readiness to submit to all these unavoidable inconveniences.... In the few cases where selfishness and unreasonableness have led to opposition the officials have considerately but firmly insisted on carrying out their instructions."[22]

Emery's rhetoric, explicitly framing cooperation with the vaccinators as a matter of good citizenship, held special resonance in a multi-ethnic metropolis such as Brooklyn, whose large immigrant communities included Germans and Poles in the neighborhoods of Williamsburg and Greenpoint, Irish in the Navy Yard, and Italians in Red Hook.[23] These enclaves presented some of the greatest pockets of resistance in the city, and the health department's use of police force was in general more aggressive toward immigrants and the poor. But it would be erroneous to understand either the discourse or the methods of Emery's smallpox control program as representing the conflation of the foreign-born with the spread of contagion. Reluctance to be vaccinated, far from being confined to immigrants, cut across a wide swath of Brooklyn society, and, as we shall see, Emery used coercive means against Brooklyn's propertied classes as well as against the impoverished and politically marginal.

Emery was able to wield power as he did because he continued to enjoy political support among important constituencies who viewed the threat of smallpox as sufficiently grave to justify drastic measures. He retained the backing of Mayor Schieren—he was Schieren's family physician—and in March, the mayor granted an emergency appropriation to the health department for the hiring of additional vaccinators.[24]

Emery was also backed by the city's Common Council, which passed a resolution in support of his actions in fighting the disease there.[25] The Kings County Medical Society passed a similar resolution, commending Emery's "energy, efficiency and zeal" in dealing with the outbreak.[26] The major newspapers of Brooklyn and New York, while they may have had qualms about some of the department's tactics, remained supportive of vaccination in general. The *New York Times* commented in an editorial that those opposed to the practice were engaged "in a futile attempt to head off human progress and to reopen a question about which pretty much all of the world has made up its mind."[27]

As winter turned into spring and the epidemic showed no signs of abating, Emery's vaccinators continued to blanket the city, focusing especially on large employers. At the Havemeyer & Elder sugar refinery, some 2,000 "big men bared their brawny arms and were inoculated," according to the *New York Times*.[28] At the Chelsea Jute Mills in Greenpoint, almost all 800 workers were scraped, while at the nearby Dunlap's hat factory, half of the 500 employees were. All the operators of the city's surface and elevated railways were to be vaccinated.[29] Such efforts were carried out not only at the health department's insistence; many companies, concerned about the devastating effects an outbreak of the disease among their employees might have on their businesses, requested that a team of vaccinators come on-site. Workers' anxiety over the threat of unemployment—the nation had plunged into a depression the previous summer, and thousands of Brooklynites were thrown out of work—probably made many of them more inclined to go along with the programs without complaint.

The use of neighborhood sweeps with police accompaniment continued, sometimes sparking civil unrest. After four more cases of the disease were discovered on Atlantic Avenue, not far from the McCauleys' house, Emery sent in a team of vaccinators accompanied by six policemen. According to a newspaper account, after a "small riot" broke out among the mostly Scandinavian residents, there were "hurried calls for more policemen and for an hour patrol wagons filled with bluecoats came scurrying in from the outlying precincts, until finally the entire two blocks were guarded by policemen."[30] Another focus of concern was the city's seventy-two lodging houses, which sheltered a transient population of some 2,400 each night. "[I]n them are gathered nightly a large proportion of those homeless and vagrant ones in our population whose unwholesome heredity and unsanitary lives render them liable not only to the commission of crime, but to the contraction of disease," a health department report noted, in language that revealed the close connection that persisted in the popular imagination between moral degeneracy and illness. "In the presence of an epidemic, such houses become strategic points in the consideration of places to prevent its spread."[31]

Meanwhile smallpox was ravaging other major U.S. cities, and their health boards were also moving aggressively to contain it, with mixed reactions from citizens. The resistance of the German immigrant community played a prominent role in events in Milwaukee, where the health department's insistence on forcibly removing patients, especially children, from their homes became a flashpoint for opposition and resulted in several violent uprisings against department inspectors and their police escorts.[32] In Chicago, teams of vaccinators accompanied by police went house to house, using quarantine as they saw necessary, which also provoked community opposition.[33] The health boards of Minnesota and Wisconsin requested that Chicago authorities be especially vigilant in ensuring that no travelers sick with the disease were able to depart by train to neighboring states, but the city had difficulty finding enough physicians to keep watch for suspects at all the railway stations.[34] When smallpox appeared in Muncie, the Indiana Board of Health banned all public gatherings in the city and ordered that no one be allowed to leave the city by rail without first being vaccinated; but due in part to agitation by the local anti-vaccination society, there was widespread failure to comply with the quarantines placed around infected neighborhoods.[35] In Providence, the state legislature voted to repeal Rhode Island's compulsory vaccination law following years of agitation by anti-vaccination activists.[36]

In mid April, Emery's teams intensified their efforts in Brooklyn's schools. Proof of vaccination upon enrollment was required for students under state law, but enforcement was desultory, and spot checks by the department discovered that in many schools, scarcely half the children were protected.[37] A team of fifty-six vaccinators was sent out and administered a total of about 27,000 vaccinations to the city's young scholars.[38] The doctors encountered an especially delicate situation in the elite schools where the children of Brooklyn's leading citizens studied. Only those students who could show a recent scar were to be spared the vaccinator's lance, but the custom among the upper classes was not to vaccinate on their daughters' arms, because the scar would spoil the beauty of a young debutante wearing a sleeveless gown. The teenage girls could hardly show an unknown health department doctor the place on their body where they had been vaccinated, and after tense consultations between Emery and at least two school principals, the department arranged to have its three female doctors verify protection among the daughters of the well-to-do.[39]

Perhaps sensing an opportune moment to capitalize on public unease about health department tactics, a group made up mostly of homeopathic doctors formed the Brooklyn Anti-Vaccination League in April 1894. In addition to demanding the repeal of all state and local laws on the practice, the league launched a number of charges against Emery, accusing him, among other crimes, of falsifying death certificates to conceal the fact that vaccination was having fatal consequences for some of those who underwent it.[40] The group was to remain a thorn in the side of Emery and the Brooklyn Health Department, especially in the courtroom, where a series of protracted lawsuits would set limits on what health officials could do in the name of protecting the community's welfare.

VACCINATION ON TRIAL

On May 2, 1894, two health department vaccinators visited a livery stable in the Greenpoint neighborhood where William H. Smith operated an express delivery and hauling business. Smith employed more than a dozen men and boys who delivered goods from factories in the metropolitan area to retail businesses and from businesses to homes, and hauled away discarded items. In addition to offices, the upstairs quarters of the stable included a parlor, where Smith sometimes spent the night after working late.[41] A case of smallpox had been discovered in the area, and the department was concerned that because of the nature of their business, Smith and his employees might be vectors for spreading infection. In making this decision, Frederick Jewett, who headed the Bureau of Contagious Disease, must have remembered a similar case during the outbreak of 1886, when he was serving as an assistant sanitary inspector, and a driver employed in the same type of hauling business had been found to spread the disease, leading to the death of at least one child.[42]

The inspectors gave Smith and an employee at the office, Thomas Cummings, twenty-four hours to be vaccinated, and when they returned the following day and found that the two men had not followed their orders, stationed a police guard at the front door and declared the business under quarantine. Smith called Charles Walters, his family physician, who— unfortunately for the health department—was a member of the Brooklyn Anti-Compulsory Vaccination League. Walters immediately hired a lawyer to seek a writ of habeas corpus from a special session of the state supreme court, demanding that the two men be released from custody.[43]

The next day Smith's lawyer managed to obtain a hearing before Judge William J. Gaynor. It is unclear whether Smith specifically sought out Gaynor to hear the case, but he could hardly have chosen a more receptive audience for his complaint. Like Emery a friend and ally of Mayor Schieren, Gaynor was a well-known figure in local political circles. As a longtime prosecutor in the Brooklyn courts, he had led crusades against municipal corruption; a libertarian mistrustful of government power, he had in his short time on the bench become well known for rulings protecting the rights of the common citizen, as well as for his brusque and irascible temperament.[44] "Each day the judge fires sharp and caustic remarks to lawyers who have not prepared their cases," according to one newspaper account, "[and] to witnesses who are slow beyond endurance or tricky in their answers."[45] Upon being presented with the case, Gaynor acted with the swift decisiveness for which he was well known. He granted Smith's writ the following day, commanding that the quarantine be lifted and the men be freed pending his decision on the legal aspects of the case.

Meanwhile, Emery continued to press his case with the public that the health department's control measures were just and appropriate. On May 7, he issued a lengthy statement, reprinted in the *Daily Eagle,* offering his rationale for strict enforcement of vaccination and quarantine. He appealed most of all to civic duty, claiming that "in the presence of imminent peril private rights must subserve to public necessity." He attempted to portray the procedure as widely accepted, asserting that the "vast majority of people have sympathized with the department and aided us in every practicable way, even where it involved considerable personal sacrifice." He invoked economic necessity, citing figures showing that if Philadelphia had adopted more aggressive control measures during its 1872 outbreak, it could have saved more than $24 million worth of lost commerce. He pointedly noted that "carriers of miscellaneous parcels, such as bedding, furniture, packages and other baggage are especially liable to come in contact with and spread the disease." Finally, he cited several cases, by name, of people who had refused vaccination and had met with predictably dire fates, including death.[46]

When Gaynor's ruling came on May 18, it proved a blow to the health department. Refusing to acknowledge that Smith and Cummings were a danger to the community, Gaynor asserted that the legislature had conferred on Emery no power to quarantine those who were not actually infected with a disease. "Arbitrary power is abhorrent to our system of government," he declared. "If the Legislature desired to make vaccination compulsory, it would have so enacted.... [The law] does not confer on the Commissioner the right to imprison any more than to take life."[47]

Emery promptly appealed the decision, hoping to obtain a ruling that would throw the weight of the law behind his actions. Testifying at a later trial, Emery revealed his motivation for pressing the case against Smith. "My motive [in appealing Gaynor's decision] was for the purpose of obtaining a ruling defining the powers and rights and the duties of the Health Boards, this Health Board as well as others. And I deemed it essential to the efficient discharge of my duty and the duty of my subordinates that my authority should be particularly defined in that crisis."[48] Notably, he was not seeking a law that would explicitly declare vaccination compulsory; rather, he wanted a more general affirmation of the right to use his discretion in how he protected the city.

Gaynor's action was widely reported in the press, garnering notices in the *Daily Eagle* along with the *Times, Daily Tribune,* and *World,*[49] and public awareness of the ruling emboldened those who were inclined against vaccination. At the end of May, one of the employees at the Standard Oil factory in the Newtown Creek neighborhood took ill, and Emery sent a squad to the plant to vaccinate the man's co-workers. When the men refused and the doctors tried to insist, one of the workers pulled out a copy of a newspaper that had printed Gaynor's decision. "You can't touch us," the men were reported as saying. "We are protected by the law."[50]

Although the imposition of quarantine had been suspended, the use of coercive measures continued. In one late-night raid, a squad of 40 physicians accompanied by 120 police officers swept into an Italian quarter of Flatbush brandishing points. The *Eagle* reported that upon seeing the policemen's badges, many "sprang through windows and doors," but they were soon caught.[51] The following night, approximately 50 doctors and more than 100 police conducted another raid. A scuffle broke out when one of the residents lunged at a doctor and attempted to stab him with a pocket knife.[52]

The Brooklyn Anti-Compulsory Vaccination League had a field day with Emery's legal troubles, and at the end of May, it publicly called for his removal.[53] Emboldened by Gaynor's ruling, which seemed to open a legal door to further action against vaccination, the league next mounted an attack on the state law requiring the practice for school enrollment. Charles Walters—the family physician who had come to William Smith's aid—filed suit against the principal of Brooklyn Public School No. 22

seeking to compel him to admit Walters's two children, who had not been vaccinated.[54] On this front, however, the group was unsuccessful. A month later a judge ruled, "A common school education, under the existing constitution of the State of New York, is a privilege rather than a right. . . . It follows that the State can certainly exercise this discretion by debarring from attendance at the public schools such persons as are unwilling to adopt a precaution which, in the judgment of the legislature, is essential to the preservation of the health of the large body of scholars."[55] The judge was careful to point out that the legal question in this case was different from that which Judge Gaynor had considered in the Smith case.

From March through August of 1894, when the epidemic finally dwindled, the health department administered approximately 225,000 vaccinations (to close to one-quarter of the city's population), in addition to an unknown number that were done by private physicians. Of the vaccinations performed by city doctors, close to three-quarters were done house-to-house.[56] Smallpox virtually disappeared from Brooklyn the following year, but the legal battles over what had occurred during the 1894 outbreak, and over the practice of vaccination more generally, continued to be waged in the courtroom.

In February 1895, Emery claimed a victory for health department authority when an appellate court overturned Gaynor's ruling of the previous May asserting that Emery had overstepped his bounds. The new ruling underscored just how ambiguous the definition of terms such as "compulsory" could be, and how much disagreement remained over whether vaccination constituted an assault or a public service. "There was neither coercion nor compulsion" in the health department's actions, the judges ruled. Smith and Cummings "were isolated and deprived of their freedom because they had been exposed to small pox and were liable to be seized therewith. . . . If they availed themselves of the privileges tendered to them, their acceptance would terminate their quarantine."[57] It was an unalloyed victory for the kinds of broad powers Emery had claimed for the department of health.

Lawyers for Smith and Cummings appealed, however, and on May 3, 1895, exactly a year after the health department had placed the quarantine on Smith's business, a three-judge panel on the court of appeals affirmed Gaynor's original ruling that Emery had overreached. "That the powers conferred upon the health commissioner by the provisions of the city charter give him the right to compel the vaccination of every citizen in the city of Brooklyn, if he would escape quarantine, seems an unnecessary and . . . unwarrantable inference in the language," the decision said. While the judges did not doubt that the law properly invested the health department with certain powers to protect the public, "Like all enactments which may affect the liberty of the person, this one must be construed strictly."[58]

Not content with Gaynor's order releasing him from quarantine, Smith had also filed suit against Emery seeking damages for lost business during his confinement. Smith's complaint alleged that the health department's action constituted an unlawful arrest without probable cause that had led to the loss of $10,000 as a result of his inability to continue his business. (The suit for damages, *Smith v. Emery*, was a separate legal action from *In re Smith*, the original suit contesting forced vaccination, although for several months during 1894–95, both were pending simultaneously in the state court system.) The second suit came to trial in the Brooklyn circuit court on the first day of December, 1895, and two weeks later, the judge awarded Smith $641.32 in damages after the jury found in his favor.[59]

The trial of the damages suit revealed the wide gap between the rationale of the health department doctors and the legal perspective of the court. To justify the attempt to force vaccination on Smith and Cummings, Emery's lawyers produced multiple types of evidence to demonstrate the rapid spread of smallpox and the grave peril it posed to the population: statistics on the incidence of the disease, city maps depicting the distribution of cases, testimony by department inspectors, resolutions from the Common Council and the medical society describing the scope of the threat. But Judge Charles Brown found all of this irrelevant. "I do not regard it as at all material that there was smallpox in the City of Brooklyn or that they had 140 cases a day," he told Emery's lawyers during cross-examination.[60] The sole relevant issue, according to Brown, was whether or not Smith himself had actually been diagnosed with the disease; failing that, quarantine was unjustified.[61] Brown's decision over the use of quarantine, like Gaynor's before him, underscored the difference between types of evidence that were persuasive to health officials and those that stood up in courts of law.

Smith's suits over quarantine were not the only legal actions arising from the smallpox outbreak. In 1895–1896, the health department faced at least three other suits charging it with either assault or wrongful death as a result of vaccination. These suits were among a handful brought during this period against private or public sector doctors by disgruntled citizens who claimed they had been harmed by negligently performed vaccination.[62] These actions partly reflected a larger legal trend around the turn of the twentieth century: a sharp rise in personal injury lawsuits. But only a tiny fraction of these personal injury suits involved medical malpractice; most were for injuries sustained in the workplace or through traffic or transportation mishaps.[63]

Although none of the cases against the Brooklyn Health Department had a direct bearing on the issue of the department's legal authority, the negative press coverage they generated fueled public unease about the safety of the procedure and, more generally, about the competence of the medical profession to protect the community from disease. At the end of 1895, a jury awarded $1,500 to Emil Schaefer, who claimed that he had come "near dying from loss of blood and shock" after being vaccinated against his will by the same health department doctors who had attempted to force the procedure on Smith and Cummings.[64] In early 1896, two suits involving the death of children during the outbreak of 1894 reached the court. The more well publicized of these involved 10-year-old Julia Burggraff, the daughter of a Williamsburg mineral water manufacturer. Within three days of being vaccinated at her school by a city doctor, "her entire left side had become swollen and inflamed," according to a press account; the muscles in her arms, legs and neck became rigid, she lost her ability to swallow, and three weeks later she died. The family doctor declared the cause of death to be lockjaw.[65] Peter Burggraff, Julia's father, filed a wrongful death suit against Emery and the vaccinator, Frank Boyden, seeking $5,000 in damages.[66] The question was one of medical negligence: had Boyden, in administering the procedure, exercised "proper care" and ensured that the site of the girl's incision was adequately cleansed?[67] Burggraff claimed that the doctor had been criminally incompetent in his work, while Boyden maintained that the girl's wound had become infected when her mother had rubbed Vaseline into it.[68] The jury was ultimately unable to reach a decision and the case was dismissed.[69]

In December 1896, the circuitous legal battles between Emery and his antagonist William Smith finally came to an end when a panel of judges in the appellate division of the state supreme court heard Emery's appeal of the damage award that Smith had won against the health department a year earlier. The court found that the judge in the earlier trial had improperly excluded from consideration the evidence Emery's lawyers had submitted concerning the prevalence of smallpox and his judgment about Smith's and Cummings's risk of contracting the disease through their work. The appeals court ruling affirmed the validity of the professional

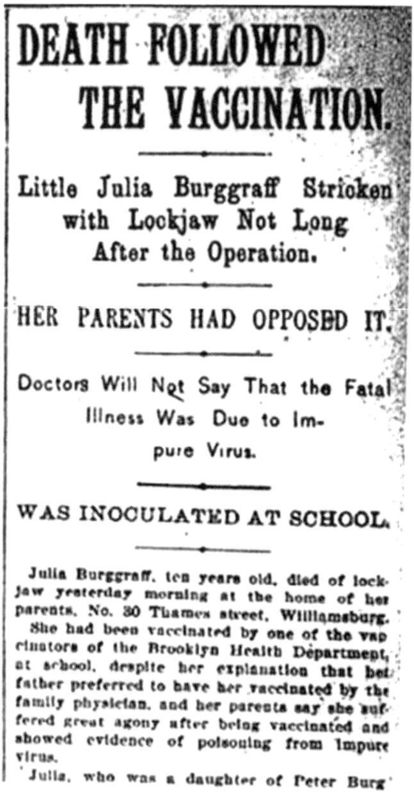

DEATH FOLLOWED THE VACCINATION.

Little Julia Burggraff Stricken with Lockjaw Not Long After the Operation.

HER PARENTS HAD OPPOSED IT.

Doctors Will Not Say That the Fatal Illness Was Due to Impure Virus.

WAS INOCULATED AT SCHOOL.

Julia Burggraff, ten years old, died of lockjaw yesterday morning at the home of her parents, No. 30 Thames street, Williamsburg. She had been vaccinated by one of the vaccinators of the Brooklyn Health Department, at school, despite her explanation that her father preferred to have her vaccinated by the family physician, and her parents say she suffered great agony after being vaccinated and showed evidence of poisoning from impure virus.

Julia, who was a daughter of Peter Burg

Figure 2. In 1894 the *New York Herald* reported on the sensational case of Julia Burggraff, the 10-year-old daughter of a prominent Brooklyn businessman. Julia died of lockjaw shortly after being vaccinated against smallpox, and her father filed suit charging that the health department doctor who had performed the vaccination had been negligent.

opinion Emery had attempted to present. "The conditions requisite to constitute exposure, and whether those which actually exist ... are not necessarily, and may not be, matters within common understanding," the judges declared, showing striking deference to the authority of scientific knowledge. "They present medical questions, and the effect of them in a given case is the subject of professional opinion."[70] With these words, they overturned the previous court's ruling.

It was at best an ambiguous victory for Emery and the health department, finding not that the attempt to compel vaccination was justified but that Emery had not had adequate opportunity to prove it so. Smallpox having passed from the city, however, the issue had lost its urgency for the moment. But the question of the limits of compulsion would resurface in a few years, in a somewhat different form, when the disease returned to the city just after the commencement of the new century.

THE EPIDEMIC OF 1901–1902

Smallpox was largely absent from New York in the final years of the nineteenth century, during which time Manhattan joined with Brooklyn and the surrounding boroughs to create the greater city, with a total population of some 3.5 million. But an unsettling outbreak of cases in the northern wards of the city in December 1900 prompted long lines to form at the health department's midtown headquarters.[71] The health commissioner, Ernst Lederle, moved swiftly against the new cases. Lederle, who held a doctorate in chemistry, authorized the allocation of $22,500 to hire seventy-five vaccinators, who over the next several months administered close to 375,000 immunizations.[72]

Over the 1890s, the stature of the New York City Department of Health had steadily risen in the eyes of city residents. It had gained an international reputation as one of the leading municipal departments in the country, thanks in large part to the pioneering work of its bacteriology laboratory, which had served as a model for similar programs around the country.[73] The laboratory's highly publicized introduction in 1895 of diphtheria antitoxin, which it was the first in the country to produce, had been a great success, dramatically reducing the death rate from the city's most common childhood disease over the next few years, especially among the children of poor tenement dwellers, who were disproportionately afflicted with diphtheria.[74]

Some of the goodwill generated by the department's success in controlling diphtheria was probably transferable to persuading people to be vaccinated. But smallpox vaccination differed from diphtheria antitoxin in two important ways. First, the antitoxin had been introduced with great fanfare and was emblematic of advances in the new scientific medicine, while vaccination predated the wondrous discoveries of the bacteriologists and remained freighted with uncertainty about its safety. Second, diphtheria antitoxin was a treatment, the success of which people could see—children who were sick became well. Vaccination, on the other hand, was a preventive, and as such, its powers had to be taken on faith, since people who underwent it and then remained free from the disease could never be sure that they would not have escaped anyway had they not been vaccinated.[75] For these reasons, suspicion and hostility toward vaccination remained among some New Yorkers who welcomed other medical innovations.

The extent to which such resistance remained among city residents was revealed by their frequent attempts to evade health department vaccination squads in their neighborhood sweeps. One such incident occurred in the Morrisania section of the Bronx. After a case was discovered in the area and the news spread that everyone would have to submit to a doctor's lance, people "fled from houses and sought to elude the vaccinators," the *Daily Tribune* reported. "Many of the men and women attempted to escape by going down the fire escapes and climbing to the roofs, but policemen were at hand at every place of egress, and appeals and entreaties were unheeded."[76]

Such aggressive measures were proving insufficient to contain the epidemic, and in 1901, just under 2,000 cases of smallpox were diagnosed, with about one out of five victims dying of it.[77] As 1902 began and the epidemic showed no signs of dying out, Lederle intensified his efforts, increasing the vaccination force to almost 200 and sending letters to all large manufacturers and businesses in the city offering free on-site immunizations.[78] In response to a request by the board of health, the city's operators of elevated trains ordered all of their motormen and conductors to be vaccinated.[79] The department also passed a regulation targeting lodging houses: every lodger at Manhattan's 105 establishments had to show proof of vaccination before being given a room, or consent to the procedure, otherwise the proprietor risked revocation of his license. The gritty nature of the vaccinators' work among the lodgers was captured in the first-person account of the young physician John Sedgwick Billings, describing a night's rounds in the winter of 1897 after a single case of smallpox had been found in the city's Bowery neighborhood:

> I cannot describe to you the filth, and dirt and rank, reeking, penetrating foulness of the place.... 180 men were there, and I vaccinated over 140 of them—one eighth too dead drunk to even remonstrate—another eighth fighting drunk.... I had one row—the fellow struck me, and I knocked him down and the policeman arrested him—I told him I would let him go if he would be vaccinated. He came around like a lamb, and all the other men in the room ... could not come up and bare their arms quick enough.[80]

Days after the new regulation was passed in 1902, health department inspectors made similar nighttime visits and vaccinated some 6,000 men.[81]

The severity of the outbreak, which was raging in major cities across the Northeast, presented the city with a frustrating paradox. On the one hand, the number of vaccinations administered by the health department was impressively large and seemed to indicate the success of its nominally voluntaristic policy. On the other hand, smallpox was spreading unabated, suggesting to some that more aggressive control measures—backed up with explicit legal authority—were needed. It was the lack of such a mandate, after all, that had stymied Emery's efforts to compel vaccination during the 1894 epidemic in Brooklyn. In May 1901, the New York County Medical Association appointed a special committee to consider the question of whether vaccination should be made compulsory and invited all the group's members to offer their opinions.[82]

After several months of study, the group prepared a recommendation in favor of a compulsory law and gained the sponsorship of State Senator James McCabe, a physician who had formerly practiced at the Long Island College Hospital. In February 1902, McCabe introduced a bill that would require each city in the state to enforce the vaccination of every citizen in any instance where the department of health deemed it necessary; anyone who refused would be guilty of a misdemeanor and subject to a fine of at least $50 and imprisonment of at least ten days. No company employing more than ten people would be allowed to hire anyone who had not been vaccinated within the previous five years.[83]

The bill sparked a fierce debate that revealed fissures within the medical profession about whether compulsion best served the ends of public health. Although the medical profession had become more uniform in its use of allopathic methods, it remained highly fractured throughout this period along lines of practice setting; doctors associated with health departments, who embraced the power of bacteriology and laboratory methods in diagnosing and treating disease, clashed with physicians in private practice, who placed greater value on the empiricism of clinical experience.[84] Private practitioners often resented health department regulations such as mandatory reporting of infectious disease, which they saw as an intrusion on the doctor-patient relationship. But the debate over compulsory vaccination did not break out along any typical or predictable lines.

An editorial in the *Brooklyn Medical Journal* spoke candidly about the politically strategic reasons for keeping the practice voluntary. "[I]t is unwise to make vaccination compulsory, for fear of arousing an antagonism to it which would defeat the very object it seeks to secure. . . . The antivaccinationists meet with very little encouragement, and their efforts to stay the onward march of the army of vaccinators amount to nothing. It is the fear of putting a powerful weapon in their hands which makes the Board of Health hesitate to endorse the bill of Senator McCabe."[85] Similarly, the *New York Medical Journal* stressed the value of retaining a policy that was voluntary—at least in name. "We have always felt that an out-and-out compulsory vaccination law ... was doomed to more or less complete failure.... Compulsion in the matter of vaccination is an unwarrantable encroachment upon personal liberty and therefore one to be resisted."[86] Instead, the journal's editors favored a strategy of what they termed "indirect compulsion" through which businesses with extensive public contact could assure compliance of their customers: "[T]here are other agencies than the government that have it well within their power to enforce general revaccination, notably the railway companies."[87] In other words, coercion was accomplished more appropriately, and more effectively, through the private sector. The editorial went on to describe with approval a plan recently instituted in Illinois, in which all the principal railway lines leading to Chicago were to require proof of vaccination for travelers embarking in localities where smallpox was prevalent.

Yet many physicians expressed a very different view of the merits of compulsion. The editors of the *Medical Record* declared that the bill "deserves the support of the medical profession." Compulsion was justified because "the good of the many is the first consideration. A person who has been exposed to the contagion of smallpox is clearly a public menace."[88] Writing in the *Journal of the American Medical Association,* a health officer with the state of Kentucky (one of the states that did have such a law on the books) declared that "compulsory vaccination and surveillance of the exposed, has never yet failed to bring an outbreak under quick control."[89]

Members of the New York Medical Association personally visited health department officials hoping to gain an endorsement of the measure.[90] But Ernst Lederle and his colleagues on the board of health ultimately came down firmly in opposition to McCabe's bill, describing it as "unwise and uncalled for" and contending that "vaccination should be taught not by force but by education"—a somewhat ironic claim given the health department's strong-arm tactics.[91] Similar legislation had been heard in the state house at least once before, in 1889. At that time, however, the health commissioner, Cyrus Edson, had endorsed the bill, further illustrating the diversity of views among municipal health officials of the day on the open use of coercion. "We have in New York City a class, mostly Bohemians, who are a source of danger to the rest of the people by reason of their prejudice to vaccination," Edson had told the state assembly's committee on public health. "They will yield only to the strong hand of the law."[92] Edson and Lederle both made extensive use of the city's police powers to regulate the actions of recalcitrant citizens, but whereas Edson was comfortable with public assertions of state authority—and indeed had used the open exercise of such power as a strategic tool to heighten public respect for the health department—his successor Lederle preferred to cloak such paternalism in the mantle of voluntarism.[93]

Lederle's position on the bill was no doubt influenced by current events in Massachusetts. Only a month before McCabe introduced his bill in the New York state legislature, anti-vaccination activists in Massachusetts, who had successfully attacked various provisions of local laws on smallpox control over the years, introduced legislation at the statehouse in Boston to repeal that state's compulsory law. The result was a protracted political fight between activists and the Massachusetts Medical Society, which supported the law.[94] In light of the controversy in Massachusetts, a compulsory law must have appeared to Lederle not so much as a means to gain greater compliance with his programs, but rather as a likely spur to resistance and a potential source of political and legal headaches. Lederle also could not have failed to notice that the Massachusetts law did not seem to be helping it greatly: smallpox was just as prevalent in that state as in New York.[95]

The wisdom of Lederle's assessment appeared to be borne out by the tepid response that anti-vaccination activists had been receiving in their attempts to generate public outrage during the current epidemic. A meeting of the New York Anti-Compulsory Vaccination League, at which the group called for an immediate end to the house-to-house sweeps by city doctors, was, according to the *Times,* attended by "nine men, one boy and seven reporters."[96] The group's message depended on two parts: first, that vaccination was unsafe and ineffective; and second, that legal enforcement of it constituted an unacceptable tyranny. The absence of a law on the books at least partially defused the second half of the message and deprived it of much of its resonance. New Yorkers might attempt to escape when they saw the vaccinator coming, but in general they declined to join any active resistance to the city's practices.

Amidst a heavy legislative schedule, the bill died in the state assembly in March 1902 without making it to the governor's desk. Within a few months, the epidemic finally seemed to have burned itself out. A total of about 800,000 people were vaccinated in 1902, almost one out of every four city residents.[97]

At the turn of the twentieth century, the question of how much a state or local government could limit the liberty of residents in order to

protect the community welfare remained unsettled. Decades of litigation by vaccination opponents had resulted in dozens of decisions
in courts around the country. Most upheld compulsory vaccination
laws, especially as they applied to school attendance, but there were
notable exceptions, such as the ruling in William Smith's suit against the
Brooklyn Health Department. Several of these cases, like Smith's, turned
on the question of whether or not the state legislature had expressly
authorized the use of compulsion.[98] These conflicting opinions set the
stage for a landmark U.S. Supreme Court ruling that established the
right of states and localities to use broad police powers in controlling
epidemic disease.

JACOBSON V. MASSACHUSETTS
AND THE ENFORCEMENT OF HEALTH

Like the rest of the Northeast, Massachusetts was hit hard during the
epidemic that struck in the first years of the new century. The state was
well known for being a hotbed of anti-vaccination activism, which had
had a ripple effect on the actions of the general citizenry. According to
the *Medical News,* many people in the Boston area, "though themselves
without pretense of being antivaccinationists, have shirked their duty to
the public health because of the amount of talk indulged in and have
put off their vaccination from year to year."[99] Between 1901 and 1903,
Boston, which had a population of roughly half a million, recorded
some 1,600 cases and 270 deaths from smallpox.[100]

It was in the depths of the winter of 1902 that the board of health of
the city of Cambridge passed a resolution requiring all citizens who had
not been vaccinated in the previous five years to undergo the procedure
again. The board did so in accordance with a state law that empowered
localities to enforce general compulsory vaccination when deemed
necessary for the public safety. On March 15, two weeks after the resolution was enacted, Dr. E. Edwin Spencer, the chairman of the board of
health, visited Henning Jacobson and offered to vaccinate him; if he
refused, Spencer informed him, Jacobson would face a fine of $5.
Jacobson's refusal both to be vaccinated and to pay the fine instigated a
series of legal actions that led over the next three years through the
Massachusetts court system to the U.S. Supreme Court.

Little is known about the life of Henning Jacobson. He was born in
Sweden in 1856 and came to the United States when he was thirteen. He
attended college in Illinois and as a young man underwent a spiritual

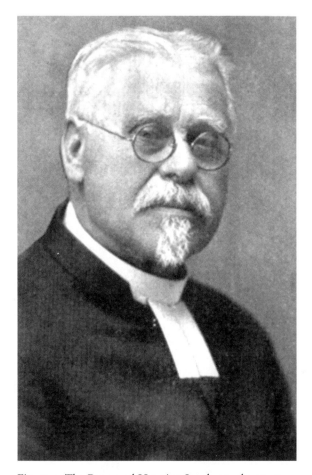

Figure 3. The Reverend Henning Jacobson, the most famous opponent of vaccination in U.S. history, in an undated photo. Photo courtesy of the Archives of the Evangelical Lutheran Church in America.

awakening that led him to travel as a student pastor in the Midwest and Northeast and pursue studies at Yale Divinity School. In 1882, he married Hattie Anderson, a student at a Lutheran college in Minnesota, and together they had five children. He was ordained as a pastor in the Swedish Evangelical Lutheran Church in 1892. The following year the church called upon him to establish a congregation in Cambridge, Massachusetts, where he would live the rest of his life. He was reputed to be a powerful orator, exceptionally devoted to his congregation.[101]

While the court case that bears his name has made Jacobson the most famous opponent of vaccination in U.S. history, it is unclear whether he ever participated in any organized anti-vaccination activities, or what events in his background led him to carry on his fight so persistently. His subsequent legal briefs indicated that both he and one of his sons had at some point "suffered severely" from being vaccinated, but we do not know when these incidents occurred and what impact, if any, they had on Jacobson's attitudes or behavior in the years prior to his confrontation with the Cambridge authorities.

For his refusal to pay the fine, Jacobson was brought in July 1902 before the third district court in the county of Middlesex, along with two other Cambridge men who had also violated the health board's order. After the district court found him guilty, Jacobson appealed for a jury trial in the county's superior court. At that trial, Jacobson argued that the state's vaccination law violated several provisions of both the Massachusetts and U.S. constitutions. He attempted to introduce fourteen facts relevant to vaccination that in his view would serve to demonstrate the unreasonableness of the law. The first twelve facts related to the general lack of safety and efficacy of the procedure; point number one, for example, contended that vaccination "quite often causes or results in a serious and permanent injury."[102] The last two facts were specific to Jacobson himself: that "he had, when a child, been caused great and extreme suffering, for a long period, by a disease produced by his vaccination," and that "he had witnessed a similar result of vaccination in the case of his own son."[103] The court, however, excluded all fourteen facts as immaterial, and at the end of February 1903, the jury found him guilty.[104] He thereupon appealed to the state's highest legal authority, the supreme judicial court, on the ground that the superior court had improperly excluded his evidence.

The following month, the supreme judicial court heard two cases, Jacobson's and a similar one brought by another Cambridge resident, Albert Pear, who had also sought unsuccessfully in lower court to overturn the vaccination law. Both men challenged the constitutionality of the statute, and Jacobson, in addition, argued that the lower court jurors should have been allowed to hear his fourteen facts. The state's high court found no merit to any constitutional objections to the law. It was a reasonable measure, the judges held, duly enacted by the legislature, to protect the people from a known hazard. Citing numerous precedents, the judges noted that other courts had been deferential to the enactment of health regulations; in the few cases that had been decided otherwise, such as *In re Smith,* it was because the wording of the contested statute did not provide sufficient authorization for the restrictions that were imposed.[105]

Turning to Jacobson's complaint that the lower court had improperly excluded evidence that he would have been physically harmed by undergoing vaccination, the judges affirmed the previous ruling that any such evidence was immaterial. "It would not have been competent to introduce the medical history of individual cases," the judges claimed. While the majority of the doctors "have recognized the possibility of injury to an individual from carelessness in the performance of [vaccination], or even in a conceivable case without carelessness, they have generally considered the risk of such an injury too small to be seriously weighed as against the benefits coming from the discreet and proper use of the preventive."[106] Thus, the court held, the "theoretical possibility of an injury in an individual case as a result of [the law's] enforcement does not show that as a whole it is unreasonable."[107] Faced with the third ruling holding him liable for the $5 fine, Jacobson filed a petition to the U.S. Supreme Court, and on June 29, 1903, his case was added to the court's docket.

The case came before the justices in December 1904. A large crowd, including officers of the Massachusetts Anti-Compulsory Vaccination Association, attended the day the arguments in the case were heard.[108] Jacobson was represented before the court by the prominent lawyer and politician George Fred Williams. A former Mugwump and activist in the free silver wing of the Democratic party, Williams had represented Massachusetts in the U.S. Congress and made three unsuccessful bids to be elected state governor.[109] The briefs submitted by Williams offered numerous examples of the ways in which Massachusetts law violated the due process and equal protection provisions of the Fourteenth Amendment. For example, the law provided an exemption for persons under age twenty-one who presented a certificate from a physician that they were "unfit subjects" for vaccination, but no such allowance existed for adults.[110] It was unreasonable for the state to interfere with Jacobson's liberty when he had not been taken with any illness, the brief claimed; although there was no doubt that the police powers could be brought to bear against "existing offensive acts or conditions," it did not then follow that such force "can be imposed upon healthy citizens, merely because as human beings they have the potentiality of contracting contagious diseases."[111]

In his brief for Massachusetts, the state's attorney general cited the numerous lower court rulings from around the country that had upheld the power of local and state legislatures to enact laws for the common welfare and to delegate the authority for their enforcement to administrative bodies. The brief asserted, somewhat misleadingly, that Jacobson "did not seek to show that in his own case the requirement of the board of health was oppressive, or that by reason of his state of health or other circumstance vaccination would be dangerous to him."[112] But, in fact, the last two points of Jacobson's fourteen points of evidence, which the lower courts had refused to hear, had concerned his own and his son's prior adverse reactions to vaccination.

On February 20, 1905, the Supreme Court handed down a seven-two decision in favor of Massachusetts.[113] Writing for the majority, Justice John Marshall Harlan declared that while the high court had never attempted to define the limits of the police powers, it had distinctly recognized the authority of the states to enact "health laws of every description" to guard the common good in whatever way the citizens, through their elected representatives, thought appropriate.[114] By the same token, the state could legitimately impose penalties such as fines or quarantine on those who refused to cooperate with such laws. Turning to the central question of whether the statute violated Jacobson's liberty, Harlan offered an unequivocal vision of the role of the individual within society:

> [T]he liberty secured by the Constitution of the United States to every person within its jurisdiction does not import an absolute right in each person to be, at all times and in all circumstances, wholly freed from restraint. There are manifold restraints to which every person is necessarily subject for the common good. On any other basis organized society could not exist with safety to its members. Society based on the rule that each one is a law unto himself would soon be confronted with disorder and anarchy.[115]

The compulsory vaccination law, Harlan contended, was consistent with what the Massachusetts constitution had laid out as "a fundamental principle of the social compact that the whole people covenants with each citizen, and each citizen with the whole people."[116] Harlan conceded that there might be instances where a public health statute would be sufficiently "arbitrary and oppressive ... as to justify the interference of the courts," such as the case of an adult who would be physically harmed by being forced to undergo vaccination; in that situation, enforcement of the statute would be "cruel and inhuman to the last degree." But, Harlan insisted, "no such case is here presented. It is the case of an adult who, for aught it appears, was himself in perfect health and a fit subject of vaccination."[117] Harlan was apparently unconvinced

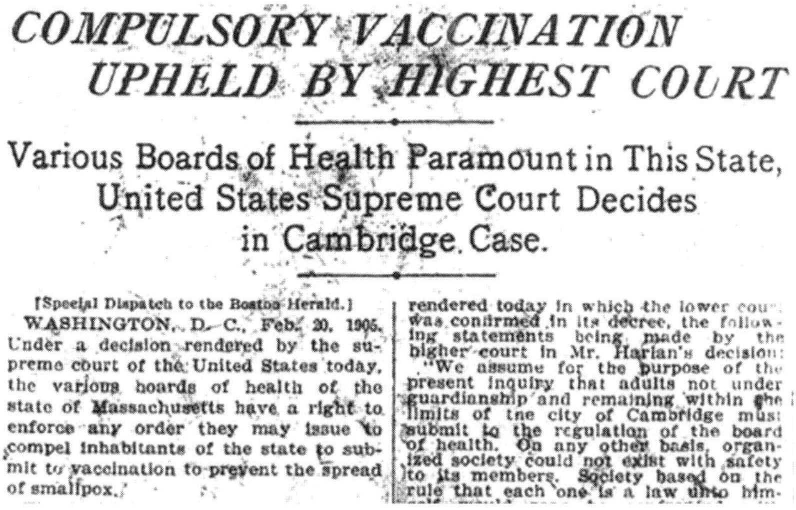

COMPULSORY VACCINATION UPHELD BY HIGHEST COURT

Various Boards of Health Paramount in This State, United States Supreme Court Decides in Cambridge Case.

[Special Dispatch to the Boston Herald.]
WASHINGTON, D. C., Feb. 20, 1905. Under a decision rendered by the supreme court of the United States today, the various boards of health of the state of Massachusetts have a right to enforce any order they may issue to compel inhabitants of the state to submit to vaccination to prevent the spread of smallpox.

rendered today in which the lower cou'' was confirmed in its decree, the following statements being made by the higher court in Mr. Harlan's decision: "We assume for the purpose of the present inquiry that adults not under guardianship and remaining within the limits of the city of Cambridge must submit to the regulation of the board of health. On any other basis, organized society could not exist with safety to its members. Society based on the rule that each one is a law unto him-

Figure 4. The *Boston Herald* of February 20, 1905, featured the verdict in *Jacobson v. Massachusetts* on its front page. The U.S. Supreme Court's ruling on the constitutionality of compulsory vaccination settled a legal issue that had been the subject of dozens of lawsuits over the previous decades.

by Jacobson's assertion that his having previously suffered from vaccination was evidence that he would have been in special danger if he underwent the procedure again.[118]

Two justices, David Brewer and Rufus Peckham, dissented from the ruling without opinion. Two months later, they were in the majority when the court handed down another opinion centering on the state's police powers and a health regulation. *Lochner v. New York,* which would ultimately prove a more far-reaching and influential decision outside the realm of public health, contrasted starkly with the court's position in *Jacobson.* The case concerned a New York State law that limited the working hours of bakers to a maximum of ten per day or sixty per week. Writing for the five-member majority, Justice Peckham rejected the notion that bakers warranted special protection under a health law: "the trade of a baker, in and of itself, is not an unhealthy one to that degree which would authorize the legislature to interfere with the right to labor, and with the right of free contract on the part of the individual."[119] By interpreting the Fourteenth Amendment's due process clause as safeguarding, above all, the right of employee and employer to negotiate the terms of their labor with each other, *Lochner* articulated a conception of liberty that was centered on the freedom of economic contract, and thus came to serve, over the next three decades, as the classic defense of laissez-faire capitalism.

In dissenting from *Lochner*, Justice Harlan argued that it was for legislatures, not courts, to decide whether a given statute warranted an infringement on individual rights. Citing his own opinion on vaccination from earlier in the term, Harlan wrote, "I take it to be firmly established that what is called the liberty of contract may, within certain limits, be subjected to regulations designed and calculated to promote the general welfare or to guard the public health, the public morals or the public safety."[120] In a separate dissent, Justice Oliver Wendell Holmes also pointed to the decision in *Jacobson* as proof that freedom may be constrained for the social good. "The liberty of the citizen to do as he likes so long as he does not interfere with the liberty of others to do the same ... is interfered with by school laws, by the Post Office, by every state or municipal institution which takes his money for purposes thought desirable, whether he likes it or not," Holmes wrote.[121]

The ruling in *Jacobson v. Massachusetts*, though it did not attract wide attention in the press, garnered favorable editorial comment in newspapers in Boston and New York. "It is too much to expect that this [ruling] will abate the obstinacy of the anti-vaccinationists," declared the *Boston Herald*, "but they will probably recognize the inexpediency of putting their obstinacy in practice as against the health authorities when the latter undertake to execute the law."[122] The *New York Times* predicted that the ruling "should end the useful life of the societies of cranks formed to resist the operation of laws relative to vaccination."[123] These confident forecasts turned out to be premature, however. Three years later, the Anti-Vaccination League of America would be founded in Philadelphia, and a diverse assortment of activists would, over the next quarter-century, redouble their efforts at combating attempts to force vaccination upon the people. These challenges to authority, embodying fundamental conflicts between democratic values and scientific expertise, are the subject of chapter 2.

Science in a Democracy

Smallpox Vaccination in the Progressive Era and the 1920s

In the summer of 1914, eleven-year-old Lewis Freeborn Loyster died three weeks after being vaccinated in the small town of Cazenovia, in central New York State. The cause of death on autopsy was determined to be infantile paralysis, and the boy's father, James, was convinced that smallpox vaccination was responsible. Spurred by grief, James Loyster began canvassing the cities and towns in the region for stories of children who had been similarly harmed, and he soon reached two conclusions: that the deaths alleged to have been caused by the vaccine far outnumbered those from smallpox itself, and that sentiment in the area ran strongly against the practice—"a feeling almost insurrectionary in its intensity," he claimed.[1] Loyster, who was active in Republican party politics in the region, collected his findings into an illustrated pamphlet, which he distributed to members of the state legislature, in an effort, ultimately successful, to overhaul the state's compulsory vaccination law for students in public schools.

The Supreme Court's 1905 opinion in *Jacobson v. Massachusetts* did not have the sweeping effects on smallpox control that might have been foreseen when the ruling was issued. Although the constitutional right to use compulsory measures in the enforcement of vaccination had been affirmed by the country's highest court, after decades of legal controversy, city and state health departments rarely—outside of school entry requirements—used the authority they had won. The incidence of smallpox continued to decline and, for reasons that remain unclear, became marked by a milder course of illness and lower mortality. Mass vaccination campaigns became increasingly uncommon, and the locus of control for the disease began to center almost exclusively on routine vaccination of students. Not coincidentally, the twenty-five years following *Jacobson* were a period of intensified advocacy against vaccination, with activists turning to their legislatures to achieve what they were unable to win in the courts.

In the Progressive Era and the 1920s, a wide range of groups and individuals articulated political, spiritual, and philosophical opposition to vaccination. In addition to questioning the value of orthodox medicine, their arguments were strongly inflected with libertarian, anti-government views, and emphasized the protection of children from state intervention. They scored numerous legislative and rhetorical victories, engaging their opponents—public health officials, physicians, and scientists—in an ongoing battle for public opinion. This heightened opposition was not a reaction against the more vigorous use of compulsion; on the contrary, the less systematically laws were enforced, the more intense was the resistance on those infrequent occasions when they were.

This chapter examines the contested status of vaccination during the first decades of the twentieth century. As developments in scientific medicine triggered debates about the role elite knowledge should play in a rapidly changing democratic society, vaccination emerged as the focal point for a broad spectrum of groups concerned about government intrusion in personal decision-making, especially related to the health and the welfare of children. In this context, opponents of vaccination brought about changes in law and policy around the country, and in so doing, they left a legacy that had profound consequences for all the vaccines that would be introduced in subsequent years.

THE STATUS OF SCIENCE AND THE REACH OF THE STATE

In the nineteenth century, the severity of smallpox was a regular spur to action, but after the turn of the century, an attack of the disease in a community no longer provoked the urgency that had once led people to seek vaccination. A milder form of smallpox, *variola minor,* first appeared in the United States in 1897 and over the following two decades became the dominant strain.[2] Although the pustular rash that spread across the body was similar to that seen in classic smallpox (*variola major*), the new form was not as severe and debilitating, and it left less scarring afterward. In contrast to the fatality rates of 20 to

30 percent that were typical of *v. major,* only rarely did a victim die from *v. minor.*[3]

An important consequence of this epidemiological shift was that vaccination came to seem more dangerous and unjustified in the minds of those who were inclined to oppose it. Adverse events arising from the procedure, long the subject of popular lore, were magnified when the disease itself came to seem less of a threat. "Dread of vaccination has been increased by the reports which fly about in regard to someone almost dying, and of arms being nearly lost, and of serious illness which is attributed to it," noted one health officer in upstate New York. "On the other hand the disease itself has been so mild that in the absence of deaths from it little real concern is felt, and it is regarded as an inconvenience rather than danger."[4] This changed perception was ironic. The U.S. Public Health Service was given the authority to license and inspect vaccine manufacturers in 1902, and most evidence suggests that the procedure became safer as a result, although the purity of vaccine continued to be a sporadic problem, and government inspection sometimes revealed contamination by tetanus bacillus or other microorganisms.[5] Public health experts increasingly insisted that vaccine-related injury was a thing of the past. "That tetanus, erysipelas and general infection have had their origin in the vaccination abrasion or sore we cannot nor do we wish to deny," conceded a 1915 editorial in one medical journal; however, it added, such unfortunate incidents "under the present federal supervision can hardly occur again."[6] A health department pamphlet assured the public that "the chance of harm to-day from vaccination is very remote when the number of ill results is compared with the great number being vaccinated."[7]

But neither epidemiological features of smallpox nor the perceived or actual frequency of vaccine injuries fully accounts for the vehemence and persistence of the anti-vaccinationists' efforts during this era to change laws and practices around the country. Anti-vaccinationism was a response to two broad and interrelated trends in the new century: first, the proliferation of biologic products for preventing and treating illness; and, second, reform efforts that expanded the reach of the state into previously private spheres. Together, these two developments fueled bitter debates about whether the government and civic institutions should use advances in scientific medicine to dictate the actions of individuals.

The pharmaceutical industry grew rapidly during this period, and drug firms became more rigorously scientific, employing larger staffs, with training in bacteriology and medicine. As techniques for research, production, and marketing all became more sophisticated, companies brought many new products to market and established close relationships with universities, pharmacists, and the medical community.[8] Vaccines were developed against several diseases, including cholera, plague, and typhoid, and by the 1910s the term "vaccine," which originally had meant only the preparation of cowpox that provided immunity against smallpox, began to be applied more broadly to any product designed to produce active immunity. The director of the U.S. Hygienic Laboratory wrote in 1916 that "the term *vaccine* has become too widely used, in its extended sense, to attempt to limit it at present to the original application."[9] The efficacy of these new preparations remained uncertain, however, and their application was largely confined to controlling scattered disease outbreaks in limited geographic regions.[10] The typhoid vaccine proved the most valuable, because of its use in the military, where it had a substantial impact on troop mortality.[11] Because the vaccine required a series of three shots over several months and conferred only short-term immunity, it was never widely used among civilians, though it was recommended for people living or traveling in areas with poor sanitation.[12]

Although the promise of scientific innovations usually exceeded their actual benefits, they attracted enthusiastic and often breathless coverage in the popular press. Newspaper and magazine articles trumpeted the prospect that other diseases would soon yield to the principles of immunization that had brought smallpox under control, expressing the hope that prophylactic "serums" to combat diseases as diverse as tuberculosis, pneumonia and cancer might soon be developed.[13] But these advances also provoked an anti-modernist backlash against the paternalistic and potentially coercive uses to which scientific medicine might be put. Anti-vaccination literature of the period reflected a pervasive fear that new vaccines and treatments—with all of their unknown and untoward side effects—would be made mandatory. The brief that Henning Jacobson, the plaintiff in *Jacobson v. Massachusetts*, filed with the Supreme Court gave voice to this concern:

> The present tendency of medical science is toward the treatment of contagious diseases by the use of serums, and it is entirely possible that public authorities and physicians may be encouraged to extend the vaccination scheme to all other contagious diseases and set up a general compulsory medical regime, which will subject a healthy community to attack by boards of health under compulsory laws. If it be justifiable to compel the inoculation of a citizen for one disease, then by a parity of

reasoning it is for the public interest that every citizen should be inoculated to render him immune against all possible contagions which may menace the community.[14]

Dovetailing with these scientific advances were broad social changes that altered the relationship between the citizen and the collective. New institutions of the administrative state and civil society expanded their purview over matters once reserved to the individual, the family, or the church. Agents of expertise and authority such as social workers, visiting nurses, and educators, employed in both the public and private sectors, represented a threat to the autonomy of family decision-making.[15] In part because of the rise of worker's compensation programs, physical examination of employees became widespread in many industries after 1910.[16] Around the same time, major life insurance companies began requiring such exams for their policyholders.[17] In previous decades, Americans might have gone most of their lives without seeing a doctor, but they now increasingly came under the scrutiny of health professionals as part of the emerging practice of preventive medicine. In 1914, New York City's health commissioner, S. S. Goldwater, announced his support for a plan (which was never instituted) to conduct mandatory annual medical inspections of all city residents for their own good. "I, for one, am not willing to cease short of a radical change in the manner of applying medical knowledge," Goldwater said. "Preventive medicine cannot do its utmost good until physicians are regularly employed by the entire population, not merely for the treatment of acute and advanced disease, but as medical advisers in health."[18] It is in the context of such bold assertions that one may better understand the claim of a leading anti-vaccinationist in 1920 that "there exists a well-laid plan to medically enslave the nation."[19] In this view, the very concept of preventive medicine represented a calculated effort by doctors to shift attention away from wellness toward sickness and foster the belief that only experts could legitimately make health decisions, moves that held obvious benefits for the medical profession.

The medical control of young people sparked the most heated reactions from anti-vaccinationists. Child welfare was a preoccupation of Progressive Era reformers, who brought about multifaceted changes in law and social policy, ranging from new systems of juvenile justice to legislation barring child labor.[20] Expert knowledge formed the basis on which these reformers based their claim to be better qualified than parents to judge the well-being of children. The medical inspection of

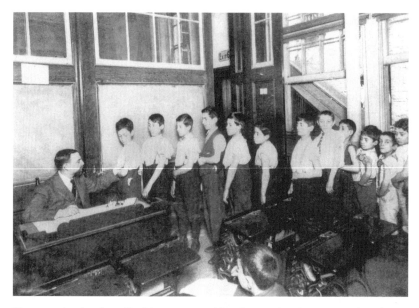

Figure 5. A school medical inspector verifies the vaccination status of students by checking each arm for a scar. Originally focused on contagious diseases, school health inspections expanded during the Progressive Era to include screening for hidden or chronic conditions such as tonsillitis and vision and hearing defects. This photo is from the 1913 book *Medical Inspection of Schools*, by the education reformers Luther Halsey Gulick and Leonard Ayres. Photo courtesy of the National Library of Medicine.

children in public schools, which had originated in the nineteenth century for controlling acute infectious diseases, was expanded around the turn of the century to include screening for hidden or chronic conditions such as tonsillitis and hearing and vision defects.[21] By 1912, about half the states had passed laws permitting or requiring medical examination in schools; under the laws, parents could be ordered to seek treatment for a child found to have a physical defect.[22] Such programs heightened anxiety that government bureaucrats were seeking to use science as a covert means of removing children from the control of their parents. "Little by little," wrote one activist, "an effort is being made to bring about the medical domination of the schools and the children attending them."[23]

Perhaps the most extreme example of the medical control of children was the tuberculosis "preventorium" movement. These specially designed sanatoria were intended to provide a better environment for

"pre-tubercular" children—those discovered through laboratory examination to be infected with the tubercle bacillus but not yet exhibiting
symptoms—than the one they would experience at home. Separation of
endangered children from their parents was the cornerstone of an overall plan to protect them from unhealthy influences, and although the
transfer of a child to a preventorium was ostensibly voluntary, coercion
by charitable organizations and health officials of the poor, often immigrant, families whom illness had struck was sometimes implied.[24]

Closely related to concerns about the overreaching efforts of child
welfare reformers were controversies over state medicine, a protean
term that encompassed a wide range of government programs to provide
for health care through mechanisms such as universal health insurance
and publicly funded clinics. To proponents of such programs, state medicine was a rational and economically efficient way of dealing with the
vagaries of illness in society; to opponents, it represented an insidious
attempt to transform the country into a socialistic state. Legally mandated vaccination, provided at public expense by city-employed doctors,
was a paradigmatic example of the evils of state medicine.

The campaign during the 1910s to establish a nationwide system of
compulsory health insurance was at the center of extensive public
debates about state medicine.[25] The enactment in 1921 of the Sheppard-
Towner Act, which provided federal matching funds to help states set
up programs to improve maternal and child health, was both the
culmination of years of efforts by Progressives and a lightning rod
for criticism of expanding government involvement in health care.[26]
Sheppard-Towner required the establishment of a state-level bureaucracy to administer the work.[27] To its opponents, it embodied the creep-
ing expansion of a distant, centralized government, a trend that was
especially threatening amid the postwar backlash against socialism.[28]
The anti-statist mood of the period was captured in the words of a
congressional representative in 1921 who attacked "Government supervision of mothers; Government care and maintenance of infants;
Government control of education; Government control of training for
vocations; Government regulation of employment, the hours, holidays,
wages, accident insurance and all."[29]

While suspicion of science and orthodox medicine and an anti-statist
ideology hostile to government intrusion in personal behavior provided common ground for anti-vaccinationists, this surface similarity
masked important differences in background and outlook. Health officials of the day generally characterized anti-vaccination activism as a

homogeneous movement, referring dismissively to "the anti's," and commentators in the popular press echoed this simplistic assessment. But it is erroneous to view the opposition to vaccination that took place across the nation during this period as representing a single, unified phenomenon. Anti-vaccination activity in the early twentieth century comprised a heterogeneous assortment of individuals and organizations who differed in their beliefs, tactics, and goals.

THE DIVERSITY OF ANTI-VACCINATIONISM

One of the most prominent groups was the Anti-Vaccination League of America, which was formed in Philadelphia in 1908 by two wealthy businessmen, John Pitcairn and Charles M. Higgins. The group described itself as a "national confederation" of affiliated societies in states around the country, and its members devoted themselves to opposing compulsory vaccination laws at the state and local levels.[30] Pitcairn, the group's president, was born in Scotland in 1841 and immigrated as a teenager to western Pennsylvania, where he eventually made his fortune in oil, steel, and railroads. He was a civic leader in the town of Bryn Athyn, near Pittsburgh, where he had an estate. He was also an active member and major benefactor of the Swedenborgian Church. Pitcairn came to the anti-vaccination cause late in life, after he became engulfed in a controversy in 1906 among church members who resisted the state's efforts to vaccinate them during a smallpox outbreak. Pitcairn's opposition to vaccination was rooted partly in Swedenborgian teachings and in his devotion to the alternative medical practice of homeopathy, which many church members embraced.[31] He was also influenced by the fact that years earlier, his son Raymond had suffered an adverse reaction after being vaccinated as a child. Yet his position did not rest primarily on grounds of theology or medical practice, but rather on a political basis: he believed that it was wrong for government, no matter how worthy its intentions, to force people to act against their will.[32] In a tract that cited, among other works, John Stuart Mill's classic defense of individual rights in the philosophical treatise *On Liberty,* Pitcairn asked rhetorically, "We have repudiated *religious* tyranny; we have rejected *political* tyranny; shall we now submit to *medical* tyranny?"[33]

After determining that Pennsylvania's efforts to compel his fellow Swedenborgians to be vaccinated were unjust, Pitcairn became politically active, lobbying the state's general assembly in Harrisburg for the repeal of the compulsory vaccination law, and in 1911, he was appointed

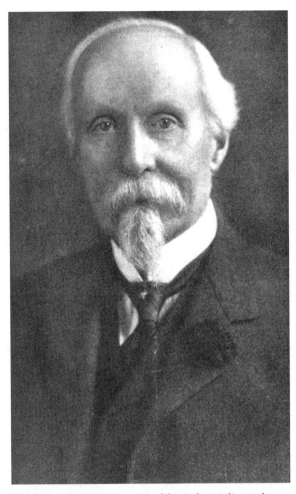

Figure 6. John Pitcairn, a wealthy industrialist and
civic leader in western Pennsylvania, co-founded the
Anti-Vaccination League of America in 1908. This
portrait appeared in the book *Horrors of Vaccination
Exposed and Illustrated*, by Pitcairn's friend and fellow
activist Charles Higgins.

by the governor to serve on a special commission to investigate the practice (after three years of study the panel recommended retaining the law,
over Pitcairn's minority objection).[34] In 1908, as part of his newfound
interest in the topic, Pitcairn bankrolled a national conference in
Philadelphia of vaccination opponents, which led to the founding of the
Anti-Vaccination League of America.

The league's co-founder, secretary, and most active member was Pitcairn's friend Charles M. Higgins of Brooklyn. Higgins had much in common with Pitcairn; he had immigrated from Ireland as a child and had made his fortune as the manufacturer of a special type of ink he had invented. Higgins was also active in civic affairs, donating money for the renovation of historic sites in Brooklyn and serving as a co-founder of the Kings County Historical Society.[35] Higgins was the group's chief spokesman and pamphleteer, writing numerous polemical tracts such as *Open Your Eyes Wide!* (1912), *The Crime against the School Child* (1915), *Vaccination and Lockjaw: The Assassins of the Blood* (1916), and *Horrors of Vaccination Exposed and Illustrated* (1920), which regaled readers with graphic descriptions and photographs of hapless victims who had been disfigured, blinded, and killed by vaccination. He made numerous attempts to overturn New York State's law mandating vacccination of students in public schools.

Another influential group in this period was the Citizens Medical Reference Bureau, founded in New York City in 1919 with the mottoes "Against Compulsory Medicine or Surgery for Children and Adults" and "Advocating No Form of Treatment but in Defense of Parental Control over Children." Rivaling Higgins in energy and devotion to the anti-vaccinationist cause was the bureau's secretary and sole paid staff member, Harry Bernhardt Anderson. Little is known about the life of H. B. Anderson (as he typically identified himself in print), but for more than two decades, his was the most prominent anti-vaccination voice in New York City, and his influence was felt nationwide by dint of his tireless letter-writing to public health officials in cities and states around the country. Anderson also published a monthly bulletin, which he sent to supporters (and opponents) and used as a lobbying tool in his efforts to get compulsory laws repealed. In addition to opposing vaccination, Anderson spoke out at public forums and meetings on a wide range of health policy issues, including the medical examination of schoolchildren, requirements for premarital syphilis tests, and increases in the New York City Health Department's budget. The common theme uniting these topics was the specter of "state medicine," which Anderson attacked in a 1920 book as "A state (or Federal) system of administration of compulsory allopathic medicine ... untrammeled in the exercise of authority, reaching down through the subdivisions of county and township to the people; ... in daily touch with every nook and corner of the state or nation."[36]

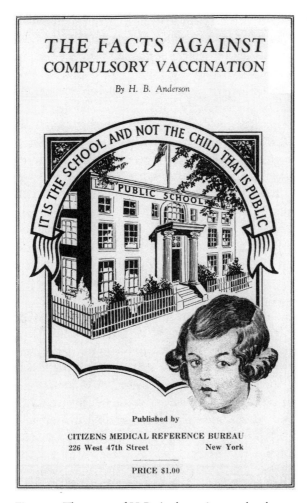

Figure 7. The cover of H.B. Anderson's 1929 book
The Facts against Compulsory Vaccination illustrates
the extent to which the protection of children against
state intervention, and the potential use of schools as a
site of coercion, were central to the concerns of anti-
vaccinationists in the early twentieth century.

The Citizens Medical Reference Bureau had a family tie to the
Anti-Vaccination League of America: its work was supported by two
of John Pitcairn's sons, Harold and Raymond.[37] The extent of the
Pitcairn brothers' substantive involvement in the work of the bureau is
uncertain; they served as directors from the 1920s through the 1940s,

and it is likely that their primary role was in providing the financial support that made possible the organization's many publications. Illustrating the extent to which libertarian ideology was a part of some anti-vaccinationists' worldview, both Harold and Raymond Pitcairn were also major financial backers of Sentinels of the Republic, a right-wing political organization founded in 1922 and devoted to opposing the concentration of government power, counteracting radicalism and Bolshevism, and "checking the growth of Federal paternalism." For two decades, the group fought against a variety of social reforms it viewed as communistic, including laws aimed at limiting child labor, a proposal for a federal department of education, and Franklin Roosevelt's New Deal program.[38]

Founded around the same time as the Citizens Medical Reference Bureau, and similar in its outlook and mission, was the American Medical Liberty League, which fought ongoing battles during the 1920s against what it saw as the hegemony of allopathic practice. The group's letterhead described it as "A citizen's movement for medical liberty on the same basis as religious liberty with the same constitutional guarantees." The league's secretary was Lora C. W. Little, who had an active and successful career as an anti-vaccination agitator dating from the turn of the century. She was the editor and publisher for five years of the *Liberator,* a "journal of health and freedom" in Minnesota, and preached a message of freedom from medical tyranny during travels in England, Scotland, and Massachusetts, before settling in Portland, Oregon, where from 1909 to 1918 she led activities against the state's compulsory vaccination law.[39] As the Liberty League's secretary and chief propagandist, Little published a monthly newsletter from the group's Chicago headquarters and sought to influence policy and law not only in Illinois but around the country; like Anderson, she conducted national letter-writing campaigns, engaging with health officials in Washington, D.C., and in state capitals. Like the Anti-Vaccination League, the Liberty League had affiliated chapters across the country, although the extent of the membership in these local societies is difficult to determine.[40]

The rhetoric of "medical liberty" groups emphasized the legal and political aspects of vaccination; it was compulsion that they found most objectionable. Other groups, however, objected to the practice because it was antithetical to their ideas about health, healing, and the body. Perhaps best known of these were the Christian Scientists. Founded by Mary Baker Eddy in 1879 in Massachusetts, Christian Science was premised on the belief that illness was a mental rather than a material phenomenon, and that, as such, it could be overcome through prayer. Its adherents rejected allopathic medical interventions such as pharmaceutical treatments and surgery (though some did consult dentists and oculists).

Christian Science grew rapidly around the turn of the century, counting roughly 40,000 followers by 1906, and experienced a corresponding degree of public scrutiny and, often, hostility. Sensational cases of children dying, especially from diphtheria, while under the care of Christian Scientist parents and practitioners drew the wrath of the public and lawmakers, who increasingly brought charges of manslaughter and unlawful practice of medicine against them.[41] In this hostile environment, the church adopted a stance that accommodation with the law wherever possible might be the better part of valor. Eddy told her followers in an official church publication in 1901, "Where vaccination is compulsory, let your children be vaccinated, and see that your mind is in such a state that by your prayers vaccination will do the children no harm."[42] Around the same time, she enjoined church members from publishing materials "uncharitable or impertinent towards religion, medicine, the courts, or the laws of our land."[43] Christian Scientists were thus not highly visible in spreading an anti-vaccination message in the early part of the century. Under frequent attack in the courts, they largely focused their advocacy efforts on changing the state laws that barred them from practicing medicine. Individual adherents of the religion evaded compulsory laws, however, either taking advantage of lax enforcement or home schooling their children when necessary,[44] and attempted to sway legislators who were considering bills related to vaccination.[45] The *Christian Science Monitor* also reported on the activities of anti-vaccination societies.[46]

Another health movement that was antagonistic to vaccination, though less based in religion and spirituality, was physical culture. Founded and popularized by the fitness guru Bernarr Macfadden, physical culture entailed a Spartan regimen of strenuous exercise, a diet of natural foods, and exposure to fresh air and sunlight; Macfadden and his followers urged periodic fasting and opposed consumption of coffee, alcohol, and tobacco.[47] The movement rejected the germ theory and contended that those who lived a clean, natural life were not susceptible to disease. Macfadden's persistent opposition to vaccination dated from early in his career. In 1901, the Physical Culture Publishing Company issued the book *Vaccination a Crime,* which portrayed Jenner's methods

as a dangerous delusion advanced to maintain the hegemony of allopathic medicine.[48]

After establishing numerous exercise schools and sanatoria and the
monthly fitness magazine *Physical Culture,* Macfadden built a media
empire, publishing tabloid magazines such as *True Story* and *True
Detective Mysteries* and the *New York Evening Graphic,* a sensational
newspaper specializing in stories of sex and crime. While Macfadden did
not devote his energies to the anti-vaccination cause as single-mindedly
as the prolific pamphleteers Charles Higgins and H. B. Anderson, he
was arguably more influential, because he was able to reach a far wider
audience. During the 1920s, the total nationwide circulation of his
publications was estimated at as many as forty million people. Both
Physical Culture and the *Graphic* ran numerous articles opposing vaccination. In a 1922 article in *Physical Culture,* for example, Macfadden
claimed that deaths from vaccination outnumbered those from smallpox itself, and that "it is now admitted by many of the ablest physicians
and scientists that the constitutional taint produced by vaccination
causes a tendency towards all pus-forming diseases like catarrh, consumption, pneumonia, etc."[49] The *Graphic* featured an article, allegedly
written by a physician, entitled "Vaccination Killed My Two Sisters"
(which Macfadden subsequently confessed was not written by a doctor
at all),[50] and ran a series of photographs of people whose ghastly skin
diseases were said to have been caused by vaccination.[51] Macfadden
also used his magazine's mailing lists to urge readers to oppose New
York's compulsory law.[52]

Ideals of bodily integrity also lay behind the opposition of another
newly prominent group of healers: chiropractors. Founded in 1895, chiropractic stressed a holistic view of health and the belief that illness stemmed
from an imbalance or interference with the flow of energy from the brain,
usually produced by misalignment of the spine. Chiropractors, embracing
drugless healing and fighting disease through natural means such as
skeletal adjustments, rejected the interventionist view of disease prevention that vaccination represented.[53] Practitioners and their devotees advocated against the procedure through their journals and pamphlets, lobbied
legislators and other public officials, and frequently made public protests
out of their refusal to comply with compulsory vaccination laws.[54] The
opposition of chiropractors may in one sense be seen as the last salvos in
the decades-long battle between alternative and allopathic physicians for
status and authority. The fight between regular and sectarian practitioners
such as chiropractors, homeopaths, and naturopaths, centering on issues

such as licensing and medical education, was coming to an end in the Progressive Era, especially after the famous Flexner Report in 1910 dealt a symbolic if not actual deathblow to the legitimacy of alternative sects.[55] Chiropractors were the most active among sectarian practitioners in their opposition to vaccination; although a vocal minority of homeopaths opposed the practice, many supported it.[56]

Because smallpox vaccine was made from the lymph of calves deliberately infected with cowpox, vaccination also drew the wrath of anti-vivisection groups. Anti-vivisectionists did not necessarily believe that vaccination was ineffective, rather that the suffering it imposed on animals made its use ethically unjustifiable. Although animal rights activism lacked the explicit libertarianism that underpinned much anti-vaccination rhetoric, it expressed a similar belief that the scientific establishment could not be trusted to act in the best interests of the public, and the two movements had a long association, dating from their origins in mid-nineteenth-century England.[57] American anti-vivisectionists experienced a heyday at the turn of the twentieth century, when they enjoyed wide public recognition and support. Their battles to end the use of animals in laboratory experimentation were largely unsuccessful, however, and the steady increase in the prestige of scientific inquiry eclipsed their efforts.[58]

As these brief sketches have shown, the anti-vaccination movement encompassed a wide range of beliefs and activities, and it is difficult to generalize about the people who made up this heterogeneous movement. Most of the authors of anti-vaccination tracts and pamphlets were men (Lora Little being a notable exception), but the officers and directors listed on groups' letterheads and publications included a few women. Many women were Christian Scientist practitioners and teachers; and the majority of anti-vivisection activists were women.[59] While some prominent anti-vaccinationists had considerable financial resources and social standing, it is also clear that many of those who spurned the practice belonged to the middle class.[60] One very significant personal characteristic shared by prominent activists was family tragedy: Henning Jacobson, John Pitcairn, James Loyster, and Lora Little all had children who had either died or suffered injury following vaccination.

Activism and lobbying represented only part of the overall picture of public opposition, of course. Far greater were the numbers of ordinary citizens who opposed the practice not because of philosophical principles but because they objected to the discomfort and inconvenience—the transient fever and swelling caused by vaccination often resulted in time missed from work—in the absence of an imminent threat of disease. For example, the crusading spirit of Higgins, Little, and Anderson contrasted sharply with the pragmatic concerns of the more than 100 residents of Van Buren, Arkansas, who in 1918 took the unusual step of petitioning President Woodrow Wilson to excuse them from the state's new compulsory vaccination law, citing both the $1 cost of the procedure and the attendant economic losses, and saying,

> it is not the cost of the Vaccination alone that we are opposed to, but also the loss of the childrens time from the field from the effect of same, as well as the uncalled for suffering, after a carefull investigation, we can find no record of there being a case of smallpox in this vicinity for the past ten years or more.... According to the Laws of this State, we are forced to send our children to School (which is right) But if we have our Children Vaccinated now, It will keep them out of the field untill School begins, Then School, and after loosing as many boys as we have, who are in the Army, it will make it impossible for us to harvest what crop we have, and sow our Wheat and other Fall crops without a loss to one or the other.[61]

The most familiar public face of the anti-vaccination movement emerged through its literature. The numerous tracts, pamphlets, and books emphasized the danger of the procedure in rhetoric that tended to be highly polemical, designed to incite outrage and public revolt. Vaccination was "barbarous medical child-slaughter,"[62] while its compulsory enforcement was "based upon superstition, commercialism and paternalism."[63] Vivid descriptions of the injuries and deaths attributed to vaccination figured prominently, and many pamphlets used photographs showing the side effects allegedly caused by the procedure: deep abscesses, scarring, and missing limbs and eyes. (Pro-vaccination propaganda published by health departments often used photos to similar effect, showing the gruesome symptoms of smallpox victims.)[64] The claim that the secular decline in smallpox was due to sanitary reforms and improvements in standards of living rather than vaccination was a recurrent theme; so too was the charge that compulsory policies were a profit-making scheme in which doctors, health departments, and vaccine manufacturers colluded to enrich themselves by forcing the public, through the threat of civil or criminal penalties, to submit to the procedure. Lora Little's early tract *Crimes of the Cowpox Ring*, for example, characterized the practice as a conspiracy perpetrated by entrenched interests: "[T]he salaries of the public health officials in this country...

reach the sum of $14,000,000 annually. One important function of the health boards is vaccination. Without smallpox scares their trade would languish. Thousands of doctors in private practice are also beneficiaries in 'scare' times. And lastly the vaccine 'farmers' represent a capital of $20,000,000, invested in their foul business."[65]

Though diverse, the groups opposed to vaccination were in regular contact with one another. They sometimes worked together in loose coalitions, as when Christian Scientists, chiropractors, and anti-vivisectionists joined in 1910 under the organizational umbrella of the National League for Medical Freedom to campaign against a federal-level department of health.[66] They distributed one another's literature, lent rhetorical support to one another's efforts, and had officers and members in common.[67] They also shared an interest in other libertarian political causes. Charles Higgins, Lora Little, and Harold and Raymond Pitcairn all campaigned against Prohibition; Higgins claimed that "religious freedom, medical freedom, and alimentary freedom are equally unalienable rights of the American people and must be kept inviolate."[68]

"SCIENCE IN A DEMOCRACY"

At the heart of the ideological battles over the legitimacy of vaccination were differing views of the role elite knowledge and scientific expertise should play in a rapidly changing liberal democratic society. The U.S. Public Health Service, state and city health officials, state and local medical societies, and the American Medical Association all sought to convince legislators and the citizenry that scientific elites should have broad latitude in making decisions about health. The AMA kept a running file on medical "dissidents," and Morris Fishbein, the editor of the *Journal of the American Medical Association,* ridiculed many of them in his book *The Medical Follies.*[69]

A lay organization that took up the cause of scientific medicine was the American Association for Medical Progress, made up of prominent academics and civic leaders.[70] Founded in Massachusetts in 1923, the group advocated on behalf of modern methods of investigation—especially animal experimentation—to counteract what it saw as the forces of ignorance and superstition. The association spoke before legislatures, community groups, and educators on the importance of research and criticized the propaganda of anti-vivisection and anti-vaccination groups, which it termed "chronic opponents of scientific medicine."[71]

The group's 1924 book *Smallpox—A Preventable Disease* collected data from countries around the world in order to demonstrate the connection between the systematic application of vaccination and the control of smallpox. Eschewing the scornful tone that Morris Fishbein took in his attacks on the medical profession's opponents, the book offered a more measured assessment of the apathy brought on by decades of steadily declining smallpox rates:

> In this complacent state of mind we become a ready prey to the propaganda of the many high-minded, but misinformed or prejudiced persons who hold that power for harm in smallpox does not exist.... Cults and societies have arisen to break down the barriers that years of scientific investigation and endeavor have set up against disease. We are told that our "personal liberty" is being impaired—and we forget that there is no such thing as personal liberty apart from the liberty of the community in which we live.... We are accused of being the dupes of "state medicine"—and we do not trouble to look back and see for ourselves what our health officials have done for the people of this country.[72]

In the essay "Science in a Democracy," the group's managing director, Benjamin Gruenberg, sought to reconcile liberal democratic values with the growing complexity of the modern world that technological advances were creating. "Most people would not venture an opinion on the feasibility of producing transparent lead, or steel-hard aluminum, or synthetic proteins," Gruenberg wrote. "Yet these same people insist upon the right to hold opinions (and to act according to these opinions) upon such highly technical questions as the efficacy of vaccination, the value of serums, or the causation of cancer."[73] With such rhetoric, Gruenberg sought to move a contentious issue—how to protect the self and the community from disease—out of the realm of popular knowledge and into the domain of the expert. The AAMP deplored the trend of "placing the decision on scientific matters on a popular vote," noting that, "By specious arguments for personal liberty, by subtle appeals to tender emotions and kindly sentiments, many voters have been led to oppose well founded measures for the protection of the public health."[74]

But anti-vaccination activists refused to be excluded from decision-making about such "technical" matters. The ongoing debate between proponents and opponents of vaccination centered on a set of related empirical questions: To what extent was the practice truly responsible for the decline in smallpox that had been observed over the previous century? Could the decline be traced instead to the improvements in sanitation and environmental conditions? Were the low rates of small-pox that were seen in some countries and in some regions of the United States due to the level of vaccination in the population? Were periodic outbreaks of smallpox attributable to the lack of vaccination? Activists such as Lora Little and H.B. Anderson attempted to meet scientific experts on their own territory. Astute in their use of statistics, they sought to persuade legislators and policymakers through the same techniques as public health officials: careful marshalling of epidemiological data. For example, both the American Medical Liberty League and the Citizens Medical Reference Bureau seized on reports of high levels of smallpox in the Philippine Islands, where vaccination was widespread, as evidence that the practice was ineffective. In the spring and summer of 1922, Little sent letters to Surgeon General Hugh Cumming and the health commissioners of several states declaring that the demonstrated failure of vaccination warranted repeal of any compulsory laws.[75]

The U.S. Public Health Service for its part offered a contrary interpretation of the data: the Philippines epidemic was the result of incomplete levels of immunity due to lax enforcement of vaccination, as well as of insufficiently potent vaccine due to prolonged storage without proper refrigeration.[76] "I would no more permit the incident in the Philippine Islands to weaken my faith in the value of vaccination than I would lose faith in the principles of engineering because a great bridge in process of construction collapsed," one state health officer wrote in response to Little.[77] Moreover, PHS officials saw a clear correlation between compulsory vaccination laws and low incidence of smallpox. A study by the service published in 1921 found that the disease was higher in central states with no such laws (such as Utah, the Dakotas, and Colorado), lower on the eastern seaboard, where the broadest requirements were in place, and increasing in western states such as California and Oregon, where anti-vaccination sentiment was on the rise. "In the absence of compulsory features in the law, or where there is no law at all, smallpox reaches a high rate," the study's authors concluded.[78] Echoing Gruenberg's concerns about the damage that the democratic process could do to public health, they declared, "Smallpox in the United States is dependent on the popular vote."[79]

Some scientists contributed contrarian voices to the debates. The eminent Johns Hopkins University biologist and statistician Raymond Pearl claimed in a controversial 1922 book entitled *The Biology of Death* that much of the work of public health officials over the previous decades had had no effect on patterns of sickness. Intended partly as a warning to his colleagues against professional hubris, Pearl's work, though it did not specifically discuss the correlation between the use of vaccination and the decline of smallpox, provided ammunition to those who claimed that there was no relationship between the two.[80] Supporters of the practice were dismayed. In a rebuttal of Pearl's claims published in the popular magazine *The Survey,* Louis Dublin, chief statistician for the Metropolitan Life Insurance Company and a champion of vaccination, ruefully predicted that medical dissident groups "will probably get a great deal of satisfaction out of the spectacle of a professor of a school of public health shattering the gods of his colleagues."[81]

Metropolitan Life, which at the time provided life or disability insurance to one out of every six Americans, was a powerful institutional supporter of scientific medicine. In response to the brouhaha over the Philippines smallpox data, Met Life issued a press release claiming that anti-vaccination propaganda was responsible for continued outbreaks of the disease, and that children were its greatest victims.[82] The company's special concern for the well-being of the young reflected an important shift in public perception in this period: vaccination was increasingly seen as a procedure not for adults but for infants and schoolchildren.

ADULTS, CHILDREN, AND THE·SCOPE OF COMPULSION

The Public Health Service's concern about smallpox was heightened by extensive political activity in states around the country during this period, as attempts were made to narrow the scope of legally permissible compulsion. Utah enacted a law in 1907 expressly forbidding the passage of any compulsory vaccination law, and North Dakota followed suit in 1919.[83] Massachusetts, which had one of the most forceful laws in place, continued to be a site of extensive protests, including efforts to repeal the law every year from 1915 to 1918.[84] Much of the activity nationwide focused on school entry requirements. Washington State repealed its mandatory school vaccination law in 1919, and Wisconsin did the same the following year.[85] But in many instances, the vote went against the anti-vaccinationists. Oregon voters in 1916 narrowly rejected a citizen initiative that would have made it a felony for schools, public agencies, or employers to mandate vaccination; a similar measure was defeated by a wide margin in 1920.[86] The latter initiative was sponsored by a group called the Public School Protective League, which the same year sought to abolish California's school entry law. The league espoused a libertarian philosophy and also opposed various other child health-related bills, including one to establish a bureau of child hygiene in the state government. On the same ballot were two other populist medical measures, one outlawing vivisection and one allowing chiropractors to practice in the state.[87] All were defeated by substantial margins.[88]

New York State's vaccination law also came under attack in this period. Charles Higgins and the Anti-Vaccination League of America made repeated attempts, all unsuccessful, to modify or repeal it in the state legislature.[89] But it would take the crusade of a political insider—and grieving parent—to achieve the goal. James A. Loyster was a lawyer active in state politics, serving as a member of the Republican state committee in his home town of Cazenovia in central New York.[90] He was not affiliated with any anti-vaccination society and claimed that he had earlier been a believer in the procedure. But in 1914 his only son, Lewis, had died after being vaccinated, and Loyster had begun a personal crusade to investigate what he saw as the dangers of the procedure. He surveyed upstate residents in towns and villages, sending out hundreds of fliers and letters to find other cases of vaccination-related injuries and deaths in the rural regions in the state, and over the next several months received reports from parents that in 1914 at least fifty children had been killed, and countless more injured—a figure that dwarfed the three deaths the state had recorded from smallpox itself during the year.[91] Loyster collected the damning statistics and heart-rending testimony from grieving parents into a pamphlet he published at the beginning of 1915, and began lobbying members of the state legislature to modify the state's compulsory vaccination law.

Although Loyster favored complete repeal, the resulting bill was a political compromise, reducing the use of compulsion in the state's rural areas, while expanding it in the largest cities. The existing law required that all public schools in the state exclude from enrollment any pupil who could not present proof of having been vaccinated. The Jones-Tallett amendment, named for the bill's two sponsors, modified the law so that it applied only to cities with populations of more than 50,000 (of which there were ten in the state). In all other cities, towns, and villages, the school entry requirement could be enforced only during a local outbreak of the disease, if the state health commissioner certified the existence of smallpox in the area in writing. At the same time, the bill expanded the scope of compulsion in the ten largest cities: under the

CASE No. 25

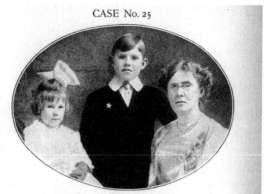

LEWIS FREEBORN LOYSTER

LEWIS FREEBORN LOYSTER, son of James A. Loyster, Cazenovia, N. Y.
Age 11.
Vaccinated Aug. 29, vaccine "E."
Commenced to complain Sept. 10,—11 days from vaccination.
Died Sept. 21.
Diagnosed "Infantile Paralysis."

This boy was the picture of health. To quote the attending physician, he was "a splendid specimen" physically. On the night of Sept. 10 he had a bad headache. The next morning at six was no better. At ten he was found by his mother unconscious. He was very constipated and slightly nauseated. Vomited once. Examination of urine showed indican in considerable quantities. The initial diagnosis was acute indigestion. Blood examined and found normal except for an excess of white corpuscles, explained as a natural sequence of vaccination. Unconsciousness continued. On Sept. 13 lumbar puncture made. Fluid from spinal cord not under pressure; perfectly transparent, subject to microscopic and culture tests; proved absolutely sterile. Case diagnosed as infantile paralysis of the cerebral type. Temperature very high, ranging from 104 to 106 rectal. About Sept. 14 throat became paralyzed. For five days could not swallow a drop. Food administered through rectum; medicine hypodermically. Paralysis of right leg and arm appeared about Sept. 17. Lungs filled with thick mucus. Respiration labored. Slight cyanosis. Small amount of oxygen administered continually after Sept. 16. Death occurred at 10:10 P.M. on Sept. 21 from paralysis of respiratory muscles. Temperature about 107 at death. Microscopic examination of spinal cord after death confirmed diagnosis as infantile paralysis.

Figure 8. One of the cases collected by James Loyster for his booklet *Vaccination Results in New York State in 1914* was that of his own son, Lewis, who died of polio three weeks after being vaccinated.

new law, private and parochial schools, which had previously been exempt, would have to enforce vaccination.

The state medical society and virtually all of the local societies lined up against the measure.[92] Abraham Jacobi, a prominent New York City physician and pioneer of pediatric medicine, spoke of the necessary function of compulsory laws. "I have met in the bulk of our population with more indifference than farsighted public spirit," he testified to the legislature. "It takes the collective thought and activity of a political center like the Legislature to instill a democratic soul into the big political body."[93] But the state health commissioner, Hermann Biggs, stunned many of his colleagues by declining to oppose the bill. Biggs had been associated with compulsion during his tenure with the New York City Health Department, where he had been instrumental in enacting laws requiring physicians to report cases of tuberculosis and venereal disease to the department and had enforced strict quarantine measures against noncompliant tuberculosis patients who would not submit voluntarily to hospitalization.[94] To many of Biggs's colleagues, his accommodating stance toward the proposed change was apostasy. But Biggs was more of a pragmatist than an ideologue; he believed in using compulsion judiciously, when it could accomplish his goals. The existing law had never been systematically enforced, he noted, and because of the decline in smallpox, it was engendering opposition that outweighed whatever value it might have. "I would rather have the sentiment of the community strongly supporting the health authorities without legislation than compulsory legislation and an antagonistic public sentiment," Biggs testified to the state legislature's public health committee, in words that echoed Lederle's position on the McCabe bill of 1902. "An attempt at the present time to enforce strictly the present law will in many of the rural communities of the State result in my judgment in much harm to the public health without any equivalent return."[95]

In part due to Biggs's measured support, the bill passed the legislature and was signed into law. But illustrating the extent to which the goals of activists could diverge, Charles Higgins of the Anti-Vaccination League of America bitterly attacked the Jones-Tallett amendment. In Higgins's view, the new law was a craven political capitulation, representing "every evil against which we had been working steadily for years and … a complete surrender to the advocates of medical compulsion."[96] The ten cities in which compulsion was expanded contained most of the state's population, Higgins pointed out. But the bill clearly accomplished Loyster's primary goal: it removed the burden of compulsion from the state's rural areas, where it was most resented.

Most of the controversy during this period centered on children and schools because adult smallpox vaccination was becoming increasingly rare. About a dozen states at this time had laws authorizing the compulsory vaccination of the general population; most of these laws were permissive rather than mandatory, that is, they allowed but did not require localities to enforce compulsory vaccination should officials deem it necessary.[97] But even places where general vaccination remained legally enforceable rarely saw concerted attempts to achieve the widespread protection of adults.

The eighteen months during which the United States was involved in World War I represented one of the last systematic and large-scale efforts to secure the vaccination of the adult civilian population. In this context, health officials reframed vaccination as a patriotic measure designed to protect the nation's wartime industrial capacity.[98] Surgeon General Rupert Blue issued a general advisory to all state public health officials urging them to work with their local officials to achieve universal vaccination, especially among workers in war-related industries and in areas near military cantonments.[99] But the campaign achieved little success. In Arizona, a state important to the war effort because of its copper mines, the health commissioner complained to Blue that the compulsory vaccination law there was a "dead letter" due to widespread opposition, and that his efforts to enforce the policy simply exacerbated resistance in the state.[100] A plant manager at a steel company in Albion, Michigan, one of many in the state engaged in war production, noted that only some plants were enforcing the order, and that in so doing they placed themselves at a competitive disadvantage: "Some laborers will refuse to be vaccinated, and will go to the other plants where vaccination is not required."[101] In Chicago, many employees in war industries refused, not on philosophical grounds, but "because they are not paid for the time lost, which amounted to from one to five days in some cases."[102]

In the context of labor shortages and bitter struggles over union organizing brought on by the war, some in government felt that vaccination was not sufficiently important to risk inflaming sensitive workplaces.[103] The War Department recommended to Blue that "this measure not be too aggressively advanced at this time or at least until the War Labor Policies Board has an opportunity to secure a better stabilization of labor matters. Numerous instances have been reported to this Branch of the loss of labor in large numbers due to the enforcement of inoculation and vaccination."[104] Similarly, the U.S. Railroad Administration expressed concern that "a very considerable numbers of employees would leave" their jobs if a compulsory vaccination policy were enforced.[105] The American Federation of Labor also fought during the war against the compulsory physical examination of munitions workers, illustrating the extent to which threats to bodily integrity could become a flash point for factory unrest.[106]

In this highly charged climate, several public health officials sought
to have anti-vaccination literature suppressed on the ground that it was
impeding the war effort—"I can see no difference between this propaganda and any other anti-war pro-German propaganda," claimed one
state health officer—but there is no evidence that these attempts were
successful.[107] Anti-vaccinationism also fell victim to the suppression of
radicalism and dissent that marked the war effort. Lora Little was
arrested in North Dakota in 1918 under the Espionage Act for attempting to cause insubordination and mutiny in the military after she distributed pamphlets attacking the compulsory vaccination of soldiers.
She was eventually freed after the state supreme court threw out the
case against her.[108]

In the postwar years, rates of vaccination among the population
dwindled steadily. Health officials often complained that physicians in
private practice were lax in encouraging their patients to undergo the
procedure on a routine basis, instead leaving the work to the overburdened and underfunded municipal health departments that sought to
control the sporadic outbreaks of the disease. "When I was a child the
family physician saw to it that his patients were immunized against
smallpox," complained New York State Health Commissioner Matthias
Nicoll in 1927. "How many do it now? Practically none. The vaccination
against smallpox has of necessity and by the consent or lack of interest
of the medical profession relapsed into a public health function."[109]
Nationwide surveys conducted around 1930 provide some indication
of the low levels of protection to which the country had sunk. A study of
child health found that in the average U.S. city, only 13 percent of
preschoolers had been vaccinated. Age five was the most common time
to have children protected against smallpox, reflecting the effect of
school entry requirements around the country; it was during that year
that almost 75 percent of vaccinating was done.[110] There was little variation in vaccination by income level, also a reflection of the public settings in which vaccination was performed.[111] In a survey of physicians
on patient attitudes toward vaccination, most reported that their patients
were favorably disposed toward it—suggesting a gap between what
people may have believed about the practice and what they actually
did.[112] (Alternatively, this finding may indicate that physicians were not
reliable judges of the attitudes of their patients.)

Another survey conducted at around the same time found a distinct
split between densely and sparsely populated regions: vaccination was
much commoner in large cities than in rural areas.[113] Regardless of

where they lived, children tended to be vaccinated only once, most commonly at age five, and almost no one underwent the procedure after puberty; very few adults heeded public health officials' recommendations to renew the protection against smallpox every seven years. The survey revealed the extent to which vaccination was becoming perceived as a procedure for children, which adults only rarely, if ever, needed to consider undergoing themselves.

APATHY, ACTIVISM, AND THE LINGERING THREAT OF SMALLPOX

The change in New York State's law under the 1915 Jones-Tallett amendment introduced considerable ambiguity into smallpox control efforts. The provision in the law that compulsory school vaccination could be enforced only after the presence of smallpox was "certified"— a determination that rested with the state health commissioner, acting on the advice of local and regional subordinates—meant that repeated judgments were necessary, in which the severity of the reported cases and the apparent likelihood of rapid spread had to be balanced in a careful calculus with political considerations about how the public might respond to compulsory or voluntary vaccination policies. As events in New York State during the 1920s reveal, a combination of factors hindered efforts to achieve vaccination of the public, including the open-ended nature of the law, public apathy and resistance, bureaucratic inefficiency, and lack of financial resources.

The surveys reported above showed a mixed picture of New York's vaccination status. New York City had the highest level of protection in the country, with 48 percent of its preschoolers vaccinated.[114] But in most other cities, levels were far lower. In rural counties, an average of only 7 percent of preschoolers were vaccinated; in Niagara Falls, Buffalo, and Elmira, all cities where anti-vaccination sentiment ran high, just 6, 4, and 3 percent of children, respectively, had undergone the procedure.[115]

State Health Commissioner Matthias Nicoll, who had succeeded Hermann Biggs upon the latter's death in 1923, was acutely aware of the political nature of public health work. A veteran of the state health department, who had served as assistant director in the New York City Health Department before moving to Albany in 1915, Nicoll was a consistent fighter for professionalization of the field of public health and worked during his tenure as commissioner to strengthen the administrative apparatus at the county level. Nicoll favored the use of persuasive measures whenever possible, but his was hardly an egalitarian commitment to community involvement in health work. On the contrary, he believed that health officials should have broad latitude to do as they saw fit—to act paternalistically in the best interest of the masses. "Those who are in a position to influence public health legislation should do everything in their power to prevent the cluttering up of public health laws with unnecessary mandatory provisions," Nicoll wrote in 1927. "It is far better to confer permissive powers on administrative officials to be used in their discretion, than to enact compulsory statutes of wide application which are anybody's or nobody's duty to enforce."[116] Such a vision, similar to that expressed by Brooklyn's Z. Taylor Emery in the 1890s, was entirely consistent with the latitude granted to Nicoll's office under the provisions of the Jones-Tallett bill.

Aware that sentiment ran strongly against vaccination in much of the state, Nicoll and his deputies were reluctant to "certify" an outbreak of smallpox too frequently, or leave the declaration in effect for too long, for fear of triggering a court challenge to the law that might weaken it even further.[117] Edward Godfrey, the chief of communicable disease control, believed that certification was a double-edged sword: on the one hand, "it does impress the general public with the seriousness of the situation and leads to the vaccination of a good many more adults than can be gotten without it"; on the other hand, he believed that more "moderate" reactions relying on persuasive measures could win over more people and help to dissipate anti-vaccination sentiment.[118]

Local health officers met with only sporadic success in getting adults to undergo the procedure. Partly this was due to inadequacy of staffing and budget. In sharp contrast to New York City, which of necessity had developed an early and forceful public health infrastructure, the upstate region in the 1920s had only minimal administrative mechanisms for carrying out health work.[119] The majority of local health officials served part time and made their primary livings through private medical practice.[120] The responsibility for conducting vaccination campaigns typically rested with one or two doctors and nurses who had been enlisted for the task and were paid with limited public funds to cover large geographic areas. Commenting on the paltry resources that local officials commanded to control a smallpox outbreak upstate, one local health officer wrote ruefully to the state health department,

"City governments are pretty cheap affairs sometimes as perhaps you have observed."[121]

Local newspapers generally supported vaccination efforts, running lengthy articles quoting authorities on the need for universal protection, and such articles usually stimulated considerable voluntary response among a city's residents.[122] But newspapers also felt an obligation to their cities' commercial interests, and alarmist coverage of a smallpox outbreak was bad for business. In Watertown, a state health official noted that in the first days of an outbreak, "the newspapers were cooperative, and much favorable publicity matter was given out, but as the weeks lengthened the harm to business was so apparent that the papers changed their policy, and little or nothing was said further on the subject."[123]

While rumors of a smallpox outbreak could damage a city's business, a full-fledged epidemic was an even worse calamity, and most business leaders could be persuaded to go along with control efforts if the threat seemed real enough. The Lockport Board of Commerce, after intense lobbying by the city health officer, sent a "Dear Employer" letter to the town's businesses, in which it cautioned that if universal vaccination were not achieved in all businesses, it was likely "that a real epidemic of smallpox will develop and as you know this would curtail business in this city and ... the state can quarantine the city and cut us off from a social and business intercourse with the outside world."[124]

The most volatile battleground over vaccination during this period proved to be schools. In some ways, the gradual shift during this era from enforcement of vaccination in the adult population to a focus on children made health officials' task easier, since students were a "captive" population to whom ready access was available. The U.S. Supreme Court in 1922 dispensed with the question of whether school entry requirements violated any constitutional rights (an issue that had not been directly addressed in *Jacobson v. Massachusetts*). The decision was handed down in a case arising from Texas, where Rosalyn Zucht, aged 15, was expelled from Brackenridge High School in San Antonio after her parents refused to have her vaccinated. In a unanimous decision relying primarily on the earlier opinion in *Jacobson*, the court determined that no constitutional right was abridged by excluding unvaccinated children from school.[125] (Justice Louis Brandeis, who wrote the opinion, subsequently claimed that he did not believe the court should have taken the case, because it presented no new constitutional issues.)[126]

The problem for New York's health officials was that beyond exclusion from school, state law provided no penalty for parents who let their children remain unvaccinated. Although parents could, in theory, be prosecuted for violating the state's compulsory education law if they kept children out of school rather than have them vaccinated, such action was almost never taken. When Nicoll certified the existence of an epidemic in Corning, a group of parents opposed to vaccination contacted a lawyer, who advised them to send their children to school every day without the required proof of vaccination, in a gesture of protest, whereupon the youth would be sent home.[127] An officer with the state health department described the parents as "very 'cocky' in their attitude toward other children and seemingly very proud of the manner in which they have avoided vaccination."[128] The attempt to enforce compulsion in this case gave opponents the opportunity to score rhetorical points by publicly flouting the law without fear of prosecution.

The law vested school districts with the charge of enforcing the entry requirement, and local health departments had no authority to intervene in the way schools conducted their affairs. School officials felt that their primary mission was educating children, not controlling epidemics, and they rarely gave priority to enforcing health laws. They also had an economic incentive to admit unvaccinated students: districts were reimbursed by the state on the basis of an "average daily attendance" formula, receiving sums based on their student census, and any district that excluded large numbers of students stood to lose a commensurate amount of money. Health officials repeatedly expressed their frustration with what they saw as the cavalier attitude of school authorities toward a potentially dire health threat. One wrote to a colleague: "I am unaware that [education officials] have done anything at all.... Unless WE make the arrangements very little is done.... Last year in four municipalities which were certified no attempt was made to exclude unvaccinated children." The resulting failure was then blamed unfairly on health authorities. "No matter how many arguments are offered to the contrary, the health officials are looked to for [the law's] enforcement and failure to do so is chalked up against us, not the educational authorities."[129]

The most thorny legal question was whether any children should be exempt from the requirement. Religious exemptions were uncommon at this time, and in New York, even unvaccinated children whose health might be endangered by vaccination could not legally be admitted to a public, private or parochial school. New York was unusual in this respect; most states with compulsory vaccination laws had provisions exempting those who were physically unfit to undergo it.[130] Vaccination supporters agreed that such provisions were desirable; even the U.S. Supreme Court had conceded in *Jacobson* that forcing the procedure on someone whose health might thereby be endangered would be "cruel and inhuman in the last degree."[131] But in New York, both health and education officials feared, correctly, that anti-vaccinationists would use the addition of a medical exemption as a foot in the door, and would push to eliminate the law entirely once they had gained the sympathetic ear of legislators on the issue of exemptions.

This was the strategy of H.B. Anderson, the indefatigable secretary of the Citizens Medical Reference Bureau. In his efforts to end compulsory vaccination in New York's largest cities, Anderson made himself a fixture at school board hearings and in the offices of the president and members of the board of education; he also sought the support of the United Parents Association, a volunteer group concerned with school betterment.[132] In 1932, he persuaded the New York City School Board to pass a resolution favoring the addition of a medical exemption— and then promptly argued before the state legislature that the board's concession that vaccination was dangerous to health in some cases was proof that compulsion should be abandoned entirely. Having to determine which students truly deserved a medical exemption would inevitably rely on arbitrary judgments, Anderson claimed; far better to simply make the procedure voluntary for all.[133] Even though both the health department and the board of education ultimately gave cautious support to the addition of an exemption, Anderson's efforts to change the law were unsuccessful.

THE WANING OF ANTI-VACCINATIONISM AND THE DISAPPEARANCE OF SMALLPOX

As the 1930s wore on, the activism of H.B. Anderson and the Citizens Medical Reference Bureau became an increasingly isolated crusade. The Anti-Vaccination League of America faded from prominence during the 1920s and vanished after the death of Charles Higgins in 1929; the American Medical Liberty League underwent a similar decline after Lora Little's death in 1931. The virtual disappearance of these organizations revealed the extent to which the movement depended on the persistence of a few dedicated leaders. Anderson continued to fight against "socialistic" medical programs during the 1930s and 1940s. He testified in Congress in 1935 against provisions of Franklin Roosevelt's Economic Security Act that provided federal grants to support state maternal and child health programs.[134] His 1945 book, *Public Health the American Way*, attacked several contemporary developments in health policy, including screening for sexually transmitted disease, mass chest x-rays to detect tuberculosis, and congressional proposals to provide universal health insurance.[135] He continued to be an energetic letter-writer, corresponding with state and local health officials in New York and throughout the Northeast.[136] After Anderson's death in 1953, the bureau fought against the fluoridation of public water supplies and the polio vaccine, but these were losing battles.

Those who advanced alternative health practices that rejected vaccination also suffered diminishing influence. A nationwide survey conducted at the end of the 1920s showed that alternative practitioners, including chiropractors, Christian Scientists, and other drugless and faith healers, cared for a scant 5 percent of all cases of illness in the country.[137] Allopathic medicine by this time had effectively won its battle for cultural status and authority over other forms of medicine, and the recommendations of physicians began to exert more influence on the health decisions of the public—a crucial factor in the ultimate acceptance of vaccination as preparations against other diseases began to be developed.

Smallpox appeared in New York City for the final time in March 1947, arriving by bus from Mexico City in a traveler named Eugene Le Bar, a forty-seven-year-old merchant who was en route with his wife to Maine. Le Bar had begun feeling ill early in the journey, and upon arriving in New York, he had gone to Bellevue Hospital's dermatological ward with a fever of 105 degrees and a strange rash on his face and hands. Three days later, he was transferred to Willard Parker Hospital, the city's contagious disease facility; two days after that, he died. The cause of his death was not immediately recognized, however, and it was not until the end of March, after smallpox was diagnosed in two people who had been patients at Willard Parker during the time of Le Bar's stay, that hospital personnel grasped the situation and notified the health department.[138]

On the afternoon of Friday, April 4, health commissioner Israel Weinstein called a press conference at his office to announce that smallpox was in the city. While assuring the public that the danger of a widespread epidemic was "slight," Weinstein nevertheless urged every

New Yorker who had not been recently vaccinated to undergo the procedure again. Newspaper and radio reports of the threat prompted lines to form at clinics around the city; meanwhile, health department investigators fanned out in an effort to retrace Le Bar's steps, and locate and vaccinate anyone with whom he may have come in contact. As the days went by, health officials grew more alarmed. They learned that before checking into Bellevue, Le Bar had been in the city for several days, staying at a midtown hotel and even shopping on Fifth Avenue one afternoon. A second person died from the disease, the wife of a man who had contracted it from Le Bar during his stay in Willard Parker. Another case traceable to Le Bar—a four-year-old boy who had also been a patient at the hospital—was diagnosed in Millbrook, north of the city. These developments, and a dwindling supply of vaccine, prompted Weinstein to visit Mayor William O'Dwyer in person on April 12 to request a special appropriation of half a million dollars to purchase more vaccine and hire additional staff to expand the campaign to protect the public. O'Dwyer agreed to the requests and called reporters to a press conference that day. As news cameras flashed, Weinstein vaccinated O'Dwyer and the mayor made an urgent appeal for all New Yorkers to take the same precaution.

O'Dwyer's announcement pushed the mass vaccination program into high gear, and over the next three weeks, New York City witnessed one of the most extraordinary mobilizations of the population in its history. Each day, hundreds of thousands of people waited, sometimes for hours in the rain, in long lines that snaked around blocks. From the time the announcement first hit the press on April 5 to when the clinics were closed a month later, 6.35 million people were vaccinated, some 80 percent of the city's residents. The majority of those vaccinated, about 5 million, sought protection in the two weeks after Mayor O'Dwyer's special plea. About half the vaccinations were performed at health department clinics and public and private hospitals, where the enormous logistical task of keeping people moving in an orderly fashion was made possible by the efforts of some 3,000 civilian volunteers, mostly from the American Red Cross and the American Women's Voluntary Services. About 1 million of the inoculations were done in the offices of private physicians, and about 1.2 million at special locations arranged by civic and fraternal organizations and at on-site workplaces organized by industries and labor unions.[139] Many of the city's large employers, such as Eastman Kodak, TWA, Union Carbide, and Wanamaker's, invited

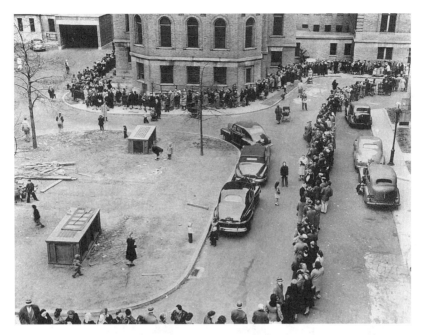

Figure 9. In mid April 1947, thousands of New Yorkers lined up to receive smallpox vaccination after cases of the disease were diagnosed in the city for the first time in over a decade. Courtesy New York City Municipal Archives.

health department doctors to come on site and vaccinate all employees; some businesses, including the Arthur Murray dance studio and Lane Bryant department store, also offered their space for use as public clinics.[140] The cooperation of employers and labor groups no doubt secured the participation of many reluctant or uncertain people who might not otherwise have taken the trouble to visit a clinic. The secretary of the Amalgamated Clothing Workers of America, for example, wrote to Mayor O'Dwyer, "We are desirous that all our members co-operate in your campaign for vaccination for small pox. However, great numbers of them for one reason or another ... hesitate."[141]

What accounts for the overwhelmingly positive response of city residents to the drive? Perhaps most significant, the willingness of so many people to undergo considerable inconvenience reflected a remarkable degree of trust in the judgment and recommendations of local health officials.[142] This faith had been built up over decades as a

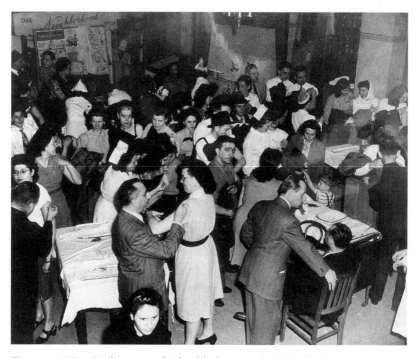

Figure 10. New Yorkers crowd a health department clinic during the 1947 smallpox outbreak. Because the immunity provided by smallpox vaccination waned after several years, and adult revaccination was rare, very few residents were protected against the disease when it was discovered in the city. Courtesy New York City Municipal Archives.

result of the department's visible presence in the city, including its extensive network of community clinics and its health education materials. A second factor was skillful management of the media. Karl Pretshold, the health department's chief of public relations, who would play a prominent role in polio campaigns a decade later, described an intensive effort to keep the press constantly updated, respond immediately to all reporters' inquiries, and track down rumors. A third factor was a general community-oriented frame of mind that the country's wartime experience had fostered; in the immediate postwar period, New Yorkers were still accustomed to cooperating with drills and other emergency measures.[143]

Only a few scattered protests were lodged about the effort. H.B. Anderson took the opportunity of the campaign to reiterate his opposition to the school entry requirement, writing to Weinstein that "so long as the Department of Health is on record as favoring compulsion as applied to one group there is always the doubt in the public mind how much farther the Department might wish to extend this compulsory attitude."[144] There was also grumbling among some private physicians about the city offering the vaccine for free. "During the recent vaccination stampede, many wealthy persons took advantage of the free service rendered by the [health department]," an irate Brooklyn doctor subsequently wrote to the health department. "If the city were to give away free meat & groceries to everybody, the butchers and grocers would protest!... Doctors did not go thru medical college to have politicians and salaried men from the [board of health] take away their patients."[145] But active opposition to the massive effort was conspicuous in its absence. "All during the drive we half expected that anti-vaccinationists and their activities would become a problem," Pretshold later reflected. "They never did. At one health center a person appeared and tried to pass out anti-vaccination leaflets. The people waiting to be vaccinated took matters into their own hands. Their protests drove him away."[146]

After the last of the special clinics closed on May 3, the drive was widely judged to have been a success; the toll from smallpox had been limited to twelve cases and two deaths. Many New Yorkers wrote to the health department to thank it for its efforts.[147] But the campaign, in addition to a price tag of some $900,000, also had a human cost. Three people were subsequently determined to have died from effects of the vaccine itself, a sixty-six-year-old man who contracted septicemia from an infected vaccination site and two infants who died of generalized vaccinia, the condition resulting when the cowpox virus spreads out of control in the body. "Tragic as these incidents were," Weinstein wrote in a report on the effort, "it must be borne in mind that had vaccination not been carried out on such a large scale, there very likely would have been thousands of cases and hundreds of deaths."[148] Health experts generally agreed that the harm that had been forestalled far outweighed the expense and even the three deaths that resulted.

The acknowledgment of the deaths foreshadowed an extended debate that would emerge fifteen years later about the risks and benefits of smallpox vaccination and the ethical acceptability of using a preventive that could have occasionally fatal consequences. But in 1947, the risk-to-benefit calculation tipped decisively in favor of vaccination's positive effects. The concept of immunization had by this time become associated with protection against illnesses other than smallpox, most notably diphtheria and pertussis, and was a largely uncontroversial practice, unburdened by the negative attitudes that had dogged small-pox vaccination during the Progressive Era and the 1920s. As we shall see in the next chapter, this shift in popular perception was accomplished through the techniques of mass persuasion rather than the enforcement of laws.

CHAPTER 3

Diphtheria Immunization

The Power, and the Limits,
of Persuasion

On a sunny spring afternoon in 1933, New York City Health Commissioner Shirley Wynne looked on proudly as nine-month-old May
McDermott received an injection at an Upper East Side clinic. May was
the city's one millionth child immunized against diphtheria, and she
smiled happily as news cameras flashed. (The one-million-and-first
child, who received her injection moments later, "screamed and scowled,"
according to the *Times*.)[1] Everyone at the clinic later joined several
thousand schoolchildren in a march three blocks to a health pageant in
Central Park, where musical performances, ethnic folk dancing, and
speeches by politicians and civic leaders drew attention to the importance of protecting children against one of the most common infectious
diseases. The day's events were emblematic of the city's approach to
promoting this medical innovation, which in just two decades had won
widespread popular acceptance.

In the 1920s, prophylactic injections against diphtheria joined smallpox vaccination as the second immunizing procedure to be widely used
by the general public. After a decade of trials in New York City schools
and institutions, health officials at the beginning of 1926 launched an
ambitious statewide effort to eliminate diphtheria by 1930. This campaign made education, not compulsion, its cornerstone. The newest
techniques of mass persuasion—newspaper advertisements, billboards,
motion pictures, staged publicity events, colorful placards using emotional appeals to parental duty and sentiment—would motivate the

public. While this approach was successful at forestalling the backlash and resistance that had developed against smallpox vaccination, the effects of advertising proved ephemeral, requiring constant reinforcement that was expensive and time-consuming.

This chapter examines the ways that researchers, state and local health officials, physicians, and child welfare advocates introduced diphtheria immunization to the public in the 1920s and 1930s and attempted to make the procedure routine. Two trends were especially important in shaping this effort. First was the rise of education as a public health approach, and, as a corollary, use of the techniques of advertising to sell immunization the way businesses sold cars, appliances, and cigarettes. Second was professional tension over the newly emerging category of preventive medical care. Immunization lay at the crossroads between public health interventions and medical practice, and private physicians were often at odds with government health departments over where and by whom the new procedure should be offered, how much it should cost, and how it should be promoted to the public.

The diphtheria immunization drives ultimately fell short of their original goal—universal use of the vaccine and eradication of the disease—but they had broad and long-lasting effects. The campaigns helped to transform the popular perception of vaccination from a potentially risky crisis-control measure into a safe, routine part of child-rearing, and in so doing helped to establish the concept of preventive care.

TOXIN-ANTITOXIN AND THE ORIGINS OF DIPHTHERIA IMMUNIZATION

Efforts to control diphtheria had been among the early success stories of the bacteriological revolution. Spread by air-borne droplets, diphtheria was a leading cause of illness and death among children throughout the nineteenth century (it rarely struck adults). It was caused by a bacterium that produced a toxin, which in turn attacked the upper respiratory tract, typically causing a thick membrane to form inside the throat, which obstructed breathing. About one in ten victims died from the disease, as a result of either inability to breathe or the effects of the toxin on other organs of the body. The New York City Health Department played a central role in the history of efforts to control diphtheria. The department's bureau of laboratories began producing a newly developed treatment—an antitoxin—in 1895, and mortality from the disease dropped sharply as doctors around the city began to give the substance to stricken children.[2]

The tantalizing discovery that antitoxin also produced a transient immunity that could provide temporary protection to household contacts who had not yet become ill spurred efforts to devise a way to confer lasting protection. Two scientific breakthroughs in 1913 made that possible. The German researcher Emil Behring developed a method of combining a small amount of diphtheria toxin with antitoxin in a formulation that appeared to provide active and long-lasting immunity against the disease. The same year, the Viennese physician Bela Schick devised a skin test that could reveal a person's immune status relative to diphtheria: after an injection of a small amount of toxin just below the skin, those who were not immune would develop a small red swelling at the site. With this pair of developments, scientists had both the means of inducing immunity as well as a simple and relatively straightforward way of measuring the efficacy of the procedure.

The director of New York City's Bureau of Laboratories, William Hallock Park, immediately moved to capitalize on these two advances. Park and his colleagues began a series of studies involving thousands of children in hospitals, institutions, and orphanages, where they administered Schick tests to determine who was already immune to the disease and gave toxin-antitoxin injections to those who were not in order to study the reliability and duration of the immunity produced by the procedure. Their work was temporarily halted by World War I, but in 1921, Park, with funding from the American Red Cross, secured the cooperation of the city's school system and began to carry out mass Schick testing and administration of toxin-antitoxin to students there. Conducting studies in public schools offered obvious strategic advantages. Students were a captive population, who, like institutionalized children, could be easily reached at specified places and times for intervention and follow-up. Nevertheless, these trials presented several logistical hurdles. Unlike the work that had been done with orphaned and institutionalized children, affirmative consent was secured from all parents of students before toxin-antitoxin was administered (a practice that was far from universal at the time).[3] To reassure wary parents whose knowledge of immunization was based mostly on their experience with smallpox control, the researchers worked closely with school principals and distributed fliers to parents in English, Italian, and Yiddish. "Children are not made sick by [toxin-antitoxin], as sometimes happens after smallpox vaccination," explained one pamphlet sent home to parents.[4]

The favorable results Park and colleagues obtained among students convinced them that toxin-antitoxin was a safe and reliable way to confer immunity. But targeting youth in schools failed to address the more pressing problem of preschool children, who were most susceptible to diphtheria and among whom the disease was most likely to be fatal. Park noted the daunting challenges to be overcome in reaching infants. "These young children are scattered in individual homes and cannot be reached like school children in large groups," he wrote. "The parents have to be seen and convinced before they will give consent. All this requires considerable effort and time on the part of the health officer."[5] The health department began to extend the service to the public by offering the procedure in its baby health stations, mailing thousands of fliers to parents of newborns, and popularizing the procedure through visiting nurses and at settlement houses.

The extensive work in New York City's public schools did not escape the notice of anti-vaccination activists, who, as we saw in chapter 2, were deeply suspicious of government-sponsored medical programs, especially those targeting children. In 1922, H. B. Anderson of the Citizens Medical Reference Bureau lodged a formal protest with the board of education in which he urged it to bar the health department doctors from using the city's children as guinea pigs. "[T]he public schools should not be used for the exploitation of a medical procedure which is of such a controversial character," Anderson claimed.[6] He was convinced that the health department was taking the first steps toward making toxin-antitoxin compulsory like smallpox vaccination.

New York State Health Commissioner Hermann Biggs, Park's mentor from their days together in the New York City bacteriology lab, had played a prominent role in developing antitoxin and was eager to make the procedure widely available. The studies in the city's schools had laid the groundwork for this, but the procedure remained little-known outside of New York City. Biggs selected Auburn, a town of 36,000 residents in the Finger Lakes region of central New York, as the site of the first citywide trial of mass immunization using toxin-antitoxin. Biggs and Frederick Sears, the district health officer in Auburn, chose the city because it had the state's highest rate of diphtheria; it would make a good test case, because it was of a manageable size but also had a diverse population. In February 1922, Auburn began a trial program to determine if the favorable results in New York City schools could be obtained there.[7]

Letters were sent to the homes of all parents of the city's seven thousand schoolchildren asking for consent to perform a Schick test and immunize those positive with toxin-antitoxin; the parents of 58 percent of children gave consent. Over the following year, local health officials reported that the public was receptive to the procedure, and by 1926, the city's death rate from the disease had dropped to zero.[8]

Communitywide deployment of toxin-antitoxin got an additional, unplanned tryout in 1924 when an unusually severe outbreak of diphtheria struck several small towns in largely rural Ulster County, along the Hudson River. Health officers in the area took advantage of the situation to try to secure broad public acceptance of the procedure. But in the attempt to branch out beyond school-based efforts, the results were mixed. "It does not seem to be possible to stir up very much interest in TAT [toxin-antitoxin] immunization," wrote a health official in Glasco, one of the affected towns.[9] Constant, labor-intensive measures were necessary to gain acceptance. "[I]t is impossible to carry on very extensive immunization work without a nurse on the ground at all time. A great deal of house to house visiting must be done.... [A]nnouncements of clinics, and sending circulars to the families and work in the schools is not sufficient."[10] In response, authorities in the town of Ulster enlisted the help of a prominent community member, an Italian-American justice of the peace named DeCicco, who was key in persuading members of the town's large Italian community. "He succeeds in securing attendance of families at the immunization clinics which could not otherwise be reached," reported the district health officer to the state commissioner's office. "Many of these families are brought in to the clinics by Mr. DeCicco in his car."[11]

The events in the area also highlighted the potentially controversial nature of using compulsion. The city's health officer, who favored aggressive legal means, including the quarantining of suspected carriers and their contacts, to compel people to have their children immunized, clashed with his superiors in Albany, who objected to "these moves which have a tendency to break down the good feeling which is an important factor in securing the immunization."[12]

The difficulty physicians and health officials had in convincing parents—even in the midst of an outbreak of diphtheria—that they should bring their children in to undergo this beneficial new procedure illustrates the halting and uneven pace at which the lay public accepted innovations in scientific medicine. Medical professionals, who were increasingly uniform and science-based in their outlooks and methods, accepted toxin-antitoxin with striking rapidity during the 1920s. A 1921 pamphlet issued by the New York City Health Department described the Schick test and toxin-antitoxin as "so new that very few physicians have had the opportunity to become acquainted with them."[13] But only five years later, a survey of state and provincial health officers around the country found that toxin-antitoxin immunization for all children was viewed as standard practice, with thirty-five out of thirty-eight responders recommending that it be done routinely.[14] The initial gains in recognition were due in large measure to the energetic efforts of Park and his colleagues, who made numerous presentations around the state and at meetings of medical societies. Their work, published in leading medical journals, drew interest from health departments around the country, which considered mounting their own campaigns on the strength of the evidence of the procedure's safety and efficacy.[15] The use of toxin-antitoxin entered standard medical texts in the 1920s. It appeared in the fourth edition of Milton Rosenau's *Preventive Medicine and Hygiene* in 1921,[16] and in the third edition of Sir William Osler et al.'s *Modern Medicine* in 1925.[17] Arnold Gesell, the Yale professor who was perhaps the most influential expert on child-rearing of his day, gave his endorsement to toxin-antitoxin as an essential procedure in a 1923 text.[18]

Public acceptance increased more slowly. In 1921, some physicians reported that only a small minority of their private patients were convinced of the procedure's value and ready to accept it for their children.[19] But toxin-antitoxin got an early boost in recognition from the Metropolitan Life Insurance Company. Persuaded by the work of Park and his colleagues in New York City's schools, the company began playing a prominent role in popularizing the results in the 1920s. Through its field agents, it distributed thousands of circulars to policyholders touting the procedure, and it ran full-page advertisements in popular magazines such as the *Saturday Evening Post* trumpeting the benefits of diphtheria immunization and urging readers to take advantage of the procedure for their children.[20]

Antitoxin also became the center of public attention in the winter of 1925 when a diphtheria epidemic broke out in Nome, Alaska. The nearest supply of antitoxin was some 600 miles away in Anchorage and had to be brought overland. Three teams of dogsleds raced through driving blizzards in a "race against death" that captured front-page headlines across the country. After the antitoxin arrived and the babies were saved, the ten drivers and their huskies were hailed as heroes, especially the Siberian wolfhound Balto, who had led the winning team.[21] New York City, which had supplied the antitoxin that was flown to Anchorage, felt a proprietary pride in the dramatic success of the adventure and responded by erecting a statue of Balto in Central Park. (H. B. Anderson of the Citizens Medical Reference Bureau formally protested the statue, telling the parks commission that antitoxin was of dubious value and thus should not be commemorated.)[22]

From the patient's standpoint, diphtheria immunization was a far milder experience to undergo than smallpox vaccination. Unlike the multiple small abrasions to the arm that were made in vaccination, toxin-antitoxin was administered through a hypodermic needle, and thus did not leave a scar. It often caused a small swelling around the injection site, and occasionally a transient mild fever, but reactions were generally negligible, and the doubts about safety that clung to vaccination never developed around toxin-antitoxin. A disadvantage from the standpoint of widespread public use, however, was that the procedure required a series of three injections over the course of one month.

The early days of diphtheria immunization were not entirely free from controversy. In 1919, five children died and dozens experienced high fever, vomiting, and inflammation of the arm and hand after they were given toxin-antitoxin from a lot that had been improperly prepared.[23] When exposed to below-freezing temperature, the toxin-antitoxin mixture could dissociate, thus returning the toxin to its active, harmful state; a 1924 incident involving such a batch in Concord and Bridgewater, Massachusetts, caused widespread inflammations in children (though no deaths).[24] But in contrast to injuries from smallpox vaccination, which many people saw as inherently risky, these incidents were clearly attributable to errors in manufacturing and administration. The flurry of negative publicity that followed the incidents did not do lasting damage to the procedure's reputation for safety.

By the mid 1920s, the widespread recognition that toxin-antitoxin had achieved among health and medical professionals set the stage for efforts to boost awareness among the general public. Mindful of the lessons that had been learned in Auburn and Ulster County, New York State Health Commissioner Matthias Nicoll pressed ahead with a statewide drive against diphtheria. Because New York City faced unique financial and logistical challenges in mounting a large-scale effort, and because the health department there was mired in internal scandal and turmoil over Tammany Hall political influence at the time, the campaign would be conducted throughout the state exclusive of New York City.[25] In its scope and methods, it would be unlike any public health campaign the state had ever seen.

NEW YORK'S "NO MORE DIPHTHERIA" CAMPAIGNS

As we saw in chapter 2, New York State devoted paltry resources to public health during the 1920s, and mounting an ambitious immunization campaign would require substantial monetary and practical support from external sources.[26] Matthias Nicoll convened a steering committee made up not only of the medical and public health experts and school officials who would necessarily be involved but also of leaders of business, charitable, and philanthropic organizations to guide the effort. The two most significant sources of funding and material support were the Metropolitan Life Insurance Company and the Milbank Memorial Fund.

Metropolitan Life, as we have seen, was an early and enthusiastic supporter of toxin-antitoxin and provided the bulk of the financial backing for the anti-diphtheria effort, donating $15,000 at the kickoff in 1926, the same amount the following year, and another $10,000 in 1928.[27] It also contributed many educational materials, including a one-reel film it produced, *New Ways for Old*.[28] Beginning in the 1910s, all three major insurance companies (Met Life, Prudential, and John Hancock) had significant involvement in public health activities, generating statistical profiles on health issues, providing disease prevention tips for policyholders, and publishing educational materials for the general public. At a time when the administrative infrastructures of most city and state health departments were scant, insurers, by virtue of their mortality information on large numbers of policyholders, served as de facto epidemiologists, and the U.S. Public Health Service turned to them when it needed statistical data.[29] By far the most active in this respect was Met Life. Lee Frankel, the company vice president who oversaw its welfare programs, articulated an expansive vision for his industry. "Insurance today is really a great social institution," Frankel wrote in 1914. "The insurance company is simply a medium through which aggregations of individuals protect themselves against the risks and contingencies of life."[30] The company's welfare division undertook an extraordinary array of activities to promote public health, most notably employing dozens of public health nurses to visit policyholders in their homes to instruct them in the latest techniques of fighting disease and staying healthy.

Frankel and Louis Dublin, whom Frankel hired as Met Life's chief statistician, were tireless crusaders for the popular adoption of advances in scientific medicine. This interest was expressed in terms of a utilitarian calculus that placed a dollar value on human life. "The infant just born is an economic asset because it has cost money to bring into the world and because if it be allowed to reach maturity, it will produce more than it cost to bring up," Dublin told the American Child Health Association in a 1927 address. "Our wealth is increasing because of the existence of human beings who have the capacity to produce more than they consume."[31] Dublin calculated that childhood illnesses such as diphtheria cost American society some $200,000,000 per year in medical and nursing costs and lost parental wages. Such economic justifications for public health intervention were hardly new—the threat that epidemics posed to commerce had been at the root of quarantines for centuries, and sanitary reformers in the nineteenth century had garnered support for their efforts by convincing local governments that disease was a drain on a city's productivity—but Dublin took this argument to new levels of sophistication through statistical analyses.

Met Life had other motivations besides altruism for supporting developments in scientific medicine. Healthy policyholders lived longer and thus continued paying money into the company's coffers, rather than drawing from them. Health-themed newspaper and magazine advertisements such as the ones urging parents to protect their children with toxin-antitoxin all prominently featured the company logo and enhanced its image as a caring, responsible corporate citizen.[32]

Major support also came from the Milbank Memorial Fund, one of the first large philanthropies created during the Progressive Era. Founded in 1905, the fund devoted itself to education, social welfare, and health causes. Milbank donated $5,000 to the statewide diphtheria campaign in 1926. More important, however, was indirect support in the form of three health demonstrations that the organization established in the state during the 1920s. The demonstrations were carried out in three cities of varying sizes in order to test the effectiveness of organizing public health work in rural, urban, and metropolitan settings. The projects devoted money and technical expertise to setting up bureaucratic structures for implementing public health interventions to control infectious and chronic diseases and were intended to convince residents of the value of biomedical advances such as diphtheria immunization.[33] The Milbank Fund thus provided an essential element in the anti-diphtheria campaigns: the administrative apparatus that brought toxin-antitoxin to the people through clinics and trained medical and nursing personnel.[34]

In the nineteenth century, fear had been a powerful motivation prompting people to seek vaccination. But as the outbreaks in Ulster County demonstrated, diphtheria did not provoke the sense of crisis that smallpox had done. It lacked the gruesome symptoms and high death rate, and it rarely struck in severe epidemic peaks that had characterized attacks of smallpox. "With a pre-school death risk of less than one in 1,500 per year per individual child," observed a physician in Schenectady, "we are not dealing with a risk of a magnitude such as usually excites the average parent to any great amount of fore-sighted activity."[35] Thus the threat of diphtheria would have to be magnified and dramatized if people were to accept the new preventive. The message underlying the campaigns would have to be subtly different from the themes used to encourage smallpox vaccination. Instead of protecting the community from imminent peril, citizens were urged to take action in order to move their community toward a state of perfect health. Because toxin-antitoxin was safe and painless, health officials could appeal more directly to individual self-interest, without asking people to subordinate their well-being, or that of their children, to the good of the community.

The campaigns were launched across upstate cities in early 1926 and continued over the next three years. Families with children, reached through house-to-house canvassing by public health nurses and mailings based on census records, were urged to ask their doctor—if they had one—for toxin-antitoxin. Special immunization clinics offering free or low-cost injections were set up in schools, dispensaries, and other locations. The campaigns were communitywide efforts involving civic and charitable organizations and local businesses. In Newburgh, Junior League members combed through census records at the county clerk's office in order to compile lists of all the city's children under age five, while the Lions Club donated the lollipops that were given to children following their shots.[36]

Virtually every state newspaper ran advertisements, articles, and editorial commentary. Radio broadcasts carried the message into homes. Billboards, posters, and placards were ubiquitous. Local schools held competitions between classes to achieve the highest rates of immunization; students entered contests for the best essay and poster demonstrating the importance of diphtheria protection. Young people were awarded gold stars and badges after receiving their injections. Parades, pageants, and publicity stunts were staged. The mayor of Yonkers posed for news cameras as his three children received their shots; in Yonkers and Mount Vernon, an army airplane scattered handbills urging immunizations.[37]

In Syracuse, the Boy Scouts stood on the roofs of downtown buildings and wigwagged an anti-diphtheria message to kick off the campaign; later, the health department restaged the Nome dog sled race through downtown streets, with one of the actual sled drivers mushing his team of dogs to city hall.[38] At a conference of the state Charities Aid Association, participants held a mock trial in which "Black Diph," a black-robed figure wearing a red mask, was tried for the murder of hundreds of children.[39]

These publicity efforts, like much of the child health propaganda of the day, emphasized the role of the mother as guardian of young people's well-being. Anti-diphtheria posters depicted bucolic scenes of happy mothers and children; parades featured troops of mothers pushing baby carriages down main streets. The state's efforts drew nationwide attention, garnering favorable articles in mass circulation magazines, especially those with largely female readerships such as the *Women's Home Companion, Ladies' Home Journal,* and *Good Housekeeping.*[40]

By late 1928, the New York City Health Department, having undergone a major management shake-up, was ready to join the statewide effort. Commissioner Shirley Wynne, working with Met Life and the Milbank Fund, convened an impressive group of business, civic, religious, and charitable leaders to guide the effort. Even for a city where splashy and expensive publicity extravaganzas were commonplace, the scope and reach of the anti-diphtheria drive that kicked off in January 1929 were remarkable. The health department sent almost a quarter of a million letters to mothers who had either recently given birth or whose babies had reached nine months of age. The Catholic dioceses of Manhattan and Brooklyn sent letters to parishioners and the principals of parochial schools and made announcements at masses. In conjunction with the board of education census, every home in the Bronx and Queens was visited and the names of all children under fifteen recorded. Leaflets were included in the city's electric and gas bills. Public schools distributed one million flyers to students.

To these individual appeals were joined exhortations through mass advertising. Two rotating billboards in Times Square and a painted sign over two hundred feet long at Broadway and Twenty-Third Street were among the largest pieces of outdoor advertising ever seen in the city. Some three hundred radio talks were broadcast. A series of four short films was shown in five hundred movie theaters. Virtually every newspaper in the city, including the large dailies, the foreign language press, local borough and neighborhood papers, and trade journals, carried articles about the importance of immunization. Subways, elevated trains, streetcars, and buses displayed placards. The city's largest department stores donated advertising space in newspapers. Posters were displayed in chain stores such as Woolworth's and the A&P. To reach the city's many immigrant groups, posters, brochures, and leaflets were translated into the ten most widely spoken foreign languages. Six "healthmobiles" (snow removal trucks converted into traveling clinics) toured city neighborhoods, parks, and beaches.[41]

A national survey conducted in 1930 of child health in one hundred fifty-six American cities revealed the effects of New York State's efforts. Of the ten cities in the country with the highest levels of toxin-antitoxin coverage among preschoolers, seven were in New York.[42] The enthusiasm for diphtheria immunization contrasted sharply with the acceptance of smallpox vaccination. In Niagara Falls, for example, which had the highest rate of protection against diphtheria, 50 percent of children were immunized against diphtheria, while just 3 percent were protected against smallpox.[43]

Unlike the rural-urban split that characterized smallpox vaccination, residents of big cities and small towns were equally likely to protect their children against diphtheria.[44] Also in contrast to vaccination, there was a distinct socioeconomic gradient in protection against diphtheria: parents in the highest income bracket were twice as likely to have it done than those in lowest three classes.[45] The requirement that children be protected against smallpox upon entering school may have evened out the income gradient: in preschool ages, higher-income children were more likely to be vaccinated and immunized, but differences were negligible in the 5-to-14 age group.[46]

The way that toxin-antitoxin was introduced into New York communities—as a dramatic crusade, with eradication of diphtheria as the goal—reflected a belief that contagious disease should and could be utterly eliminated. The dramatic changes in understanding of illness that occurred in the wake of the bacteriological revolution, and the many successes that followed from the application of scientific medicine, held out the promise of absolute mastery of contagion. Thus in framing the purpose of New York's anti-diphtheria drive, Shirley Wynne proudly quoted Pasteur's proclamation, "It is within the power of man to make germ diseases disappear from the face of the earth."[47] The idea of eradication was also consistent with the social and political milieu of Progressivism, which posited the perfectibility of human affairs through the systematic application of knowledge and expertise.

The anti-diphtheria efforts had a model in other ambitious eradication campaigns made possible through philanthropic largesse: the Rockefeller Sanitary Commission's ambitious drive to eliminate hookworm infection from the American South, which was launched in 1909, and the Rockefeller Foundation's campaigns in subsequent years to wipe out yellow fever in Latin America.[48]

Just as the rhetorical creation of a crusade with diphtheria eradication as its goal was rooted in a particular set of beliefs about the existence of illness and the relationship between human and microbe, so too the techniques that were marshaled to carry out the effort reflected a professional ideology. This new perspective located the source of disease within the individual, rather than the environment, and saw persuasion rather than compulsion as the most appropriate and powerful tool for effecting change.

THE POWER OF PERSUASION: THE RISE OF A NEW PUBLIC HEALTH IDEOLOGY

"The key-note of modern public health work is public health education—not compulsion," Hermann Biggs asserted in 1915, explaining to the New York legislature why he supported the Jones-Tallett amendment limiting the use of compulsory vaccination in the state's small towns and rural areas. "Success comes from leading and teaching; not from driving people."[49] Biggs's stance, which reflected lessons learned from decades of frontline health work in the nation's largest city, typified a new ideology of public health that emerged during the Progressive Era. The anti-diphtheria campaigns in New York were emblematic of this shift in professional culture.

This approach began to take shape in the late nineteenth century in campaigns against tuberculosis, when health departments and voluntary agencies began to distribute brochures designed to teach people how they could protect themselves from the disease. But health education truly flowered during the Progressive Era, when it was recognized as a distinct discipline encompassing specialized knowledge and skills and moved to the forefront of the profession's activities.[50] The New York City Department of Health established the first bureau of health education in the country in 1914, and in 1923, the American Public Health Association established a health education and publicity section for members.[51]

The belief in education as a force for moral uplift and social melioration, especially as directed by elite reformers toward the working and lower classes and the immigrant poor, was a prominent theme of Progressive Era policy and politics. The change in public health methods also reflected a conceptual shift that accompanied the bacteriological revolution, as leaders in the profession came to identify the source of disease as lying within the individual rather than in the environment. This new perspective engendered a focus on personal behavior rather than social change, and the development of vaccines contributed to and reinforced the tendency to focus disease-control efforts at the individual level rather than on broad social conditions such as poor housing or economic inequity.[52]

One of the principal areas in which the new educational methods were applied was maternal and child health, as public health officials sought to reform the practices of mothers—especially poor, immigrant ones—along the lines of current scientific knowledge. This work was embodied in institutions such as the United States Children's Bureau, which distributed millions of health education pamphlets on enlightened and modern methods of child-rearing.[53] In addition to publications, health education took the form of individual tutelage by public health nurses and didactic displays and exhibits at fairs and community gathering places. One of the most notable manifestations of the new method was the popularity of "health weeks," during which entire communities would come together to address a particular issue. These events, which combined public health reform with civic boosterism, proliferated during the 1910s and 1920s. The events gave businesses, chambers of commerce, fraternal organizations, and the general public the chance to express municipal pride through the melioration of health problems and in so doing compare their city's status favorably to that of other cities of similar size and situation.[54] Improving child welfare and reducing infant mortality were among the most popular themes of health weeks.[55]

The rise of health education was strongly influenced by a broader trend that was transforming American civic life during this period: the growth of advertising, marketing, and public relations. Spurred by technological changes in printing and photographic reproduction and the mass distribution of commodities, new forms of persuasion penetrated into all areas of daily life, creating a cultural ethos in which comfort and consumption began to replace the older values of abstinence and frugality.[56] New ways of shaping attitudes and behavior—vibrantly illustrated advertisements in newspapers and magazines, store window displays, staged publicity stunts—were a natural companion for health education, and public health professionals were quick to see the potential of these methods. The relationship between health and advertising ran in both directions: just as health officials adopted the techniques of mass marketing, so makers of consumer goods exploited the supposed healthful benefits of products such as toothpaste, household disinfectants, and detergents, attempting to lend the credibility of scientific medicine to their wares.[57] Indeed, pharmaceutical companies had been in the vanguard of using new techniques of persuasion, developing lantern slide shows and motion pictures to promote diphtheria antitoxin to boards of education and medical colleges, and their efforts exemplified the ways that modern advertising could be placed in the service of scientific innovation.[58] Signaling the new importance of mass circulation magazines, the American Chemical Society in 1919 became the first scientific organization to hire a professional science writer to communicate its work to the press and the public, and over the next two decades, other such associations began to use public relations to educate laypeople about the importance of their work.[59]

Proponents of health education self-consciously modeled their efforts on the work of those who placed the latest consumer goods in millions of American households. "Health is a saleable commodity," asserted Herman Bundesen, the president of the American Public Health Association, in 1927. "Mere laws to enforce health do not create health. A desire for good health must first be aroused, stimulated by knowledge of its value and means of attainment. Then the health salesman must come in."[60] This spirit pervaded New York's anti-diphtheria efforts. "This idea of diphtheria immunization had to be 'sold,'" New York City Health Commissioner Shirley Wynne declared in 1929, "almost in the same manner as chewing gum, a second family car or cigarettes."[61] Health education specialists urged their colleagues to adopt modern methods of visual persuasion. Instead of drab pamphlets dense with small, monochromatic type, modern health messages should feature attractive layouts, colors, and typefaces for maximum impact; publicity should be dramatic, entertaining, and carefully planned.[62] The stunts used by cities across New York to stimulate interest in toxin-antitoxin exemplified the staged "pseudo-events" pioneered by the public relations maven Edward Bernays, who famously promoted Lucky Strike cigarettes to female consumers by placing a contingent of proudly smoking women in New York City's Easter Parade.[63]

What effect the new health promotion techniques actually had on behavior remained uncertain, however. A subsequent evaluation of

New York's "No More Diphtheria" drives suggested that splashy publicity was, by itself, insufficient to spur the public to action; intensive
canvassing and in-person contact were essential. The "dog teams,
posters, lectures, letters, postcards, merely served as a background;...
it took face-to-face talk and the existence of a free clinic to get children
to a clinic or the family doctor in appreciable numbers."[64]

Public health leaders during the Progressive Era explicitly characterized the new techniques of persuasion as a repudiation of the coercive
tactics of previous generations. "The great public health progress of the
past has been made without the active co-operation ... and even against
the opposition of the average man and woman in the community," said
Iago Galdston of the New York Tuberculosis and Health Association in
1929. "Far too often, the average man's appreciation of public health is
confined to the begrudging conformity with laws that are a nuisance to
him, the significance of which he does not understand."[65] Health education was framed not only as an advance over past methods, but also
as a uniquely American innovation—reflecting strong traditions of liberty and autonomy—that made this country's public health work superior to that of its European counterparts. Charles Bolduan, director of
health education for the New York City Health Department, had been
born in Germany and had spent several years there on special assign-
ment after World War I; "The German seems to like to be bossed," he
wrote wryly. In contrast, the American preferred to act based on an
understanding of the value of various interventions.[66] The uniquely
American flavor of health education was captured in a 1933 article in a
British public health journal analyzing anti-diphtheria campaigns in the
United States. The American methods were "altogether more intensive
and more spectacular than our sober-minded ideas," the Britons contended. "We in this country are apt to look askance at the flamboy-
ant methods of propaganda used by our brethren on the American
continent.... Our respectability rebels and our insular pride stands
aloof from importing into our professional problems the methods of
the marketplace and the habit of mind of the huckster."[67]

While many in the field framed the rise of health education in teleological terms—as an inevitable advance toward ever more enlightened
means of accomplishing their goals—the use of compulsory measures
hardly vanished from either the rhetoric or the practice of public health,
and the new techniques of education stood in a somewhat uneasy relationship to the older, more coercive tools of law. An editorial in the
American Journal of Public Health, noting with approval the Supreme

Court's 1922 ruling on compulsory school vaccination in *Zucht v. King*, acknowledged the necessity of backing up persuasive measures with the force of law. "[I]t is always better to have people carry out preventive measures willingly and through a fair knowledge of the principles which underlie these measures. Where this cannot be done the police power of the State must be resorted to," the *Journal* opined. "Occasions arise when an appeal to reason is of no avail and the strength of the law must be invoked. There are certain people who cannot be educated nor reasoned with."[68] Similarly, an editorial in the *New York State Journal of Medicine* noted, "People are willing to submit to law in the presence of danger that is evident and immediate; but not everyone is willing to submit to procedures which involve annoyance, discomfort, and expense.... There are those who do not believe in the preparation of vaccines and antitoxins for use in the warfare against contagious diseases. The acceptance of modern methods of disease prevention depends on education [but] Law is necessary for the ignorant, in order to compel obedience."[69]

Coercion thus remained as a less-touted companion to modern propaganda. Quarantines were still enforced against contagions such as scarlet fever and polio, even as health departments distributed pamphlets to teach people how to avoid these illnesses.[70] One of the most high-profile public health efforts in the years during and after World War I, the campaign against venereal diseases, featured the latest persuasive techniques such as posters and films, but also relied on several coercive measures, including compulsory premarital screening for syphilis, mandatory reporting of cases by physicians, and control of prostitution.[71] And "Typhoid Mary" Mallon, the Irish cook who achieved notoriety as a "passive carrier" of bacteria, remained incarcerated on an island in the East River throughout the time that health educators extolled the virtues of changing behavior through education.[72]

Much of the rhetoric that characterized health officials' efforts to sell the public on diphtheria immunization was inflected with strong undercurrents of parental culpability for the sickness of unprotected children.[73] A pamphlet published by the Orleans County Committee on Tuberculosis and Public Health, a charitable organization that assisted with anti-diphtheria efforts in upstate New York, declared, "Hereafter, any baby or any older child who suffers or dies from diphtheria will suffer or die needlessly and because someone has failed to do his or her duty."[74] At its most extreme, the rhetoric of blame sought to attach charges of criminal negligence to uncooperative parents. "The time will come when every case of diphtheria will be an indictment against the intelligence of the parents," claimed a representative of the American Child Health Association in 1926, "and it will not be many years before every death from diphtheria will be referred to a coroner's jury for investigation to fix criminal responsibility."[75] This quasi-coercive rhetoric was typical of much of the "educational" language targeting mothers' child-rearing practices and was not limited to the health professions; advertisers of commercial goods also realized that guilt and shame could be powerful tools in persuading potential consumers to buy a product, and they exploited the fears of parents—especially mothers—who might see themselves as failing to do all they could for their children's health if they did not purchase the best vitamins or toothpaste.[76]

Threats of criminal prosecutions were not entirely far-fetched, in light of the legal actions against Christian Scientists who refused to give antitoxin to treat sick children who later died from diphtheria, but there is little evidence that charges were brought against parents for failure to give toxin-antitoxin prophylactically. New Jersey's health commissioner sought to have several people prosecuted under the state's child welfare law on the ground that their failure to have their children immunized before entry to school was neglectful, but most of these attempts were unsuccessful.[77]

Some parents, however, were unwilling to accept the implication that protecting their children was entirely a matter of personal responsibility. "I have read in several of the papers that if children have not been inoculated against diphtheria its the mothers fault," a woman in Queens wrote to New York City Health Commissioner Shirley Wynne. "Now I would like your advice concerning my 4 small children and at least 7 or 8 other young children on this block. We have no Board of Health station in Queens Village and the nearest one is at 148 St Jamaica which is at least a 2 hr trip (going and coming) on the trolley or bus so on account of this my children and several others have not been taken care of."[78] In response to this request, Wynne arranged for the health department to give injections at a temporary clinic at a local school—a move that brought a sharp rebuke from the neighborhood's physicians, who saw it as trespassing on their professional territory. The incident exemplified the uneasy dynamic during this period between health departments and private practitioners, tension that had significant consequences for immunization programs.

PUBLIC HEALTH VERSUS PRIVATE MEDICINE

Raising knowledge and awareness among the public about the importance of immunization was only one aspect of the process by which the procedure became mainstream. Equally important was providing the means for people to obtain toxin-antitoxin once they had been convinced of its value. The campaigns against diphtheria threw into sharp relief the extent to which immunization, more than any other preventive intervention, straddled the boundary between a public health program and a medical procedure, and the amount of disagreement that prevailed over who should be responsible for providing it.

As preventive medical care such as regular physicals, "well baby" exams, and screening for chronic diseases became more common in the 1920s, tensions grew between municipal health departments and the medical profession over who would deliver these services. Many physicians saw publicly funded health clinics as encroachments on their turf and a potential threat to their incomes, even though some conceded that rank-and-file doctors had been slow to take on responsibility for new preventive measures, stepping up only when they saw health departments moving to assume these duties.[79] Such tensions had coalesced around the publicly funded maternal and child programs created under the Sheppard-Towner Act, which had drawn the wrath of the American Medical Association.

During the 1920s, parents of all social classes increasingly turned to the family physician for guidance on the proper, "scientific" ways of rearing children.[80] But, as we saw in chapter 2, health officials complained that doctors did little to encourage their private patients to undergo vaccination against smallpox, seeing the procedure as a function of city governments. These charges were renewed when toxin-antitoxin became available. "The great majority of the medical profession," New York State Health Commissioner Matthias Nicoll charged bluntly, "has done little or nothing to bring about immunization against diphtheria among their private patients."[81]

New York's statewide anti-diphtheria drive involved a collaboration among local medical societies, health departments, and business and charitable organizations. Although each group publicly endorsed these cooperative partnerships and offered at least pro forma praise for the agencies with which it worked, such surface politeness masked considerable tension. One of the most contentious areas was the extent to which toxin-antitoxin should be "sold." The ethical canons of the medical profession forbade doctors to advertise or promote their services, a taboo rooted in aversion to the quackery and charlatanism of the past. But such a posture was in conflict with the goals of preventive medicine, which required urging people to take actions they might not otherwise have taken in order to safeguard their health. Matthias Nicoll attributed the tepid response of the state's doctors in the anti-diphtheria crusade to "hesitancy and delicacy on the part of our best practitioners to take any action among their patients which would seem to leave them open to the charge of commercialism by seeking to increase their practice."[82]

The differing views about whether immunization should be advertised and whether the injections should be publicly available was especially evident in Schenectady. When the statewide drive kicked off at the beginning of 1926, the Schenectady County Medical Society broke with the program recommended by the state that other cities were following. The steering committee there, dominated by doctors, declined to open special clinics, insisting instead that all immunizations be carried out in private physicians' offices. The doctors disdained the "revival meeting methods" of publicity that other cities were adopting; instead of flashy advertising and publicity stunts, they insisted that education consist solely of physicians giving talks to civic groups and their own patients and by canvassing of homes. The Schenectady doctors also declined to use the state health department's educational materials, because they felt that terms such as "Schick test" and "toxin-antitoxin" were confusing to the public.[83] The Schenectady plan resulted in fewer immunizations than in other cities where clinics were established.[84] Eventually, the city began a second phase of its campaign and in June 1927 opened a public clinic where, three days a week, people could bring their children to be immunized.

Such professional tensions were also evident in Syracuse, which had a highly successful program of free immunization clinics in schools and the town dispensary until some doctors objected. C.-E. A. Winslow, the Yale professor who evaluated the Milbank health demonstration in Syracuse, offered this dry assessment of what happened in the city in 1928:

> In this year there was some opposition to the immunization clinics on the part of certain elements in the medical profession. As an experiment the school campaign was discontinued in order to give the private practitioners an opportunity to perform the immunization themselves. Known immunizations dropped from 10,003 in 1927 to 188 in 1928, with no evidence of active immunization by private physicians; and the clinic program was therefore resumed.[85]

For their part, doctors blamed their low immunization rates on people's unwillingness to spend money on their health, and insisted that the proper response was to convince people of the value of such services—not to offer them for free. "The abuse of official and semi-official facilities for free treatment by those who can afford to pay has made appreciable inroads upon the income of the private practitioner of medicine," lamented an editorial in *New York Medical Week,* the official journal of the New York County Medical Society, in response to the large number of parents seeking immunization for their children through city clinics.[86] Public health officials saw the ease with which city residents could obtain the procedure for free as a good thing, since their goal was to achieve universal coverage, but to the city's private physicians, this ease opened the door to abuse of free services.[87]

In response to this alleged abuse, a physician in Queens urged Shirley Wynne to delete any mention of free clinics from the city's anti-diphtheria publicity, saying:

> I feel quite confident that those people really deserving of charity medical service will, in spite of this deletion, secure proper medical attention for their children, and at the same time many who can afford to pay a doctor will not be tempted to avail themselves of a service to which they are not entitled.... It is only human to try to get for nothing whatever one can; but usually it is not fair. It is the duty of every agency having to do with public health to see to it that only those get medical service free who are entitled to get it free.[88]

Wynne replied sharply that "many private physicians have not done their part" in fighting diphtheria, and that the number of immunizations performed in doctors' offices had declined since the start of the campaign.[89]

Morris Fishbein, the editor of the *Journal of the American Medical Association,* who had attacked the opponents of immunization in his book *The Medical Follies,* was scarcely more sympathetic to the public health bureaucrats who, he believed, were advancing communistic health care schemes. A vehement opponent of socialized medicine, Fishbein criticized public provision of immunization in a *JAMA* article, which included the following "typical conversation" between a mother and her family doctor:

> "Doctor, do you believe in giving of toxoid to prevent diphtheria?"
> "Yes, indeed."
> "Do you use the same serum that the health department uses?"

"Yes, indeed."

"What do you charge, doctor?"

"Five dollars."

"Doctor, does the health department give the same treatment that you give?"

"Yes."

"Do they charge anything?"

"No. They take the funds out of the taxes."

"Well, doctor, wouldn't I be a simpleton to pay you $5 when I can get the same service from the health department for nothing?"

Fishbein concluded his discussion with a plea for "individual mutual responsibilities between patient and physician."[90]

The Depression increased attendance at public clinics. Many parents of narrow means preferred them even to doctors who offered a discount rate; a health department official noted that "the public was less willing to accept gratuitous service from private physicians, than to go to stations of our Department and accept city service. They felt they were entitled to the latter."[91] But the *Medical Week* saw the hard economic conditions of the early 1930s as all the more reason to curtail the abuse of free services. "With the municipal budget badly in need of paring, the time has never been more auspicious for the restoration of individual prophylaxis to the private practitioner," an editorial urged in 1933. "The duties of the city to its indigent are too pressing to permit of gifts of medical care to those who can afford to purchase it themselves."[92]

The antipathy toward free medical care for those able to pay reflected deeply held American attitudes about charity. The belief that monetary and other forms of assistance should be given only to the "deserving" poor had been central to social welfare policy since colonial times, and it was reflected in the nature of government relief, which was limited to categories of people thought to be worthy, such as widows, orphans, and war veterans. Charity, it was thought, would simply sap the able-bodied of initiative and pride.[93] An editorial in the *New York State Journal of Medicine* exemplified this outlook when it claimed that free medical care "does not improve the morals of the recipient. It not only fails to arouse an aggressive spirit of selfhelp [sic], but on the contrary it encourages laziness and dependency."[94]

Throughout the toxin-antitoxin campaign in New York City, one of Shirley Wynne's most delicate tasks was securing and maintaining the cooperation of the city's physicians. Wynne was not a proponent of state medicine and repeatedly insisted that the health department's goal was to direct New Yorkers into doctors' offices.[95] But he also realized that the city could never achieve high levels of immunization coverage through these means alone. Wynne thus charted an uncertain course between public and private medicine. In May 1929, he sent a form letter to the city's twelve thousand physicians asking them to set aside special hours for the injections and to offer them for a special rate of $2 each ($6 for the standard series of three shots).[96] Thousands of physicians agreed to adhere to the price structure, and in 1930, Wynne followed up with a plan to have all the city's physicians establish a "children's hour" during which they would provide well-child care at a set fee.[97]

In spite of the cooperation Wynne received, the proportion of children immunized by private physicians declined from 37 percent in 1930 to 24 percent in 1931.[98] "The private physicians have not risen to the occasion as much as we had hoped," wrote a disappointed Wynne in 1932. "Their *proportion* of the immunizations should have increased from year to year as the work progressed. Especially in view of their feeling that the free immunizations by the Department of Health trespassed on their legitimate rights."[99] By the end of 1934, the proportion of immunizations performed by private physicians remained at only one-quarter, and the overall number had declined.[100]

THE LIMITS OF PERSUASION

Active resistance to the toxin-antitoxin campaigns was negligible. By the late 1920s, the anti-vaccination movement had faded considerably, and what protests there were came from non-allopathic practitioners and other long-standing opponents of the medical establishment. The *Chiropractic News*, in a front-page article headlined "Torture of the Innocents," offered a contrarian interpretation of New York City's drive: "Perfectly healthy children are brought by unwise mothers to have their blood streams polluted with virulent disease 'culture'—the result of medical trust propaganda—a crime against health in the name of 'public welfare.'"[101] The New York Anti-Vivisection Society distributed leaflets urging parents to "Beware the Schick Test" and shun the use of toxin-antitoxin. The society deplored the use of horses and guinea pigs in the manufacture of the substance and urged parents not to "immolate the little ones on the altar of immunization."[102] But such objections were muted in comparison with the widespread and vociferous protests that compulsory smallpox vaccination had aroused.

In spite of the enormous fanfare during 1929 that made toxin-antitoxin ubiquitous throughout New York City, by the middle of 1930, health officials were already complaining that public attention was wandering, and that the number of infants immunized in the city was running well below that of the previous year. As before, an immunizing procedure became the victim of its own success: in 1930, the number of cases and deaths from the disease dropped precipitously from the previous year, and this very success made it more difficult for the health department to claim an urgent threat was at hand. Thus the rhetoric of health officials portrayed a threat barely held at bay. "[U]nless checked by immunization there is a strong possibility of diphtheria being more prevalent this winter than it has been for some years," Wynne told the press. "Every child who has not been immunized by the time it arrives will be in grave danger of being stricken with the disease and probably carried off by it."[103]

While complacency bred by diminishing disease burden was clearly a factor in the failure to achieve universal acceptance of toxin-antitoxin, so too was a somewhat more complicated mixture of reluctance and confusion among the public about the nature and meaning of immunization. One Brooklyn resident was wary about having the procedure done, "because of the warm weather and the fact that the baby has been teething."[104] Another believed that "well fed well kept children do not get diphtheria."[105] Having long been told the importance of smallpox vaccination, parents were often unsure about whether the two procedures were contraindicated or redundant, which one should be done first, and how much time should elapse between the two.[106] Some parents believed that smallpox vaccination provided protection against all diseases.[107] A Brooklyn mother worried that having her son vaccinated against smallpox only three months after receiving his diphtheria immunization might "prove to be too much of a strain for him."[108] Another worried whether eczema, a well-known contraindication for vaccination, also rendered a child unsuited for diphtheria immunization. "I have had the advice of two 'Baby Specialists' who advised 'no inoculation' and three ordinary physicians who advise me to give my boy the treatment for anti-diphtheria," wrote the confused mother to the health department. "Those who said no, gave the reason that the reaction to one suffering from eczema was too dangerous and that the dreaded disease of diphtheria was a milder thing to combat."[109] Even though the germ theory had long since been accepted as orthodoxy throughout American society, suspicions of scientific medicine remained. A Queens woman wrote to Wynne that she believed that "the use of antitoxins are [*sic*] still in the experimental stages, and ... I do not believe they are or ever will be satisfactory substitutes for personal cleanliness, proper food or hygienic living conditions."[110]

Doctors themselves held divergent opinions about these matters. Some physicians also believed that toxin-antitoxin was inappropriate for children who were teething or underweight.[111] A Manhattan physician wrote to Wynne in 1930, "During the months of May and June a great many children are vaccinated against Smallpox and many physicians including myself, advise against any other ACTIVE immunization at this time.... Will you therefore inform me whether or not the immunity developing against diphtheria or vaccinia is interfered with in any way, when immunization is carried out against these diseases within a period of less than FOUR months."[112] (The department's policy was that the two procedures did not interfere with each other, but that it was preferable not to immunize for diphtheria when the pustule that appeared after vaccination was still present.) In 1931, there was a downturn in the number of immunizations against both diphtheria and smallpox because of the polio epidemic. Not only parents but many physicians as well feared that any form of immunization might temporarily lower children's resistance and make them more susceptible to polio.[113]

There was also varying acceptance of toxin-antitoxin among different ethnic communities. Jewish immigrants were more likely than other groups to embrace the applications of scientific medicine and had the lowest rates of infant mortality among New York's immigrant communities.[114] Italian Americans were most likely among ethnic groups to hold negative attitudes toward both smallpox vaccination and toxin-antitoxin, and also suffered from the highest rates of diphtheria.[115] An informal survey by nurses working in the city's child health stations also revealed the existence of a gender bias against the procedure: the most common reason for a refusal to have a baby immunized was that the father didn't want it, even though the mother was willing.[116] Some fathers objected because of bad experiences they had had with smallpox or typhoid vaccination in the military. The nurses suggested that the department develop more attractive literature to appeal directly to the fathers, and especially to those of Polish, Lithuanian, and Italian descent, who were more likely to be opposed. There is no evidence that the department ever developed promotional materials aimed at fathers. Indeed, the following year, Wynne wrote to a local medical society, "We must continue and intensify the educational campaign directing this especially to mothers of young infants, so that as far as possible such mothers will come to have their children immunized as a routine measure."[117] Wynne did, however, attempt to reach out to fathers by arranging presentations to labor unions.[118]

Some of the early confusion among the public and medical professionals was due to the evolving science of immunization. In the early 1920s, French scientists discovered that diphtheria toxin neutralized by a chemical agent, usually formalin, stimulated an immune response without causing illness. This preparation, called a toxoid, offered several advantages over the use of the toxin-antitoxin mixture. It appeared to provide longer-lasting immunity to larger percentages of children, was more stable than toxin-antitoxin, and was unaffected by freezing. Toxin-antitoxin was made using animal (typically horse or goat) serum, which could lead to adverse reactions, and in rare instances anaphylactic shock, in persons subsequently injected with other vaccines containing serum. Toxoid contained no animal serum.

Most important from the standpoint of widespread public use, toxoid seemed to require only one or two injections instead of three— though whether a single dose was in fact efficacious would remain the subject of controversy.[119] One important disadvantage was that toxoid tended to cause adverse reactions, especially high fevers, when given to children older than five or six. British researchers made an additional refinement by mixing the toxoid with alum, which appeared to boost its strength and thus lessen the number of doses needed. But the alum-precipitated formulation required a larger needle and caused local reactions more frequently.

The use of both toxin-antitoxin and toxoid in varying doses caused considerable confusion among the general public and private physicians about whether boosters were needed and whether children were being adequately protected by one, two, or even three shots. When the New York City Health Department began recommending just one dose of alum-precipitated toxoid for infants, a representative of the Queens Medical Society complained to Wynne that the policy change "gained wide publicity much to the embarrassment of the physicians who have not heard about it previously, and many of whose attention was first called to it by the mothers."[120] By 1935, the department had reversed itself and was again recommending two shots instead of one, even though it continued to mail out reminder cards that urged parents to get "a single, painless treatment."[121]

Around the country, discrepancies in practice prevailed through the 1930s.[122] During this period, there was no single advisory body that provided definitive guidelines for practitioners about which vaccines should be used, at what ages they should be given, and under what circumstances; new research findings and laboratory developments were interpreted differently by those who administered vaccines. The American Academy of Pediatrics, which was formed in 1930, issued its first set of official recommendations for the routine immunization of children in 1934 and subsequently published updated editions of the so-called Red Book every two years.[123] The American Medical Association's Council on Pharmacy and Chemistry published a list of "New and Non-Official Remedies," which also served as an advisory to help physicians make decisions about therapeutics.[124] The American Public Health Association's Committee on Administrative Practice issued guidelines as well. But matters such as timing, dosages, and risks were all subjects of considerable variation based on the professional judgment of individual practitioners and public health departments.

Over the course of the 1930s, the incidence of diphtheria plummeted even as rates of immunization remained flat or declined.[125] The rate of diphtheria had been dropping slowly for decades before toxin-antitoxin came into use, and even supporters of the practice conceded that it was difficult to state definitively how much of the reduction was attributable to immunization and how much to overall improvements in hygiene or a natural decline in the virulence of the disease.[126] Given the small number of cases each year—New York City recorded just over one thousand cases in 1936, out of a total youth population of some 1.6 million—and the fact that chronic illnesses such as cancer and heart disease were rising ominously, health officials began to question how much effort it was worth expending to promote immunization. Private sector funding sources who had contributed to anti-diphtheria campaigns turned their attention to more pressing issues. "We are somewhat uncertain," the Met Life company replied to a solicitation of further funding, "as to whether diphtheria continues to be a sufficiently important project to justify a special expenditure."[127]

While the rhetoric of the immunization campaigns in the 1920s had stressed eradication as the goal and universal use of toxin-antitoxin as the means of achieving it, in the 1930s, health officials began scaling back their expectations about what should be done in the control of diphtheria. House-to-house surveys around the city revealed that about two-thirds of children under six years old had received their shots—a level of immunity that was apparently high enough to keep the disease at insignificant levels. "It would, of course be possible to increase this percentage by more intensive work," wrote John Rice, who succeeded Shirley Wynne as New York City's health commissioner in 1934, "but the expense and effort would, in my opinion, be out of proportion to the result achieved."[128] In the late 1930s, when a slight upturn in the number of diphtheria cases prompted the city to initiate special immunization programs, these efforts were concentrated in just a handful of neighborhoods whose rates of diphtheria greatly exceeded the citywide average; all had high population density and high rates of infant mortality and other contagious disease such as tuberculosis.[129] These narrowly targeted efforts relied more on house-to-house canvassing than on advertising or publicity events.[130]

The continued presence of diphtheria in concentrated pockets around the city and the persistent level of just two-thirds of the city's children immunized—though the rate was considerably lower in some districts—clearly revealed the limits of persuasion. "The citizens in the areas requiring most attention have been found to be the ones who pay least attention," one deputy commissioner wrote, "and are most antagonistic to our efforts to accomplish diphtheria immunizations."[131]

One suggestion that repeatedly arose to the problem of low levels of coverage was to enact some sort of legal mandate for the procedure. As early as 1921, some public health and medical experts were suggesting that immunization against diphtheria be made compulsory for school entry.[132] Similar proposals were advanced over the following two decades as use of toxin-antitoxin gained popularity.[133] The health department consistently declined to support such suggestions. This was due in part to an institutional preference for education over compulsion, a position that was articulated most frequently and eloquently by Charles Bolduan, who was an important figure in departmental policymaking and a visible public spokesperson for the virtues of persuasion. But even more salient than such philosophical rationales were pragmatic concerns. Diphtheria struck preschool age children most frequently, so a school entry requirement would do nothing to enhance the protection of the majority of children who were at risk.[134] Furthermore, officials feared that such a law would encourage parents to postpone the procedure until children reached school age.[135] There was a sound empirical basis for this fear: surveys indicated that parents generally waited until children entered school to have them protected against smallpox, even though physicians and public health officials universally recommended that vaccination be done during infancy.[136]

While the predominant view within the New York City Health Department was that a legal mandate would be unwise, this position was not universal. In 1932, the declining number of immunizations prompted an assistant superintendent of health to declare, "No time seems more plausible than now to establish compulsory protection as a pre-requisite to school admission."[137] His stance was rooted in frustration over the Sisyphean task of persuasion in a city where so many children were born annually: "We have 125,000 new borns per year who make perpetual effort mandatory even if all other vulnerable children were protected." A decade later, a health department statistician made a similar plea to the commissioner on grounds of efficiency. The recurring campaigns urging diphtheria immunization "will continue to require special efforts on the part of each District Health Officer in the City each year until there is some legislative requirement"—a waste of valuable time that could be better spent.[138]

New York's stance toward compulsory diphtheria protection was typical of states around the country. In contrast to the extensive legal activity following the introduction of smallpox vaccination, just a handful of states moved to make diphtheria immunization compulsory in the two decades after its use became widespread. North Carolina adopted the most far-reaching law, requiring the immunization of all children between six months and one year of age, and of all children between one and five years old who had not been previously immunized. Four states made the procedure mandatory for school attendance, while another four required it under special circumstances, such as in institutions or in the face of an epidemic.[139]

THE LEGACY OF DIPHTHERIA IMMUNIZATION

The popular perception that diphtheria immunization was safe and effective would greatly influence the acceptability of new vaccines against other illnesses. A nationwide survey in 1941 revealed high levels of confidence in the principles of immunization.[140] About three-quarters of all adults believed that the diseases could be prevented through vaccines; less than ten percent of those surveyed expressed disbelief or active resistance. But there was also lingering confusion: some parents believed that immunization was necessary only after exposure to the disease, while others thought that six years of age was the proper time to immunize against both smallpox and diphtheria, rather than in the first year of life as physicians recommended. There was widespread ignorance about the need for boosters—confusion that mirrored ongoing professional disagreements over this issue. A survey commissioned the following year by the pharmaceutical company Sharpe and Dohme found similar results. About seventy percent of respondents thought that immunization could protect children from diphtheria, though many believed that it could not completely prevent the illness, only lessen its severity.[141]

In addition to fostering a favorable public impression of vaccination, the use of diphtheria toxoid provided coattails to other vaccines. In the mid 1930s, scientists at the Pasteur Institute in Paris began experiments with a single preparation combining diphtheria toxoid with a vaccine against pertussis, a common and often fatal childhood illness, more widely known as whooping cough. During the 1940s, experiments also began on adding the recently developed toxoid against tetanus to the mixture. Evidence suggested that double- and triple-protection vaccines had a synergistic effect, providing higher levels of immunity than any of the vaccines administered singly. More important was the logistical advantage: children could be protected against more illnesses with fewer clinic visits.[142]

The development of combination formulas was especially important for the adoption of the pertussis vaccine, which had long been plagued by doubts about its efficacy. Attempts to develop a vaccine against pertussis began as soon as the causative agent was identified in 1906. By 1931, at least fourteen different vaccine preparations against pertussis had been developed, but there was little uniformity of opinion about which was the best formulation, or when or how the vaccine should be administered.[143] "It seems that amongst the physicians each one gives a different amount of injections," wrote a confused Brooklyn mother who sought advice from the New York City Health Department in 1934.[144] Such inquiries placed the department in an awkward position. Health Commissioner John Rice and his colleagues believed that most of the pertussis vaccines had no value, but by saying so to members of the public, the department risked appearing to denigrate the professional judgment of those physicians who had decided to offer one. In response to the mother in Brooklyn, Rice instructed one of his bureau chiefs to "draw up a diplomatic reply to this letter so that we may not be criticized by physicians and yet satisfy the writer."[145]

In the absence of a single authoritative source for vaccine recommendations, partisans of the various vaccines under development advanced competing claims for the value of the new procedure. A pertussis vaccine developed by Louis Sauer, an Illinois pediatrician and researcher who had tested his formulation widely in public schools in Evanston, attracted attention in the popular press after Sauer published promising results in medical journals.[146] In the March 1935 issue of *Good Housekeeping,* Josephine Kenyon, a physician who wrote the magazine's medical advice column, strongly recommended the Sauer vaccine.[147] After Kenyon's article appeared, the New York City Health Department was inundated with inquiries from the public wanting to know where they could obtain the vaccine.[148]

Around the same time, another promising preparation was developed by Pearl Kendrick, a microbiologist at the Michigan Department of Health. Among those impressed by the Kendrick results was the Met Life Company, which remained an important force in promoting the adoption of advances in scientific medicine. In early 1941, Met Life undertook an effort to encourage its policyholders to obtain the pertussis vaccine for their children. John Rice, who remained unconvinced by the Kendrick data, was disturbed by the company's recommendation. "It is my impression that the general consensus of opinion is that there is no vaccine or serum for whooping cough of demonstrated value," Rice wrote to Donald Armstrong, the head of Met Life's welfare division, "and while you leave it up to the doctor to determine whether it should be used, your advertisement gives the reader the impression that vaccine for whooping cough is hot stuff."[149] Armstrong replied that after extensive consultation with pediatricians around the country, he had concluded that "contrary to the general attitude of public health and laboratory men, the clinical men in the pediatric field are almost universally favorably impressed with the vaccine."[150]

The American Academy of Pediatrics ultimately gave its stamp of approval to both the Sauer and Kendrick vaccines in 1943, prompting additional attention in the popular press.[151] Paul de Kruif, the most well-known medical journalist of the day, wrote a highly laudatory article in *Reader's Digest* in 1943.[152] While more private physicians and hospitals began offering the vaccine in light of the new findings, many experts remained equivocal in their endorsement. Child health guides during this period described smallpox and diphtheria vaccines as "musts," while the pertussis vaccine was considered a "may."[153] In 1946, the most popular child-rearing guide in the postwar years, Benjamin Spock's *Common Sense Book of Baby and Child Care,* strongly endorsed vaccination against smallpox and diphtheria but conceded that "scientists haven't completely decided yet how much protection a child gets [from the pertussis shot]."[154]

Nevertheless, the pertussis vaccine gradually became commonplace—almost exclusively as part of a combined injection with diphtheria toxoid. It thus piggybacked on the latter's greater efficacy and public acceptance. More broadly, favorable public attitudes toward the concept of immunization, fueled in large measure by advances in scientific medicine during and after World War II, set the stage for the most high-profile medical saga of the twentieth century: the development of a polio vaccine.

CHAPTER 4

Hard Cores and Soft Spots

Selling the Polio Vaccine

Assessing the country's level of protection against polio in late 1960, five years after the first vaccine for the disease had been licensed amid unprecedented fanfare, Alexander Langmuir, the country's leading epidemiologist, offered a mixed verdict. "Immunization acceptance has been far from uniform," Langmuir said. "Large 'islands' of poorly vaccinated population groups exist—in our city slums, in isolated and ethnically distinct communities, and in many rural areas."[1] Especially discouraging was the picture among adults: less than one-third had gotten the recommended series of four shots for full protection. The situation Langmuir described would have been inconceivable just a few years earlier, when overwhelming public demand for the vaccine had swamped the ability of manufacturers and the government to meet it.

The nationwide testing and subsequent licensing of Jonas Salk's polio vaccine were watershed events in the history of vaccination in America, bringing the value of the practice to the forefront of popular culture to an extent unequalled before or since. But in spite of the mythology that surrounds the vaccine's development, the story of its deployment in the community was hardly one of unalloyed triumph. The initial demand proved short-lived, with severe shortages of the vaccine soon giving way to surpluses in many areas. Health officials shifted from tight rationing to aggressive salesmanship in order to persuade people to receive the full course of injections. The licensing in 1961 of a second polio preventive, Albert Sabin's oral vaccine, offered hope for more widespread acceptance because of its greater ease of administration. But the vaccine could in rare cases produce the very paralysis it was meant to prevent, obliging policymakers to weigh the benefits of vaccination against its inherent risks. These thorny ethical questions had been largely absent from view since the early years of the century, when injury and death allegedly caused by smallpox vaccination had ignited acrimonious public debates.

This chapter examines how the fight against polio changed vaccination programs. New actors who would have a profound influence on policy and practice entered onto a stage that had previously been dominated by public health departments and medical societies. The National Foundation for Infantile Paralysis, a charitable organization that led the development of the Salk vaccine, brought to bear its sophisticated public relations capabilities to shape popular attitudes toward vaccination. The public's demand for protection from polio also forced the federal government to take reluctant steps into vaccine distribution and promotion, ultimately leading to legislation in 1962 that resulted in a permanent home for immunization programs within the U.S. Public Health Service bureaucracy. As a result, campaigns to promote vaccines began to take on more uniformity and become national in scope.

Even more significant, epidemiologic surveillance and social science research began to guide the promotion of vaccines. This research explained the propensity to get vaccinated according to behavioral, psychological, and sociological variables and generated a new discourse about the "hard core" of the unvaccinated—people who remained without protection and were least likely to be motivated by traditional health education campaigns. The most salient characteristic of this population was low socioeconomic status, and to a large extent, the term "hard core" was simply a new name for an old phenomenon: people of higher income and formal education responded much more readily to calls for vaccination than the poor. But in their efforts to remove barriers of cost and access, public health officials ran up against long-standing tensions with the medical profession over the extent to which vaccination should be made available outside of private physicians' offices.

THE ADVENT OF THE SALK VACCINE

Poliomyelitis, like smallpox, sparked a popular terror far out of proportion to the number of deaths it caused. It appeared in the United States at the end of the nineteenth century and first struck in epidemic form in the northeast United States in 1916. The causal virus was identified in 1908, but the disease's mode of transmission and pathogenesis remained in dispute for decades, frustrating the ability of medical researchers to combat it.[2] Although the most common symptomatic form of the disease was a flulike illness that resolved without complication, it was most well known, and feared, for the full or partial paralysis that occurred in about 1 percent of cases (hence its original name, "infantile paralysis"). The emblematic image of polio was the quadriplegic victim dependent on an "iron lung" respirator to stay alive. At a time when other contagions were yielding to advances in scientific medicine, polio presented a frightening anomaly, increasing in incidence as the century progressed. Annual rates spiked sharply upward in the 1940s, with 1952 the worst year on record; polio paralyzed more than twenty-one thousand people that year. The average age of those struck most frequently rose over time as well, from infancy to school age.[3] Unlike many other infectious diseases, its victims were children of the middle and upper classes as often as the poor. The disease returned every year during the summer months, peaking in August and September. Fearful parents kept children away from playgrounds, and public swimming pools closed.

Polio's most famous victim, Franklin Roosevelt, played a pivotal role in shaping popular impressions of the illness. Roosevelt was a politician with a promising future when he was struck with polio in 1921, and his experience symbolized the vulnerability that Americans felt to the disease. Roosevelt suffered paralysis as a result of the illness, but he kept his condition hidden from the public, giving the impression he had regained the use of his legs, and the story of his rise to New York governor and then U.S. president shaped a cultural narrative about the terror of polio and the potential to triumph over it.[4]

Even more important was Roosevelt's effect on the course of scientific research into polio. In 1938, Roosevelt, along with his former law partner Basil O'Connor, created the National Foundation for Infantile Paralysis (NFIP), a philanthropic organization that provided rehabilitative care for victims and funded scientific research into a cure or vaccine for the disease. The NFIP represented a new, democratic model for charity: unlike foundations based on family wealth, the organization drew its funds from direct appeals to the public, using the enormously successful and influential "March of Dimes" campaign, in which citizens from all walks of life were encouraged to contribute small amounts of money that in the aggregate would finance a national crusade against polio.[5]

These fund-raising appeals used the most sophisticated techniques of advertising and public relations—films, radio, and print media, the brave "poster child," the celebrity spokesperson, all playing upon parental sentiment and fear—and made the disease an object of extraordinary public concern.

During the 1940s, NFIP-funded scientific research laid the groundwork for the development of a vaccine. In an era when most biomedical research remained small-scale, the NFIP was able to bring together the nation's leading polio investigators to share their knowledge. A team of researchers convened by the NFIP in 1946 identified three types of the virus (labeled types I, II, and III) in a breakthrough with major practical implications: any successful vaccine would have to be effective against all three types, since antibodies were specific to each type and did not protect against the others.[6] In 1949, John Enders, a Harvard University researcher who would later develop one of the first measles vaccines, successfully cultured polio virus in non-nervous tissue, demonstrating that the disease did not attack only the central nervous system, as had been thought, but spread systemically.[7] These advances in basic science led to two competing types of vaccines. One was a killed virus vaccine developed by Jonas Salk, in which the virus was inactivated by formalin (the chemical that was used to neutralize diphtheria toxin to make toxoid). At the same time, several researchers, most prominently Albert Sabin, were working to develop a live, attenuated vaccine. In this process the virus was weakened by serial passage through culture until it had lost the ability to cause disease but could still produce an immune response. Which type of vaccine would offer the better protection was the subject of protracted debates, often polarized, acrimonious, and driven by personal animosity among the scientists involved. The NFIP's panel of experts ultimately judged Salk's to be the most promising of the vaccines in development and moved forward with planning a large-scale trial in humans.[8]

The developments in polio research occurred against a backdrop of dramatic advances in the fight against infectious disease. New treatments for malaria and tuberculosis, new uses for the blood product gamma globulin, and, most famous, mass production of the antibiotic penicillin were widely hailed in the popular media during and after World War II. Financial investment in biomedical research in both the public and private sectors rose quickly in the postwar years.[9] To an unprecedented extent, scientific medicine came to be viewed as a valuable national asset and force for the betterment of humanity.[10]

It is within this context that one must understand the Salk vaccine trial that was launched in the spring of 1954. The largest medical experiment conducted in the world up to that time, it riveted the public attention like no other scientific event of the twentieth century.[11] In the spring and summer of 1954, investigators enrolled some 1.8 million children around the country—"polio pioneers," as the National Foundation dubbed them—to receive either the vaccine or a placebo injection or to serve as "observed controls." Stories covering the progress of the trial were a staple in the media, and the announcement of the results, timed for release on the tenth anniversary of Franklin Roosevelt's death, April 12, 1955, captured the front page in newspapers and the lead in television and radio broadcasts across the country. According to public opinion polls, some 97 percent of the population had either read or heard about the vaccine.[12]

The initial euphoria over the favorable trial results quickly turned into confusion over how people would be able to obtain the new preventive. Spurred by decades of dread and a full year of continual publicity about the imminent arrival of the vaccine, people wanted it for their children immediately, as the summer polio season loomed. But it would be impossible for the six manufacturers of the vaccine to gear up their production to generate enough vials of vaccine for the nation's twenty million youth. The initial supplies were to go exclusively to the NFIP; confident that the vaccine would be a success, the organization in early 1955 contracted with all six manufacturers to buy $9 million worth of vaccine, which it planned to distribute to states so that they could offer it free to first- and second-graders, the age group that polio struck most frequently.[13]

The severe shortage raised several difficult policy questions. Once the NFIP's order had been filled, what portion of the vaccine should be made commercially available—sold to drug firms, who would in turn sell it to private physicians—and what portion retained for use by city and country health authorities for public provision? Should children receive their shots solely, or primarily, through mass clinics, especially in schools, or should the offices of private pediatricians be the main venue? The vaccine required three doses to deliver optimal protection, but a single shot could provide sufficient protection for a period of several months. With the summer polio season fast approaching, should cities provide a single dose to a larger number of children in order to protect them during the summer, or multiple shots to fewer children?

In New York City, overseeing the vaccine's deployment—a task in equal parts public health and public relations—fell to Leona Baumgartner. A physician with a doctorate in immunology, Baumgartner assumed leadership of the department at the beginning of 1954, the first woman to hold the position. She had headed the city's bureau of child hygiene in the early 1940s and later done a stint in the U.S. Children's Bureau, and she had a long-standing interest in vaccination, having authored the 1943 report on nationwide attitudes toward the practice.[14] She also had an intuitive understanding of the political nature of public health—an invaluable attribute when she confronted the often chaotic events following the licensing of the Salk vaccine.

Ongoing confusion about how much vaccine would be available, and when, was exacerbated by fear that the distribution would unfairly favor those with money or political connections. One of the vaccine manufacturers, for example, sent letters to its shareholders offering priority access to the vaccine for their children and grandchildren.[15] Rumors circulated about stolen vaccine turning up on the black market and physicians giving shots to their own or friends' children. Elected officials made public statements, often purely speculative, about how the vaccine should or would be distributed; such pronouncements, though intended to alleviate public concern and give the impression that competent authorities had the situation well in hand, generally had the opposite effect.[16] "I urge you STRONGLY not to get into further questions about the Salk vaccine," Baumgartner advised New York City Mayor Robert Wagner Jr. one month after the vaccine was licensed. "Every non-medical person who has done this has borrowed a lot of trouble.... Various governors, the President and other people who have taken on questions have inevitably been asked and have answered questions in a way that has caused more confusion."[17]

On April 29, partially in response to the rumors about unethical distribution of the vaccine, the city amended the sanitary code requiring physicians to record the name, address, and age of anyone receiving an injection; detailed records had to be kept of all vaccine distributed, and any theft was to be reported immediately to the health department. Unauthorized sale or possession of the vaccine was made a misdemeanor punishable by up to a $500 fine and a year in jail.[18]

The volatile situation was thrown into further confusion just two weeks after the announcement of the trial results, when reports began to come into the Public Health Service of paralytic polio occurring in people who had recently received an injection of the Salk vaccine.

Government investigators quickly traced the infections to vaccine lots from one manufacturer, Cutter Laboratories, and on April 27, Surgeon General Leonard Scheele asked Cutter to recall all outstanding lots. A special surveillance program was established in the federal Communicable Disease Center (CDC), which over the following two weeks traced dozens of cases of polio to Cutter vaccine that had been insufficiently inactivated during the manufacturing process. Ultimately, 204 cases (79 in children who had received injections and 135 in family and community contacts) were traced to the defective Cutter vaccine; 11 people died.[19]

In the course of tracing lots of the Cutter vaccine in New York City, investigators discovered that several doctors had given injections to patients outside of the priority age range (children five to nine were at highest risk) in violation of the voluntary agreement by the local medical societies. The names of the offending doctors were turned over to the health department, which promptly gave them to the medical societies for follow-up and disciplinary action. One doctor, it seemed, had given shots to his two teenage children; others to pregnant women and people who were about to travel to areas abroad where polio was widespread. The medical societies suggested that the doctors' actions represented ignorance and confusion rather than malfeasance, and although at least three doctors were reprimanded and one suspended for the actions, the societies determined that there had been no black marketeering or fee gouging.[20] The public attention that these cases attracted underscored the extent to which distribution of the vaccine had become freighted with significance far beyond the medical. Decisions about vaccination were, according to Baumgartner, "a kind of moral test of doctors and the public to see whether they can forget individual interests and cooperate to try to give vaccine to those in the gravest danger."[21]

During the second week in May, the national program was halted as government inspectors checked the safety at all manufacturers' plants.[22] Meanwhile, a fierce debate raged among scientists over whether the incident was anomalous or whether the methods Salk had devised to inactivate the virus were inherently ineffective.[23] After intensive daily meetings, a presidential advisory committee recommended that the program go forward. "Many of our immunizing substances have hazards connected with their use," wrote New York State Health Commissioner Herman Hilleboe to physicians after the recommendation. "As an example, we may point to smallpox and whooping cough vaccines, which occasionally cause serious reactions and even deaths. However, with these vaccines, the benefits and lifesaving effects so far outweigh the possible hazards that we use them unhesitatingly."[24] Hilleboe's frank admission of the balance between risks and benefits was unusual for this period. This trade-off, which had figured prominently in debates over smallpox vaccination, rarely surfaced in public and professional discourse about vaccines during the middle decades of the century.

The Cutter incident shook, but did not destroy, public confidence in the vaccine. That no massive turn against the vaccine occurred was a measure of the overall public faith in the competence of the scientific experts who were making decisions and recommendations. Very few New York City parents—less than 1 percent of those who had signed up, according to a health department survey—withdrew the permission they had given for their children to receive the shots.[25] (Accurately predicting the public demand that would ensue once the trial results were announced, Baumgartner had sent a request form to all parents of students in the city's schools earlier in the year asking them to indicate whether or not they wanted their children to receive the vaccine should it be licensed.)[26] The cancellations occurred primarily in Spanish-speaking communities, in which press coverage of the incident had been highly critical, and in schools where the principal was either indifferent or hostile to the vaccine.[27] A month after the incident, a "sidewalk interview" feature in New York's African American newspaper the *Amsterdam News* showed respondents evenly split over the question, "Do you think the Salk vaccine is safe enough for young children?" "It's not perfected yet," said one respondent. "I wouldn't risk my kid with it." Another interviewee declared that the vaccine "may harm five but will save thousands of others."[28]

Continued public confidence in the vaccine can also be attributed to the efforts of the National Foundation for Infantile Paralysis, which undertook an aggressive campaign "to get as many children back to the clinics as possible."[29] The organization had a large public relations staff in its New York City headquarters, and a national network of 3,000 chapters with a staff of 90,000 volunteers who could be mobilized in their communities on behalf of promoting the vaccine.[30] The foundation worked with local and national media outlets and city and state medical societies and health departments to "get and publish as many reassuring statements on the vaccine from prominent health and medical authorities and, if possible, get pictures published of children of prominent parents getting their second shot."[31] But even as the foundation was making this push, the ability of the public to obtain the vaccine, once they had been persuaded of its safety, was in considerable doubt.

"SOCIALIZED MEDICINE BY THE BACK DOOR"?

The shortages and delays in getting vaccine into the arms of vulnerable children pushed to the forefront the question of what role, if any, the federal government should play in assuring equitable distribution while supplies were scarce, and whether it should pay for vaccine for poor children in cities and states where free clinics were not available. Since the development and testing had been made possible through money the public had donated to the NFIP, many felt the vaccine belonged to the people and should be controlled by them, through their elected representatives. When the NFIP announced that it would only provide enough vaccine for the first two shots, rather than the full course of three, in order to make the vaccine available to more children, many of the organization's chapter heads were outraged at what they saw as a "breach of faith" and threatened to refuse to participate in future foundation activities.[32]

The day after the announcement of the Salk trials, New York's Mayor Wagner sent a telegram to President Dwight Eisenhower urging the creation of federal supervisory guidelines for the distribution of the vaccine, as had been done in the early days of penicillin and gamma globulin.[33] With Wagner and Baumgartner publicly calling for federal control of vaccine allocation during the initial phases of its release, numerous civic and political groups and parents' organizations in New York passed resolutions and held public meetings demanding that the government provide equitable and prompt access to the vaccine for all children regardless of family income.[34] Editorial writers nationwide lambasted the federal Department of Health, Education and Welfare for failing to have foreseen the demand for the vaccine and taken action to assure its adequate and orderly distribution.[35]

The calls for Washington to step forward reflected the belief, shaped by the expansive programs of Roosevelt's New Deal, that it was appropriate for the federal government to intervene in urgent matters of domestic policy. But in the intensely anti-communist mood of the Cold War era, the label "socialism" was a powerful rhetorical weapon for those seeking to counter such suggestions. Indeed, the debates over how to handle distribution of the vaccine revealed the nation's somewhat contradictory feelings about the role of the government. While many people opposed socialism in the abstract, they embraced what might be considered a "socialistic" solution—federal control of the limited supplies—when it was in the interest of their own children.

Eisenhower had campaigned explicitly against socialized medicine in the 1952 presidential election, and his administration, ideologically disinclined to interfere with the free market, viewed polio vaccination programs as a concern of the states.[36] The American Medical Association, which had invoked the specter of socialized medicine as a truncheon with which to beat back Harry Truman's plan for national health care in 1949, was predictably hostile to suggestions that federal bureaucrats might control access to this medical breakthrough. At its annual meeting in June 1955, the AMA passed a resolution opposing any government effort to purchase and distribute the vaccine except for those unable to pay. Testifying before Congress, the group's secretary noted that "we do not look with favor upon proposals to inject the Federal Government into the immunization program beyond its presently established responsibilities" and assured lawmakers that the nation's physicians would cooperate in giving the vaccine only to children aged five to nine until it was more widely available.[37] Similarly, the American Drug Manufacturers Association warned against any federal controls over distribution and opposed universal provision.[38]

Although there was bipartisan support for government intervention, the charge in Congress was led by Democrats, who advanced a proposal to use federal money to provide free vaccine for all children under age nineteen—a plan that Secretary of Health, Education and Welfare Oveta Culp Hobby labeled "socialized medicine by the back door."[39] The administration resisted any role in distribution, proposing instead to provide $28 million to the states to help them purchase vaccine. The plan called for free vaccine only for youth whose parents could not afford to pay but left it up to the states to determine how they would use the funds. Hobby contended that there was "no reason to think" that the majority of parents could not afford to pay to protect their children.[40] The plan ultimately approved by Congress called for funds to be allocated to states on the basis of a complicated formula designed to take into account the number of children in the state and its per capita income. Vaccine was to be limited to persons under twenty years old and pregnant women of all ages. The act explicitly forbade use of means testing to determine the eligibility of those receiving the vaccine.[41]

Monetary assistance to the states, however, did nothing to speed the supply coming from the six vaccine manufacturers. Stringent new testing procedures put in place after the Cutter incident, with NIH inspectors assigned to check the manufacturing process at each plant, further delayed production of the vaccine, already inadequate to meet the huge public demand, and no new vaccine was released for almost a month during the summer.[42]

With the ongoing shortages of vaccine, Leona Baumgartner and her counterparts at the state health department in Albany found themselves caught between insistent and irreconcilable forces. On one side were parents demanding quick and convenient access to the vaccine for their children. School parent associations, civic groups and individual parents deluged government officials with letters complaining about the uneven distribution of the vaccine and the exclusion of certain age groups of children, and urging more forceful intervention to assure adequate supplies.[43] Some insisted that no vaccine be given to private physicians until all children had had the opportunity to receive their shots at school or in free community settings.[44]

On the other side were disaffected doctors who demanded that they be given the vaccine in order to satisfy the needs of their paying patients. Physicians accustomed to operating with complete professional autonomy bridled at having to observe the cumbersome administrative procedures needed to obtain the vaccine. To ensure that vaccine was distributed according to age guidelines agreed on by the state advisory committee, the city requested each doctor to submit the names, addresses, and ages of all children under his or her care, and vials of vaccine were distributed accordingly.[45] Doctors were also upset that they could give the vaccine to some children in their care but not others and blasted as "socialistic" Baumgartner's decision in the fall of 1955 to continue vaccinating five- to nine-year-olds in city schools, where children whose families could afford to pay for vaccine would get it free.[46] In January 1956, the Brooklyn Academy of Pediatrics adopted a resolution condemning the city's school vaccination program as "a violation of the American principle of non-interference by a third party, governmental or otherwise, in the physician-patient relationship" and urged the city to discontinue it immediately.[47] "It is not our purpose, and I have repeatedly said so," Baumgartner responded to the group's president, "to carry on mass immunization programs after we had got the bulk of the most susceptible children immunized."[48]

Availability of the vaccine continued to be limited and uneven throughout the winter and spring of 1956. Manufacturers made shipments at irregular intervals and with little notice to states and cities.[49]

This uncertainty placed those promoting the vaccine in an awkward position. "Unless we watch our timing," wrote Dorothy Ducas, the NFIP's director of public relations, in February 1956, "we can create ill will toward the National Foundation, by indicating action is desirable in most places it is not widely possible."[50] Soon, however, action would be widely possible, and the NFIP, along with health officials around the country, would be devoting their energies to convincing people that getting vaccinated was desirable.

"DON'T BALK AT SALK": SELLING THE VACCINE

By the summer of 1956, vaccine production and supply stabilized and public uptake began to level off. In an early sign of slackening demand, seventeen states returned part of their federal allotments of the vaccine; thirteen of these were in the South, where response to vaccination programs had in general been more sluggish than elsewhere.[51] In August, when federal funding came to an end, all age restrictions on the vaccine were lifted, and health officials turned their attention to age groups that had previously been excluded. Youth aged fifteen to nineteen were the next-highest risk group in terms of incidence, but the vaccine was recommended for all adults under age forty (polio rarely struck those over that age). But even after the vaccine became widely available, large majorities of these age groups had not gotten a single injection of the vaccine. In a remarkably short time, the availability of the vaccine seemed to dispel the sense of urgency about the threat of polio, even among those who had not themselves been vaccinated.

Lagging acceptance of the vaccine did not reflect active opposition, which gained little prominence in public discourse. In general, the dissident voices that were raised against the vaccine melded anti-communist ideology with suspicion of the growing prominence of scientific medicine in public life. Just as mistrust of "socialistic" health care schemes had fueled anti-government animus during the Progressive Era, Cold War paranoia about subversion of American ideals found targets in mass health programs. Many of the groups opposing vaccination were also active in the fight against another highly publicized scientific advance in this period: fluoridation.[52] The advent of the Salk vaccine coincided with efforts by cities across the country to add fluoride to municipal water supplies to prevent tooth decay; both innovations touched on central concerns of liberty, autonomy, and bodily integrity, and opponents of the measures attacked both as communist plots to

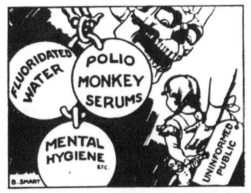

Figure 11. This flyer from a group identified as the "Keep America Committee" revealed the extent to which anti-communist paranoia during the Cold War dovetailed with anxiety about developments in scientific medicine. The polio vaccine, fluoridated water, and new psychiatric methods were all viewed as communist plots to poison Americans.

poison Americans.[53] The Citizens Medical Reference Bureau, one of the most active anti-vaccination groups in the 1920s and 1930s, testified before Congress against fluoridation.[54] The fact that Jonas Salk was Jewish (as was Albert Sabin, the other polio researcher whose name was well known to the public) also lent an overt and virulent anti-Semitic

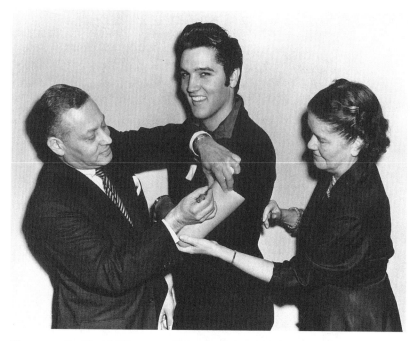

Figure 12. Dr. Harold Fuerst and New York City Health Commissioner Leona Baumgartner gave a polio shot to Elvis Presley in the fall of 1956 when he came to New York to appear on the Ed Sullivan show. The public relations staff of the National Foundation for Infantile Paralysis came up with the idea for the photo opportunity as part of its efforts to increase vaccination among teenagers. Courtesy New York City Municipal Archives.

cast to the anti-vaccination cause.[55] One flyer described the scientists running the Salk trial as "the forces of '*anti-Christ*' fighting '*Christianity*' in their sneaking attempt to *violate* and *contaminate* the bodies of MILLIONS of innocent little children with FRAUDULENT polio vaccines."[56] But such opposition remained a fringe movement.

Instead of active opposition to the polio vaccine, then, health officials were forced to counter what Leona Baumgartner labeled "general apathy about the whole situation."[57] The health department's public relations adviser felt that getting older adults vaccinated would require "heavy, concentrated salesmanship."[58] Such salesmanship was the natural purview of the NFIP, which geared up its public relations network in the fall of 1956, planning a new round of television, radio, and print publicity and pushing to persuade major businesses to promote vaccination among employees and their families.[59] In addition to the millions of brochures, flyers, and posters it distributed through chapters around the country, the NFIP had significant connections with national media and was highly skilled at getting articles placed in newspapers and magazines.

In one of its more ambitious "pseudo-events," the organization arranged to have all residents under the age of forty in the town of Protection, Kansas (population 800) receive vaccination over two days, an event that was picked up by national wire services and featured by newsreels, television, radio, and the print media.[60] The NFIP and the New York City Health Department coordinated a publicity stunt in October 1956 in which Elvis Presley was vaccinated when he visited New York to tape an appearance on the Ed Sullivan show.[61] The foundation subsequently capitalized on the event by contacting the 600 Elvis Presley fan clubs around the country and offering an autographed photo of The King getting his injection to any club in which all members were vaccinated. Dozens of clubs around the country responded.[62] The foundation's president, Basil O'Connor, met with the heads of the country's three news wire services to convince them of the importance of ongoing coverage of the need for vaccination.[63] But vaccine news had saturated the nation's media outlets since the beginning of the trial, and it was increasingly difficult to interest editors, writers, and television producers in running stories.[64]

As the stunt with Elvis indicated, reaching teenagers was a prominent focus of the NFIP's efforts. In 1957, the foundation invited approximately fifty teenagers from around the country for a three-day conference in New York City, in which it held discussion groups with the youths to learn what methods they thought would be most effective at reaching their peers. Suggestions from the teens included holding special youth-focused events such as "Salk hops" (playing off the name of the popular teen dances called "sock hops") and using teen slang in promotional materials. The young people, it was reported, especially liked a slogan that had been used in a campaign in Phoenix, Arizona: "Don't balk at Salk—Roll up your sleeve, Steve—It's the most!" But participants conceded that teens generally did not make the decision themselves, and that the primary reason for getting vaccinated was that their parents demanded it.[65]

In addition to ratcheting up publicity, health officials increased their efforts to make the vaccine available in community settings. But this strategy raised tensions with the medical profession, which disapproved of people getting their shots outside of private physicians' offices. In 1956, a tenants' group at the Boulevard Houses, a middle-income housing project in East New York, arranged for an on-site vaccination clinic. The group secured the services of two local physicians who agreed to donate their time; residents would be asked to pay $2 to cover the cost of the vaccine. When the Brooklyn Medical Society got wind of the plan, it ordered the two doctors to desist and threatened them with censure, claiming that the program violated the ethical proscription against third-party solicitation. Since some of the tenants were able to pay the customary doctor's fee, the medical society argued, the tenants' association's plan constituted unethical competition.[66] As a sop, the medical society requested that its doctors offer to give the vaccine for the cost of their minimum average office fee during regular office hours.[67] The clinic was eventually held several months later after the health department brokered an agreement between the tenants' group and the medical society.[68]

As this episode suggests, financial barriers complicated efforts to combat lagging use of the vaccine. Private doctors' fees averaged $3–$5 per shot, but the health department received many complaints from parents that doctors were charging higher fees.[69] At Baumgartner's urging, the five county medical societies, invoking the spirit of cooperation shown by the profession during the city's drive against diphtheria in 1929, agreed in late 1956 to a plan under which they would urge all of their members to offer the vaccine for $3 per injection, including the cost of the vaccine.[70] The societies also arranged for interested doctors to go on-site to conduct special immunization drives for industrial groups, labor unions, and tenant groups.[71]

Tensions between public health and organized medicine also played out at the national level. In January 1957, the NFIP and AMA leaderships met to discuss plans for a coordinated publicity effort to stimulate vaccine use. The NFIP was disappointed by the AMA's tepid response and failure to commit resources to a plan. "Purchase of vaccine with either NFIP or federal funds was unacceptable to the A.M.A. because of 'socialized medicine,'" wrote an NFIP official after the meeting. "Although the use of clinics for vaccinations was not actually ruled out in the general meeting, it was precluded in conversations prior to the meeting for the same reason: socialized medicine."[72] At the beginning of 1958, the NFIP managed to persuade the AMA to sponsor "dollar clinics" at which people could receive low-cost vaccination in community locations on special days and times.[73] The AMA's announcement helped to burnish its image at a difficult time: it was preoccupied with influencing the shape of a proposed federal health insurance plan for the elderly, which had a far greater potential to affect the income of the nation's doctors.[74] In urging local medical societies to set up the programs, the AMA appealed to their members' self-interest, noting that in the past, community clinics had actually increased doctors' business.[75]

Throughout this period, the many organizations and individuals involved in promoting the vaccine frequently disagreed about which population groups should be targeted and which approaches were most effective. Some criticized the NFIP's use of fear-based approaches. One advertisement depicted a young man in a wheelchair with the caption, "So you don't scare easy?" In another ad, a man in an iron lung was shown with the tag line, "They all got it [the vaccine] except Dad." Critics of these materials felt that young adults, especially young men, simply shrugged off such warnings.[76] Some state health directors thought too much emphasis was being placed on older age groups, and that the campaign should target immunization of preschoolers and youth. Others believed that the greater severity of the disease in adults—the fatality rate was about four times higher than in youth, and older persons who contracted the disease were much more likely to suffer severe paralysis—argued in favor of such a focus.[77]

To increase the effectiveness of their promotional efforts and ensure that their appeals were informed by the best empirical evidence, the NFIP turned to a technique that was increasingly used for gauging public attitudes: opinion surveys. In the fall of 1956, discussion began among NFIP staff members about the possibility of a nationwide survey in order to better understand the failure to be vaccinated. Melvin Glasser, a sociologist who was the NFIP's director of planning, enlisted the aid of the American Institute for Public Opinion (the polling organization run by George Gallup) and the Bureau of Applied Social Research at Columbia University for analysis.

The survey found that there was little active resistance to the vaccine, but rather "lack of definite, positive influences which might direct [people] to a clinic or doctor's office."[78] There was a widespread belief that "victory over polio had been achieved." Many people believed that adults and teenagers did not need to be vaccinated because polio was a disease of young children, a consequence of the disease's original name, "infantile paralysis," and of the iconography of crippled children that had dominated the NFIP's publicity for two decades. The recommendations of family physicians played a key role in decisions. The Cutter incident did not appear to have had a lasting impact on public perceptions; doubts about the safety of the vaccine were not a major factor in

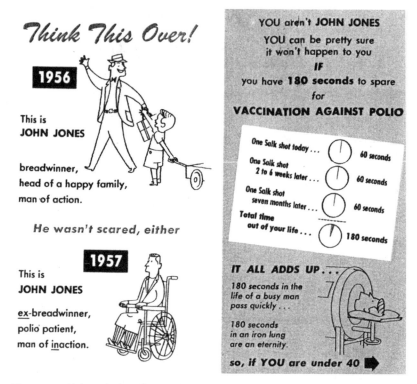

Figure 13. Although the advent of the Salk vaccine prompted widespread demand for the vaccine for children, a large percentage of the adult population had not received a single shot more than two years after the vaccine was licensed. Brochures such as this one created by the National Foundation for Infantile Paralysis were designed to encourage adult men to seek vaccination. By permission of the March of Dimes.

decisions not to be vaccinated. The lack of a sense of personal susceptibility and perceived danger of the disease were important. But financial rather than psychological factors were paramount, the survey found: low annual income, more than any set of beliefs or behaviors, best predicted failure to be vaccinated.

When the article describing the results of the NFIP survey was published in 1958 in the *American Journal of Public Health*, it joined a growing body of academic literature examining the phenomenon of "vaccination status." Beginning with studies analyzing the characteristics of parents whose children participated in the national field trial,[79] polio vaccination attracted remarkable and sustained attention from social science researchers over the following decade.[80] These inquiries reflected the burgeoning in the postwar decades of survey research by sociologists and psychologists in academic centers and commercial polling organizations. The expansion of the field resulted in a proliferation of studies analyzing, describing, and quantifying attitudes about current events and politics, consumer behavior, and diverse aspects of American society.[81]

The social science research on polio formed a mosaic portrait of those who had not taken advantage of the vaccine. Some studies emphasized psychological factors, such as perceived susceptibility to polio and the mistaken belief that polio was less severe in adults than in children. Others foregrounded sociological explanations, such as the fact that those who had been vaccinated were much more likely to have discussed the vaccine with some kind of social group, such as a church, PTA, or group of friends. Of all the correlates that were identified in this literature, the one that had the most significant effect on both the discourse and the practices of those who managed vaccination programs was socioeconomic status (SES). A measure that typically included family income, educational attainment, occupation, or some composite of the three, SES—or "class," a term it partially supplanted—was to become a dominant focus of vaccination programming.

THE (RE)DISCOVERY OF THE SOCIAL GRADIENT

The nationwide incidence of polio declined steadily after the vaccine was licensed. Total cases dropped from some 38,000 in 1954 to about 29,000 in 1955 and 15,000 in 1956. Some experts were wary of attributing the trend to vaccination, since the annual incidence of polio had fluctuated widely over the years, and use of the vaccine had been far from universal during the post-trial period. When cases declined to a new low of just 5,500 in 1957, however, there remained little doubt that the vaccine was responsible.[82] But the downward trend did not continue. Cases rose in 1958 and 1959, and a new epidemiological pattern emerged that differed markedly from the old.

A harbinger of the new pattern occurred in the summer of 1956, when an especially severe epidemic struck Chicago. Several features of the outbreak were distinctive: the highest incidence rate was among infants, not school-age children; rather than spreading throughout the city, it remained heavily concentrated in just a handful of predominately African American census tracts on the west and south sides. Rates of the disease for nonwhites was seven times higher than for whites, and whereas polio had formerly struck fairly evenly among all the city's socioeconomic groups, it was now concentrated almost exclusively among the poor. Data collected by the CDC's Epidemic Intelligence Service revealed a sharp inverse relationship between incidence of polio and measures of family income and the head of household's educational attainment and occupational level.[83]

In 1958, cases nationwide rose by about 10 percent to about 6,000, with the worst outbreaks concentrated in central city areas marked by poverty and crowded, deteriorating housing stock. The most severe outbreak occurred in Detroit; also badly affected were several cities in northern New Jersey, including Newark, Jersey City, and Bayonne, and a mountainous region of twenty-nine counties on the Virginia–West Virginia border.[84] Although New York City was not among the hardest-hit places, there was a higher than expected number of cases, almost all concentrated among Puerto Rican children.[85] Even worse was the experience of 1959, when cases rose almost 50 percent over the previous year. The proportion of cases that resulted in severe paralysis also rose, to more than double the figure for 1957. Urban ghettoes in Baltimore and Providence were epicenters; crowded slums and public housing developments were struck, while the surrounding suburbs remained free of the disease.

The partial success of vaccination efforts nationwide had shifted the epidemiology of the disease: whereas it had formerly struck first- and second-graders most frequently, it now attacked one- and two-year-olds; rather than being spread out among all social classes, it was concentrated among the poor; and nonwhites rather than whites were hardest hit. Most of all, the disease was confined to those populations in which immunization rates were the lowest: "the pattern of polio," a CDC official noted in 1961, "is the pattern of the unvaccinated."[86]

The ability of health officials both to track epidemics closely and to correlate them with vaccination status was due largely to the increased surveillance activity of the CDC. In 1958, the CDC's Epidemic Intelligence Service began regular monitoring of vaccination in 125 cities, using a sampling method in which a proportion of residents within individual city blocks were surveyed; blocks were grouped into four socioeconomic classes, based on census data.[87] Whereas in the past, the local variation in vaccine acceptance could only roughly be apprehended, and low rates in poor neighborhoods were often based on anecdotal reports, the new sampling system enabled public health officials to identify where cases were occurring, and who remained without protection, with greater precision. The CDC's expanded surveillance activities dovetailed with the burgeoning use of surveys by social scientists to determine the correlates of vaccination status. Together, these two forms of inquiry constructed a new representation of the unvaccinated.

Differential acceptance of vaccination among groups of varying class, ethnic, and economic backgrounds was not new, of course. Health officials in the nineteenth century had complained about the fecklessness of immigrants and the poor, and the first nationwide surveys of vaccination status in the 1930s had found a gradient along the lines of income.[88] But the survey findings struck an especially resonant chord in the 1950s, a time of relative economic prosperity and cultural homogeneity in the United States. The "discovery" of the unvaccinated coincided with a new concern about poverty, which was reemerging during the late 1950s as a political issue, and to a striking extent, the discourses of the two problems ran parallel.[89] The economist John Kenneth Galbraith, in his widely read 1958 analysis *The Affluent Society*, identified "islands" of poverty in an otherwise prosperous country.[90] Public health and medical journals described people who had not received the Salk vaccine as "islands" or "pockets" of unvaccinated. They were the "hard core" least likely to respond to health messages; they were "hard to reach" or "unreachable." Just as poverty in the midst of an affluent society was an anomaly requiring explanation, so too was the failure to protect oneself and one's family from polio when a preventive was readily available. Both phenomena represented isolation from mainstream American society and the material goods it had to offer.

While those planning promotional efforts locally and nationally agreed on the need to better appeal to the groups least likely to have been vaccinated, there was no unanimity about the best way to accomplish this. Some studies, for example, suggested that face-to-face contacts with friends and neighbors were the most important determinant of an individual's decision to be vaccinated, while others indicated that this was not the case. An assistant to Leona Baumgartner contended that "evidence emphasizes that the 'educational approach' and heavy reliance on newspapers, pamphlets, signs and television do *not* reach these people."[91] Although most officials stressed the need to communicate through the ethnic press, a survey following an outreach effort in an almost exclusively African American neighborhood in Pittsburgh showed that the daily metropolitan newspaper had been a more important source of information about the program than the African American weekly.[92]

Although a dichotomous conceptualization of race (black and white) was central to the discourse of the "hard core unvaccinated," there was also concern about ethnic subgroups, especially Puerto Ricans. In an effort to learn how to motivate what it termed "nationality groups," the NFIP interviewed leaders of various ethnic communities in New York City. Although NFIP interviewers conceded that there was considerable diversity among the groups, they felt able to generalize. "Many [ethnic minorities] have a real horror of anything connected with hospitals and doctors," one wrote. "[A]mong the Spanish-speaking and Italian population of New York, for instance, there is a current belief that when you go to a city hospital, 'they put you out of your misery with a little black pill.' Doctors are called only as a last resort. Obviously, to approach these people with high-level vaccine material is a waste of time."[93] To overcome such cultural barriers, the foundation considered plans to use the ethnic press, fraternal societies, and settlement houses to reach out to these groups.

Some cities and states considered—but most rejected—the enactment of laws requiring people to be protected. In 1959, a civic group urged Leona Baumgartner to make polio vaccination mandatory in New York City.[94] One of Baumgartner's bureau chiefs drafted a reply asserting: "I doubt if it is right to compel people to do things, even for their health, if the failure to do them does not seriously endanger the health or lives of others. We have demonstrated in this city that persistent health education may be as effective a tool as compulsion."[95] Reviewing the draft, Baumgartner queried in the margin: "? fluoridation"—a reference to the city's long and thus far unsuccessful struggle in the face of often bitter community opposition to add fluoride to the city's water supply.[96] Fluoridation was an example of a situation in which authorities did, in fact, believe that it was right to compel people to accept a health intervention for their own good. In the response that was ultimately sent, the bureau chief's comments on compulsion were removed.[97] But no law was enacted, and most cities and states in this period continued to rely on a voluntaristic approach.

Instead of compulsion, New York City relied on its decentralized network of child health clinics and traditional outreach and promotional methods to draw people to them, an approach that had been the hallmark of the anti-diphtheria efforts two decades earlier. The department recruited dozens of schoolchildren in Harlem to parade down the streets wearing sandwich boards that urged: "Get your free polio shots now."[98] The department also began a program to give shots to young children at

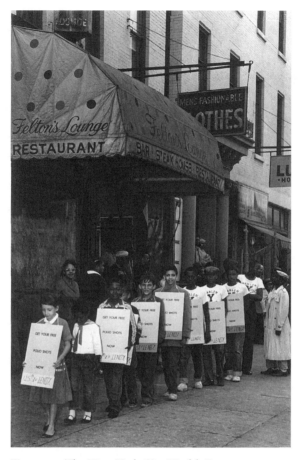

Figure 14. The New York City Health Department recruited schoolchildren in Harlem to parade through
the neighborhood wearing sandwich boards that urged
"Get your free polio shots now." Courtesy New York
City Municipal Archives.

Sunday school classes in African American churches in Harlem. At the
recommendation of the department's public relations counsel, ever alert
to photo opportunities, Baumgartner attended the kickoff of the program
and gave the first shots to churchgoing children "dressed in their Sunday
best."[99] (The event, with photo, made the next morning's *Times*.)[100]
The department stationed two specially equipped buses borrowed
from the department of civil defense in low-income neighborhoods.[101]
While efforts such as these had served the city well over the years,

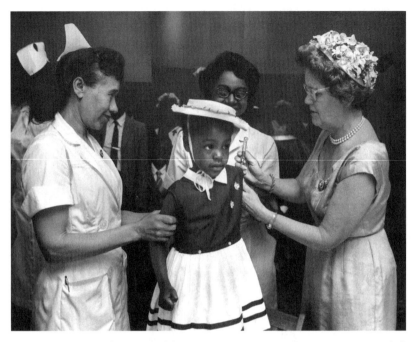

Figure 15. New York City Health Commissioner Leona Baumgartner attended
the kickoff of an outreach program in 1960 to give polio vaccinations to children attending Sunday school at African American churches. Allyn Baum/*The
New York Times*. Reprinted with permission.

they raised their own challenges. One health educator described the difficulties that sometimes arose:

> There are many problems to surmount in being "on the firing line" in
> crowded, congested areas of Brooklyn on a hot summer night. Crowds
> gather around the polio bus that are, at times, difficult to control. On
> one occasion ... the police had to be called because of the unruly actions
> of teenagers. Many of the residents who crowd around the polio bus are
> there merely out of curiosity. Although the health educators make every
> effort to convince them to take polio shots, they get many refusals. "We've
> had polio shots" is a stock answer to these appeals.[102]

At the national level, the shift from universal promotion to more
specifically targeted efforts was signaled when Surgeon General Leroy
Burney convened a special meeting at the end of 1958 of the country's
major medical and public health organizations to discuss ways to
increase use of the Salk vaccine. "Until now, programs have been aimed
principally at the general public," Burney noted. "It is proposed now

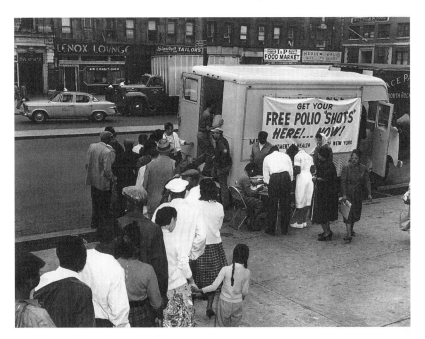

Figure 16. To increase vaccination rates among people of low socioeconomic status, the New York City Health Department deployed vans around the city. Courtesy New York City Municipal Archives.

that in addition we seek to pinpoint our targets, finding as precisely as possible what segments of the population in each community have not been reached, and devising programs to meet their special needs."[103]

Two nationwide programs reflected the new perspective. In 1959, the National Foundation established a fund that would enable local chapters to purchase vaccine for the purpose of setting up clinics in low-income neighborhoods of selected cities. Those who remained unvaccinated were "the ill-educated, the poor, the least health-conscious segment of our society," according to an announcement of the program for local chapters, and "they can only be reached by literally bringing a vaccine clinic to their door. They represent the 'soft-spots' in the vaccination picture which must be eliminated if we are ever to eliminate epidemic polio."[104] Local chapters in thirty-five cities with populations between 400,000 and one million would be eligible for the fund provided that they gained the approval of their local health departments to set up the clinics. But reflecting the numerous challenges in establishing such clinics—especially the difficulty of gaining the cooperation of local medical

societies—only six of the thirty-five eligible cities had applied for and
been awarded funds by the summer, and the foundation had expended
less than one-fifth of the $500,000 it had allocated.[105]

A focus on those of lower socioeconomic status also dominated a
1961 national campaign, "Babies and Breadwinners." Sponsored by the
Committee on Poliomyelitis Control, an advisory group convened by
the surgeon general, the promotional effort was devised by Dorothy
Ducas, who had headed the National Foundation's public relations
activities for over a decade. "Babies and breadwinners" were judged to
be the groups most in need: polio incidence was now highest in infants
rather than school-age youth; a case of the disease in a family wage-
earner could have devastating consequences, and men were much less
likely to have been vaccinated than women. Beyond these age brackets,
however, was an additional focus that was explicitly identified in the
campaign guidelines but was not to be so named in the campaign itself:
the poor. The program sought to "involv[e] the lower socioeconomic
groups without naming them as such," according to a planning booklet
for the campaign.[106] People in these groups generally had no family
physicians and distrusted officials; they lacked the money and means to
travel to clinics outside their immediate neighborhood, and "their lives
are so full of problems ... that the danger of polio seems to them relatively remote."

In addition to the familiar techniques of advertising and marketing,
the campaign gave special emphasis to enlisting the help of people within
affected communities. Drawing on research from surveys that suggested
that the behavior of friends and neighbors was a strong determinant of
vaccination status, the campaign urged communities across the country
to recruit "neighborhood leaders." The idea of gaining the cooperation
of community leaders was not a new one; during an anti-diphtheria
drive in 1924, health officials in the small upstate New York town of
East Kingston had benefited from the services of an Italian-American
justice of the peace named DeCicco, who persuaded his neighbors to
accept toxin-antitoxin. But survey research findings gave the imprimatur of social science to the idea of enlisting laypeople to persuade
their neighbors, and it assumed new prominence in the U.S. Public
Health Service's recommendations. *"Don't be put off by seemingly
inappropriate individuals,"* the *Babies and Breadwinners* booklet urged
those planning polio vaccination campaigns. "What counts is how influential they are in their own neighborhoods. The corner druggist may be
regarded as a sage. The union organizer may be the opinion-maker in

his district. The bartender may be the 'neighborhood psychiatrist.' *Any of these has the advantage of not being official.*[107]

In spite of the increasing focus on the "hard core" of the unvaccinated, it was clear that the lack of enthusiasm for the Salk vaccine cut across a wide swath of American society. By 1960, only about half of children aged five to fourteen, and about one-third of children aged one to four, had received the full course of vaccine doses. Rates among adults were even lower. More troubling was the fact that most vaccine distributed was being used for additional shots administered to people who had already had one or more; relatively little was reaching those who remained completely unprotected.[108] After several years of aggressive promotion by the National Foundation, exhortations by leaders of the U.S. Public Health Service, the AMA, and other professional groups, the outreach efforts of health departments around the country, and the advice of private doctors, acceptance of the Salk vaccine seemed to have hit a ceiling. This was the backdrop against which a new and often acrimonious debate emerged about whether to switch to a new vaccine that promised greater popular acceptance and better control of polio.

FROM SALK TO SABIN

Whether an inactivated or a live attenuated vaccine was superior had been the subject of intense disagreements within the scientific community since the mid 1940s. After the NFIP moved ahead with the Salk preparation as the most promising, several researchers continued to pursue work on a live attenuated vaccine, which, they contended, offered immunologic and practical advantages over an inactivated one. A killed vaccine such as Salk's prevented the virus from spreading from the bloodstream to the central nervous system, but vaccinated individuals could still harbor the virus in their body and thus pass it on to others. The live vaccine, on the other hand, induced immunity to infection within the alimentary tract, the common locus of virus multiplication, and thus prevented vaccinated individuals from spreading the disease. As an added benefit, recipients of the live vaccine excreted the attenuated virus in their feces and thus indirectly passed along immunity to close contacts who had not themselves received the vaccine.[109] Whereas Salk's vaccine was slow to stimulate antibody production and required repeated boosters to produce full immunity, a live vaccine produced strong immunity almost immediately (usually in days instead of months);

it could therefore be used to control an outbreak of disease that was just beginning or already in progress.

Perhaps most important, the attenuated vaccine was given orally in a spoon or on a sugar cube, obviating the need for hypodermic needles. Reluctance to come back for the additional injections was widely considered a major barrier to getting more people to accept vaccination.[110] This problem was worsened when some health officials suggested that four shots, not just three, were needed to assure protection. Although a national advisory committee convened by the Public Health Service had decided against recommending a fourth shot in 1958, Jonas Salk himself said publicly that if he were a practicing physician, he would give the fourth shot as "an added precaution."[111] Other expert panels decided in favor of urging four injections.[112]

These debates occurred amid troubling indications that even a full course of the Salk vaccine might not be protective. In Dade County, Florida, in 1959, seven of the forty-six people who contracted paralytic polio had previously gotten three shots.[113] Worse still was the experience that year of Massachusetts, where almost half of the 137 cases of polio had received three or more injections of Salk vaccine.[114] While some of the blame was laid to low potency of some lots due to poor manufacturing, partisans of a live vaccine such as Sabin's insisted that the Salk preparation was inherently limited because it was ineffective against Type III polio and would never fully control the disease.

Live vaccines had one significant drawback that cast a shadow over their potential use: the possibility that an attenuated strain could "revert to virulence" once inside the body and cause the disease it was intended to prevent. This phenomenon had been observed in trials, including a disastrous one in Belfast, Ireland, in 1956, in which numerous recipients contracted paralytic polio from an experimental live vaccine.[115] Nevertheless, by the late 1950s, several investigators had demonstrated the safety of their attenuated strains in small field tests and were ready to proceed with large-scale trials.[116] Because the widespread use of the Salk vaccine rendered it impossible to conduct such an investigation in the United States, the research was conducted abroad. By far the largest was a massive trial of Albert Sabin's vaccine, which, in an extraordinary instance of Cold War cooperation, was carried out in the Soviet Union in 1959. Some ten million children in eleven Soviet republics received the Sabin vaccine, and a subsequent evaluation found it to be highly effective and completely safe, with no vaccine-induced paralysis reported.[117]

The promising results of overseas studies, especially the Sabin trial in the Soviet Union, fueled a debate about whether the live vaccine should be introduced in the United States to either complement or completely replace Salk's killed vaccine. For all the concern over the remaining reservoirs of infection in communities across the country and the poor level of acceptance of the Salk vaccine, incidence of polio was at its lowest level ever.[118] Thus many experts were skeptical as to whether a new vaccine was needed in this country, particularly given the lingering doubts about the live vaccine's potential reversion to virulence. But a product that was cheaper, easier to administer, and more likely to gain community acceptance was at hand, with immunologic properties that promised better long-term control of polio. Preventing its use in this country seemed inconceivable.[119]

Pharmaceutical companies who stood to gain financially from the new product were strong advocates of the changeover, of course. At the end of January 1961, as the Public Health Service debated the merits and drawbacks of a live attenuated vaccine, a representative of Chas. Pfizer & Co., one of the three firms developing the product, wrote to Baumgartner asking her to consider offering the vaccine in the city's child health clinics.[120] Besides Jonas Salk himself, the most notable dissident in the changeover was the National Foundation for Infantile Paralysis. Senior managers there felt that support for an oral preparation would undercut Salk's achievement, which the agency saw as its crowning glory.[121] With the dramatic decline in polio, the organization had already begun to turn its attention to other health threats, shortening its name to the National Foundation in 1958 and announcing that it would henceforth devote its energy to combating arthritis, rheumatic disease, and birth defects.

No one in the Public Health Service or Congress wanted a repeat of the experiences of the spring and summer of 1955, when demand for the Salk vaccine had blindsided the Department of Health, Education and Welfare. In March 1961, a U.S. House of Representatives subcommittee held two days of hearings to determine the status of the anticipated live vaccine and what the Public Health Service was doing to assure its safety, efficacy, and distribution upon availability. Surgeon General Luther Terry assured lawmakers that the PHS was taking every possible precaution to avoid a repetition of the problems with safety of the Salk vaccine.[122] Days later, Terry licensed the Type I oral polio vaccine. (Each live vaccine was specific to a single type of polio; thus three vaccines would have to be licensed.) Around the same time,

communitywide trials in Ohio and Connecticut were providing additional evidence that the oral vaccine could be used in mass campaigns,
and that its ease of administration was a strong selling point.[123] Terry
licensed Type II vaccine for nationwide use in October 1961, and Type III
in March 1962.

Enthusiasm for the vaccine was soon tempered, however, by reports
suggesting that some people, especially those over age thirty, might be
contracting paralytic disease from it. In September 1962, just nine
months after he had licensed the Type III Sabin vaccine, Surgeon General
Terry recommended that its use be limited to infants and school-age
children because of the suspected risk in adults. Terry convened a special advisory committee of scientists to examine the apparently vaccine-
induced paralysis. The members conducted exhaustive analyses, including
laboratory examination of the virus type and biological evidence of the
nature of the patients' neurological damage and course of illness, and
after several months of study concluded that eighteen reported cases
were "compatible with the possibility of having been induced by the
vaccine." Because the majority of these were in people over thirty years
old, the oral vaccine "should be used for adults only with the full recognition of its very small risk," which the committee concluded was about
one per million overall and higher for those over thirty years of age.[124]
The risk was highest for the Type III vaccine, which accounted for eleven
of the eighteen cases. At the same time, however, the committee determined that the benefits of the vaccine outweighed the risks and urged
communities across the country to move ahead with any plans they had
for mass immunization programs.

The announcement threw planned campaigns around the country
into confusion. State and local health departments and medical societies
reacted differently to the committee's warning: Some communities suspended their Sabin programs altogether, while others opted out of using
the Type III vaccine but continued using I and II; still others considered
the risk so negligible compared to that of the disease that they pressed
ahead with their plans unchanged.[125]

In communities that did move forward with Sabin, the campaigns
were often able to attract far greater participation than had been typical with the inactivated vaccine. Promotional campaigns played up the
ease of administration; the depiction on posters and in newspaper
articles of a smiling child happily popping a sugar cube into her mouth
was a far more inviting image than that of someone receiving a hypodermic injection. More important, far greater numbers of people could

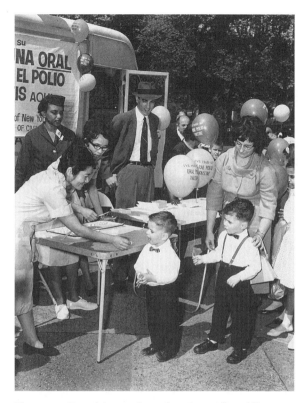

Figure 17. Requiring no hypodermic needles, Albert
Sabin's oral polio vaccine could be administered more
quickly and conveniently and in more varied locations
than the Salk vaccine. Cities around the country held
campaigns in community settings, such as this one in
New York City. Courtesy New York City Municipal
Archives.

be immunized much more quickly with the oral preparation, in virtually
any community setting that could accommodate tables and a freezer
unit to store the vaccine. Especially popular were communitywide
"Sabin on Sunday" events, which were highly successful at reaching
large percentages of the population.[126]

Given the professional confusion and disagreement about the risks of
the Sabin vaccine, the continued public enthusiasm for the product may
seem puzzling. Unlike the aftermath of the Cutter incident, when the
scientific community had closed ranks around the safety of the Salk vaccine and the National Foundation had driven home the message with a

public relations counteroffensive, the Sabin vaccine's potential danger—though remote—was openly acknowledged. This was, moreover, the period when the scandal over thalidomide, an anti–morning sickness drug that resulted in an epidemic of deformed newborns, made headlines and prompted a series of high-profile congressional hearings into drug safety. It is a measure of the high esteem in which the scientific enterprise was held that even such widely publicized examples of the potential dangers of pharmaceutical products barely dampened the public's appetite for the fruits of biomedical research.

The first year that the Sabin preparation was available, its use was generally confined to mass community campaigns run by health departments, while most private pediatricians continued to provide Salk's, but the oral vaccine soon became standard in private practice as well. The oral vaccine's superiority became even greater in mid 1963, when the government licensed a trivalent formula, which provided protection against all three types of polio. In the years that followed, Sabin's vaccine almost completely supplanted Salk's.[127] The Sabin vaccine also seemed to be more acceptable than Salk's to the "hard to reach" population of lower socioeconomic status. One survey showed that while a social gradient persisted in uptake of the Sabin vaccine, the gap in coverage between high and low income groups was less than it was for the Salk vaccine or the diphtheria-pertussis-tetanus vaccine, also given via hypodermic injection.[128]

Aside from its effects in controlling polio, the introduction of the Sabin vaccine had two far-reaching consequences for the ways that vaccination programs were run in the United States. Victims of vaccine-induced paralysis filed the first lawsuits against the makers of the oral vaccine in 1962, and in so doing, they set the stage for a fundamental transformation in how professionals and the public thought about the risks and ethics of vaccines. The ramifications of this litigation would not be felt for several years, however. More proximally, the arrival of a new agent against polio opened a window of opportunity in which CDC officials saw the potential to capitalize on the heightened public attention to immunization and boost levels of protection against other diseases.

THE VACCINATION ASSISTANCE ACT

On the heels of the House of Representatives hearings in March 1961 about planning for the Sabin vaccine, CDC employees began to plan how they might leverage the enhanced visibility of vaccination and the anticipated influx of federal funds.[129] Diphtheria, pertussis, and tetanus were "of relatively minor importance in this country" and there was no imminent danger of their resurgence, James Goddard, the head of the CDC, explained, but because reliable preventives were so widely available, "these are diseases about which you could say that *one* [case] is too many."[130] CDC officials believed that as city and state health departments around the country expanded programs to deal with the rising incidence of chronic diseases such as heart disease and cancer, mass vaccination campaigns would become impossible without federal support.[131] The planned initiative would focus on preschoolers, especially those in poor inner-city and rural areas where routine preventive health care was rare.[132]

The Public Health Service found a receptive audience in the Kennedy administration, which was far more amenable to federal involvement in health care than Eisenhower's had been.[133] The epidemiological patterns of vaccine-preventable diseases also fitted with the new administration's interest in programs for the poor. In his State of the Union message in January of 1962, Kennedy said that he would propose a "mass immunization program" in an upcoming message to Congress.[134] The following month he put forward a $1.2 billion legislative package on health care, which included a program of grants of $35 million to states for intensive programs against diphtheria, pertussis, tetanus, and polio.[135] The primary focus of the program was on "intensive community immunization programs," defined in the bill as programs "of limited duration ... to achieve, with the cooperation of practicing physicians, official health agencies, voluntary organizations, and volunteers, the immunization over the period of the program of all or practically all susceptible persons in the community."[136]

Although appreciative of new federal money coming into the state, New York Health Commissioner Herman Hilleboe was skeptical about both the purpose and the methods of the legislation. In a letter to the CDC, Hilleboe suggested that "the idea of a crash program be abandoned. We are not in the midst of an epidemic and immunization is not a one time affair but must be part of an ongoing public health program. If Federal aid is needed now its need will not end in 1965."[137] He further questioned devoting money to these diseases: "there are other features of the total health program that badly need promotion and ... the death rate among children under five from diphtheria, tetanus and whooping cough is zero as a result of existing programs."

In spite of this skepticism, congressional hearings on the bill in May 1962 produced little controversy; no one questioned the benefits of a program to protect children from disease. What dissent there was centered on concerns about the potential use of compulsion. A Christian Scientist who testified was uneasy about the language in the bill urging that programs target "all or practically all susceptible persons in a community" and sought an explicit assurance that programs funded by the program would not be compulsory.[138] CDC officials pointed out in response that nothing in the bill referred to compulsion, and that indeed the federal government had no authority to make vaccination mandatory, since health law fell under the jurisdiction of cities and states.

Although the AMA testified in support of the bill, the American Academy of Pediatrics looked with suspicion on the prospect of an expanding federal bureaucracy concerned with vaccination. "Pediatricians and other private practitioners wish to be assured," the AAP's president wrote to the CDC's Goddard, "that there is no intent to wean their patients away from their regular care into the expectation of community wide programs."[139] CDC officials portrayed their work as supporting, not competing with, that of private practitioners. "[T]he balance between immunizations given privately and publicly does not change when a community steps up its immunization activities," a CDC official argued. "Where a health department or medical society actively promotes immunization, both groups experience an increased demand for services."[140]

The Vaccination Assistance Act was significant not just because of the financial support that it made available to states but because it established a permanent presence within the CDC that would provide leadership to vaccination programs around the country.[141] In the past, activist surgeon generals had used the office's bully pulpit to encourage nationwide use of vaccines, most notably during the two world wars, and there had been considerable interstate transfer of ideas that lent some uniformity to the programs that were mounted around the country. But for the most part, individual states and cities conducted their campaigns based on local needs and priorities, without material or programmatic support from Washington, D.C. Even when the Public Health Service had stepped in to fund the Salk vaccine in 1955 and 1956, it had refrained from engaging in any education or promotion, believing that such activities were a concern of state and local health departments.[142]

The new federal leadership took a variety of forms. In 1963, for example, the CDC published *Achieving Public Response,* a manual designed to help local health officials mount more effective education and promotional programs. In 1964, the CDC's immunization program held the first of what would become annual conferences that brought together medical and public health professionals from around the country to share ideas and receive feedback and support from each other and the CDC about their vaccination efforts.

An additional development that was not a direct result of the Vaccination Assistance Act, but represented the growing attention to immunization within the Public Health Service, was the formation in 1964 of the Advisory Committee on Immunization Practice (ACIP), a permanent group made up of scientists and clinicians that would coordinate guidelines on schedules, doses, routes of immunization, and contraindications, and, to a lesser extent, on practical issues such as achieving high public response. The ACIP's recommendations were aimed primarily at public sector providers and as such would complement the recommendations of the American Academy of Pediatrics, whose guidelines were aimed at physicians in private practice.[143]

THE DISAPPEARANCE OF POLIO

Over the course of the 1960s, the incidence of polio experienced a steep decline nationwide that startled even those who had expressed high hopes for the oral vaccine's ability to provide superior control. Before the Salk vaccine, cases nationwide had numbered in the tens of thousands annually, but after 1967, there were never more than one hundred cases in a single year. Overall vaccination rates did not correlate neatly with the rapidly dwindling number of cases: the percentage of the population immunized against polio peaked in 1964 at around three-quarters, and then hovered at around two-thirds for the rest of the decade.[144] Whether the remarkable decline was due to the ability of the Sabin vaccine to spread attenuated strains to unvaccinated members of the community or was the result of some other epidemiologic phenomenon remained a matter of speculation.

When Surgeon General Terry had recommended at the end of 1962 that the nation continue to use the oral vaccine in spite of its very slight potential for causing paralysis, he had asserted that the risk of the product was outweighed by the ultimate benefit it promised. "We can, I believe, look forward to the day when poliomyelitis is finally eliminated in this country," Terry had claimed, and the experience of subsequent years seemed to justify this confidence.[145] The decline of polio helped to fuel a new ambition among public health professionals to seek not merely the control of disease but its complete eradication. This spirit had been implicit in the 1962 Vaccination Assistance Act, which was premised on the belief that even tiny numbers of cases of diphtheria, pertussis, and polio were no longer acceptable. Eradicationism would become a guiding force of immunization campaigns for the rest of the decade. But as we shall see in chapter 5, the path to eradication of infectious disease would be a complicated and mostly fruitless one.

Eradicationism and Its Discontents

In the fall of 1971, more than two decades after the last case of smallpox had been recorded in the United States, the Public Health Service recommended that vaccination against the illness be ended in this country. The decision marked the first time that complete freedom from a disease had resulted in the discontinuation of a routinely given vaccine, but the mood among health officials at this moment was far from celebratory. A nationwide anti-measles campaign had foundered, with the number of cases of the disease climbing and immunization rates stagnant. "A host of excuses and administrative problems with changing priorities have come up to block our progress," noted one postmortem on the effort. "But no scientific reason has yet arisen to make us believe that eradication of measles is not possible."[1] Another, less sanguine analysis contended that "the outlook for the ultimate prevention and elimination of measles is bleak."[2]

In the 1960s, the elusive dream of utterly eliminating one or more infectious diseases came closer to being a reality than ever before, and a spirit of "eradicationism" took center stage in vaccination policy. An ideology that held that disease should be completely and permanently banished rather than merely controlled at low levels, eradicationism found fertile ground amid the ambitious social programs of the Great Society. The Communicable Disease Center launched a national campaign to eradicate measles in the fall of 1966 with the same confidence that animated the federal war on poverty. This enthusiasm was also fueled by the dramatic decline in the incidence of polio, which provided an example of the power of vaccines to vanquish illness. But the predictions of imminent eradication soon boomeranged. Intractable social conditions and fundamental limitations of the health care system led to resurgences of measles, heavily concentrated among the poor.

The most prominent new policy initiative during this period, and the anti-measles campaign's most lasting legacy, was the enactment in every state of compulsory laws requiring measles and several other vaccines as a condition of school entry. Between 1968 and 1981, the legal infrastructure supporting immunization underwent its most thorough transformation of the century. Although these laws did not spark the kind of sustained political opposition that legal compulsion had provoked during the Progressive Era, they were the subject of several court challenges focusing on the question of whether and to what extent people with religious objections to the procedure should be exempted from the requirements. In addition, the new laws triggered debates over the efficacy and ethics of the rubella vaccine, which was universally recommended for children in order to protect pregnant women.

This chapter examines the national efforts to eradicate measles, rubella and other contagions during a period when faith in the power of vaccination—not just as a method of disease control, but as a force for social melioration—was at its apex. New vaccines and expanded federal support drove infectious diseases to record low levels, but the goal of eradication remained out of reach. At the same time, the very success of immunization programs had unforeseen and unwanted consequences, as the declining incidence of smallpox threw into sharp relief the small but measurable risks arising from the vaccine itself.

THE MEASLES VACCINE AND THE SOCIAL GRADIENT

Measles was a virtually universal experience for children in the United States before the introduction of a vaccine in 1963, and its ubiquity, more than its severity, made it an attractive target for public health action. An extremely contagious airborne viral disease, it caused high fever and a rash that began on the head and spread across the body over the course of several days. The disease's epidemiology followed a fairly regular pattern of alternating high- and low-incidence years. Close to 100 percent of youth fell ill with it at some point, usually around the time they entered school; the total number of cases that occurred annually could only be estimated, since many children with the disease never came under the care of a physician. While fatalities from the disease were relatively rare, complications could be severe and included pneumonia, ear infections, sometimes resulting in deafness, and, in about one of every one thousand cases, encephalitis (swelling of the brain), which could lead to mental retardation.[3] But in sharp contrast to polio, measles was widely seen as a mild nuisance rather than a feared killer.

Development of a measles vaccine in the 1950s grew out of the pioneering research by the virologist John Enders and his colleagues, whose work on culturing polio virus had earned them the 1954 Nobel Prize in medicine. Two vaccines were licensed in March 1963. Enders and Samuel Katz developed a live attenuated vaccine, which appeared to provide long-lasting protection with only a single injection, but it often produced high fevers as a side effect; it was therefore generally given with a simultaneous injection of gamma globulin, a blood product that mitigated the reaction. (Unlike Sabin's oral polio vaccine, the live attenuated measles vaccine had never been known to revert to virulence and cause disease.) At the same time, a killed vaccine that was less reactogenic but also less potent—requiring two booster shots—was licensed. A "further-attenuated" live vaccine was made available in 1965, which provided better protection without the troublesome side effects of the Enders-Katz preparation and soon became the vaccine of choice.[4] The killed virus vaccine was later withdrawn from the market after the discovery that it provided only short-term immunity and in a small number of cases predisposed recipients who later came in contact with measles to an especially severe course of illness.[5]

Although they had been eagerly anticipated by the medical community, the new measles vaccines did not generate the public excitement or demand that had greeted the Salk vaccine, and their use was relatively limited the first two years after they were licensed. Besides the unthreatening image of measles, financial barriers contributed to the low uptake: a dose of one of the measles vaccines cost almost $3, about double the price of the oral polio vaccine; the cost to parents to have one child immunized against measles, including the doctor's fee, a possible shot of gamma globulin for the live vaccine, or three doses of the killed vaccine, averaged around $10.[6] Thus the vaccines' initial use was largely confined to children whose parents could afford the services of private physicians; few public clinics made them available (New York City, where between 50 and 70 percent of all vaccinations were given in public clinics or in voluntary and charitable agencies, was one of the few cities to do so).[7] Public response to the vaccines remained lukewarm in spite of pharmaceutical company promotion. Merck, the maker of the attenuated vaccine, with the brand name Rubeovax, aggressively marketed the product to parents with full-page advertisements in popular magazines, especially those aimed at women, such as *Good Housekeeping* and *McCall's*.[8] But it was not until federal funding to the states became available through the renewed Vaccination Assistance Act in 1965 that use of measles vaccine began to become routine.

As we saw in chapter 4, the original Vaccination Assistance Act had specified funds for polio, diphtheria, pertussis, and tetanus when it was introduced in 1962. The act also stipulated that funds could be used for the control of other diseases at the end of its initial three-year funding period—a provision written with the imminent licensing of the measles vaccine in mind. The question of how the new measles preventives would be most effectively deployed in the community was a central concern when the act came up for renewal in 1965. Testifying before a U.S. House subcommittee on the renewal of the Vaccination Assistance Act in January 1965, New York State Health Commissioner Hollis Ingraham recommended eliminating language from the bill that called for "intensive community vaccination efforts" of "limited duration," arguing that such a change would "help to develop orderly, regular, continuing programs rather than simply 'short-term' and hence sporadic campaigns."[9] In this matter, Ingraham echoed the concerns of his predecessor, Herman Hilleboe, who had expressed similar reservations when the original Vaccination Assistance Act was proposed in 1962.

Given the disparity in vaccination rates among children of differing socioeconomic backgrounds that had become apparent during the polio campaigns, health officials were especially eager to raise coverage rates for those who did not have regular contact with a private physician. But there was continued disagreement about what types of programs were most suitable for the "hard to reach." Mass campaigns in community settings—shopping malls, recreation centers, schools—had been highly successful for oral polio vaccine, but many officials expressed concerns about the failure to sustain programs that would ensure the ongoing protection of new birth cohorts once the campaign had ended. "Crash programs are simply too extravagant for the permanent good they may accomplish," commented a physician with the Communicable Disease Center (CDC) in 1965. "Unless maintenance programs are planned, immunization tends to degenerate into a series of crash programs which eventually lose their efficacy and which are followed by hangovers of lethargy and inertia."[10]

The federal Advisory Committee on Immunization Practice concurred. "Rarely would there appear to be a need in the United States for mass community immunization programs," the ACIP declared in 1964. "Immunization should be carried out as indicated by private practitioners and through well-child [clinics] of established public health programs."[11] Even though the committee's recommendations were geared toward public sector providers, the group was clearly sympathetic to the reasoning of the major medical societies, which had traditionally stressed the primacy of private practitioners in any immunization effort. The committee reconsidered its position the following year, however, conceding that mass campaigns might be desirable in some cases "in communities or segments of communities in which immunization levels achieved through routine practice are known to be low."[12]

The merits and drawbacks of crash programs were also prominent in New York in March of 1965 when Seymour Thaler, head of the state senate's committee on public health, held hearings to examine the state's measles control efforts. Prompted by the imminent influx of federal funding into New York, the hearings sought to determine what types of programs would be appropriate, how such efforts were to be funded, what populations would be targeted, and what levels of vaccination coverage would be desired and feasible.[13] There was broad agreement that new programs were needed to take advantage of the new vaccines, but views differed on the best ways to accomplish this. Ingraham reiterated his preference for a "steady strengthening" of immunization programs rather than crash efforts.[14] The CDC's chief, James Goddard, whom Thaler had invited to Albany to testify, stressed the importance of "reaching those individuals who constitute the 'hard core' of nonresponders to health programs.... Special efforts must be made to motivate these people, including the availability of immunization at low or no cost in readily available public or private facilities."[15] These efforts, Goddard concluded, should also include special mass campaigns.

Finally, New York City Health Commissioner George James looked ahead to an even more ambitious goal: "The control and even eradication of measles is a distinct prospect assuming universal childhood immunization with one of the live virus vaccines now available," James told the committee. "Such control ... can be accelerated by a crash program comprising the majority of susceptibles in the population."[16] James's optimism reflected an ideology of infectious disease control that was ascendant among public health professionals during this period. "Eradication must always be our long-range goal," James told the

National Tuberculosis Association in 1964. "It establishes our end point, our finish line, and the only finish line we can afford to contemplate. It gives us also a perfect denominator for our success, so that we can compute the proportion of our progress toward *zero* mortality, *zero* morbidity."[17] This philosophy would have a profound effect on measles vaccination programs at the local, state, and national levels in the coming years.

THE ERADICATION OF MEASLES

The idea that vaccination might completely eliminate a disease, not just reduce it to negligible levels, had a long and somewhat checkered history. Local health officials sought to eradicate smallpox from cities and states during the nineteenth century, and New York's "No More Diphtheria" campaign in the 1920s had a comparable goal. The term "eradicate" expressed both a literal belief, born of the advances of the bacteriological revolution, in the possibility of human mastery over contagion; it also served the rhetorical function of sparking enthusiasm and motivating the public to accept vaccination. Belief in the feasibility of regional or national, as opposed to merely local, eradication programs waxed and waned over the course of the twentieth century. The Rockefeller Foundation mounted an ambitious effort to eradicate yellow fever through mosquito control in Latin America during the 1920s, but that campaign foundered after unexpected reservoirs of the disease were discovered in Brazil, and many international public health experts soured on the idea.[18]

In the years after World War II, however, several factors served to increase the preference for eradication over mere control, and to expand the geographical scope of proposed efforts. Perhaps most significant, advances in scientific medicine during the war years provided new tools for projects that were fundamentally technocratic. The Pan-American Sanitary Bureau (PASB), a nongovernmental international health organization, mounted efforts to eradicate malaria in various regions of the world through the use of the pesticide DDT to kill the mosquito that carried the disease. The dramatic decline in malaria in the Americas and elsewhere resulting from these efforts sparked enthusiasm about targeting other diseases. In the early 1950s the leadership of the PASB set its sights on eliminating smallpox from the Americas through diligent application of vaccination, and in 1959, the World Health Organization passed a resolution calling for a global smallpox eradication campaign, premised on a theoretical model of achieving a specified level of herd immunity.[19] Health officials in Europe and the Soviet Union had observed that when 80 percent of the population was well vaccinated, transmission of the disease could be permanently interrupted.[20]

It was against this international backdrop that eradicationism began to take hold in the United States. At its annual meeting in 1956, the American Public Health Association passed its first resolution supporting eradication as a method of preventing infectious disease.[21] Leading figures such as Alexander Langmuir pointed to several factors that made it a more feasible goal than it had been in the past: the increasing sophistication of epidemiologic methods, the development of better surveillance systems that enabled close tracking of disease incidence and prevalence, and the enhanced understanding of the pathogenesis of various illnesses.[22]

Armed with new knowledge and skills, health officials felt new confidence against old scourges. Tuberculosis, the nineteenth century's leading killer, had been brought to such low levels that some experts began to consider the possibility of eliminating it from the United States completely.[23] In 1962, the U.S. Public Health Service launched a campaign to eradicate syphilis from the United States within ten years using the techniques of surveillance and thorough tracing of patients' sexual contacts to offer them treatment.[24] The use of the Sabin oral polio vaccine, with its ability to halt the spread of polioviruses circulating in the community, also held out the promise of imminent eradication. The prevailing mood was such that a 1961 article in the journal *Science* could declare that "we can look forward with confidence to a considerable degree of freedom from infectious disease at a time not too far in the future."[25]

This optimism reflected the widespread sense that communicable disease had become a vestigial source of illness and death. Chronic, noninfectious conditions—especially the "big three," cancer, heart disease, and stroke—had steadily increased in incidence and moved to the forefront of medical research during the postwar period. The enormous strides in vaccine development, exemplified by Enders's work in measles virus attenuation, and the widespread deployment of antibiotics, fostered impatience with infectious disease control. In a typical expression of the new optimism, the 1962 annual report of the New York City Health Department declared that the country was "at the end of the great era of the battle against infectious disease. We are entering the great era of cold war against chronic diseases for which we do not have biologic cures."[26]

Eradicationism had its skeptics, most notably the eminent Rockefeller University bacteriologist René Dubos, who wrote widely on the subject of the precarious symbiosis between human and microbe. Dubos saw hubris in the idea that any organism could or should be utterly eliminated, and he was suspicious of the way the grand and expensive ambitions of eradication campaigns could serve as a distraction from mundane but ultimately more valuable public health activities. "The popular appeal and fervid ring of the word *eradication* is no substitute for a searching analysis of the manner in which limited supplies of resources and technical skills can best be applied for the greatest social good," Dubos wrote in his 1965 book *Man Adapting*.[27] He conceded that a utopian view of perfect health could serve as a positive force, "because, like other ideals, it sets goals and helps medical science to chart its course toward them." But, he wrote, "The hope that disease can be completely eradicated becomes a dangerous mirage ... when its unattainable character is forgotten. It can then be compared to a will-o'-the-wisp luring its followers into the swamps of unreality."[28]

Eradicationist ideas flourished in the social and political climate of the 1960s, a time of great faith in the meliorating power of state action. Ambitious crusades targeting entrenched problems—poverty, hunger, disease—were the outgrowth of a coherent ideology in which government officials, guided by social science research, would provide the technical know-how and funding to assist targeted local efforts.[29] This philosophy provided the impetus for the extensive legislative activity that included the enactment of Medicaid and Medicare in 1965 and a host of social programs targeting the conditions in which society's vulnerable members—the aged, children, racial minorities, the urban and rural poor—lived.[30] The creation in 1967 of Early and Periodic Screening, Diagnosis and Treatment (EPSDT), a Medicaid benefit intended to ensure access to preventive care for poor children, reflected the strong political interest in child welfare and the belief in the need for state intervention.[31]

As the problem of infectious disease became increasingly coterminous with the issue of socioeconomic disadvantage, the federal war on poverty provided an ideal conceptual framework for the fight that would soon be launched against measles. "The susceptibles [to measles] are concentrated in a central core, lower socioeconomic area of the city," claimed F. Robert Freckleton, chief of Immunization Activities at the CDC, shortly before the eradication effort began nationwide.[32] Just as the "discovery" of unequal vaccination coverage had dovetailed with emerging notions of wealth and deprivation in the latter part of the 1950s, so too Great Society ideals shaped the ways in which vaccination programs were conceptualized. Epidemiological patterns provided a clear indication that vaccination was an issue of social justice. In Erie County, in upstate New York, children of upper-income families in urban, suburban, and rural areas were all more likely to have received the measles vaccine than those from middle- or lower-income families; in urban areas, children of the well-to-do were twice as likely to have been vaccinated as those of the poor.[33] In New York City, 90 percent of children in the highest income bracket were fully immunized against diphtheria, pertussis, and tetanus, compared to just half of children in the lowest category; two-thirds of the highest income children were protected against polio, while less than one-quarter of the lowest-income children were.[34] A nationwide study showed that children in the highest income bracket were more than three times as likely to be seen by a pediatrician than children in the lowest.[35]

Even before the first measles vaccine had been licensed, the idea emerged that immunization would not simply reduce the disease to negligible levels, but instead completely eliminate it in the United States. Measles, like smallpox, was an attractive candidate for eradication because it had a short incubation period (so that victims had limited opportunity to spread the disease before becoming too sick to move about) and no nonhuman hosts (thus obviating the need to attack insects or other animal vectors). Nor were there any asymptomatic or inapparent cases of the disease, as there were with diphtheria and polio. Alexander Langmuir boldly declared in 1962 that eradication of measles from North America "can be anticipated soon," and when the first two measles vaccines were licensed in 1963, Surgeon General Luther Terry asserted that the disease might, "under ideal conditions," be eliminated from the United States in as little as two years.[36] James Goddard told attendees at the national immunization conference in 1965 that the CDC's "next immediate goal is the eradication of measles."[37] Other public health and medical groups, convinced by the promise of the vaccine and the CDC's optimistic stance, gave public support to the plan.[38] At the beginning of 1966, Rhode Island undertook the first statewide effort, centering on mass one-day campaigns in community settings, with the goal of eliminating the disease within its borders.[39]

The nationwide call for measles eradication was officially made at the annual meeting of the American Public Health Association in November of 1966, where the CDC's head of immunization programs,

Bruce Dull, read a paper he co-authored with CDC chief David Sencer and Alexander Langmuir. According to the CDC's vision, four elements would be essential to the effort: routine immunization of all infants at one year of age; immunization at entry into school of children who had not received an injection in infancy; ongoing surveillance at the local, state, and national levels to quickly detect cases and monitor progress; and control of outbreaks through emergency "crash" programs wherever a case was detected. With diligent attention to all four of these elements, they claimed, measles could be eradicated from the country by the end of 1967.

Its nationwide scope and ambitious timeline set the anti-measles effort apart from eradication efforts of previous eras. Also new was the extent to which epidemiological theory would provide specific target levels of immunization coverage as a guide.[40] Researchers had begun early in the century to formulate statistical theories about how contagious diseases spread, among the most important of which was the concept that the progress of an epidemic in a given community depended on the balance of those immune (either through vaccination or previous infection with the disease) to those susceptible.[41] The term "herd immunity" first appeared in a 1923 journal article,[42] and a leading 1935 epidemiology textbook elaborated on it.[43] Some health officials had begun to informally incorporate the concept of herd immunity into their immunization programming around that time; Edward Godfrey, a New York State health administrator, had posited in 1932, for example, that certain critical levels of immunization had to be obtained in different age groups in order to keep diphtheria under control, but he cautioned that this was "a mere hypothesis."[44] Because of limitations in the available data—health departments typically had only the most general idea what percentage of a city's population had been vaccinated against a given disease—it was difficult to validate the theory empirically.[45] Over the years, a level of about three-quarters was widely accepted as a desirable threshold for vaccination coverage, but this figure remained an informal target. A county health commissioner wrote in 1960:

> The goal of 70 per cent immunization of the preschool and school age population against diphtheria, pertussis, tetanus, and smallpox has become a magic number, and a figure of 80 percent for poliomyelitis is apparently becoming just as well entrenched. Whether or not these are the proper percentages needed to control the disease under consideration has never been completely proved. However, they are the levels generally accepted, and for lack of any other we must perforce accept them until some future controlled study gives us a definite answer.[46]

One of the few systematic communitywide investigations had been done early in the century in Baltimore, where the city health director had carefully tracked the incidence of measles over several years and calculated the ratio of susceptible children to those who had already had the disease and were thus immune. Based on the evidence from the Baltimore study, when immunity to measles was higher than 55 percent, epidemics did not develop.[47] The CDC's assumption about the feasibility of measles eradication was based upon the findings of the Baltimore study.

The surveillance techniques developed in the 1950s by the CDC overcame the crucial limitation in data. The ongoing survey of vaccination coverage in selected American cities allowed for vaccination programming to be guided by precise, up-to-the-minute information. Although they conceded that the exact percentage of coverage needed might vary from city to city, Dull and his colleagues were confident that the level of immunity needed was "considerably less than 100 percent."[48] For the first time, then, quantifiable goals would guide a national immunization effort; the detailed and ongoing surveillance activities of the CDC's Epidemic Intelligence Service would enable officials to chart their progress and to determine whether and when the goal of eradication was at hand.

With financial and material support from the CDC, the eradication effort debuted with great fanfare in cities around the country during 1967. At the beginning of March, Lyndon Johnson gave the program the presidential imprimatur with a statement issued from his Texas ranch.[49] The activities in New York City were typical and much about them would have been familiar to those involved in the anti-diphtheria campaigns of the 1920s. Billboards and posters blanketed the city. Health Commissioner Edward O'Rourke taped a series of television commercials and radio announcements in which he urged parents to take their children to their family physician or one of the city's neighborhood health centers.[50] All the city's major newspapers ran articles publicizing the effort. Health fairs—or "health happenings," as the department dubbed them in the slang of the day—were held in low-income neighborhoods such as East Harlem and the Lower West Side, featuring toys and games as prizes for the children attending.[51] The department staffed a telephone line to field inquiries from the public about why the vaccine was important and where it could be obtained.[52] The cartoonist Charles Schulz devoted a week of his popular *Peanuts* comic strip to Linus and Lucy's visit to the pediatrician's office for a measles shot. The CDC

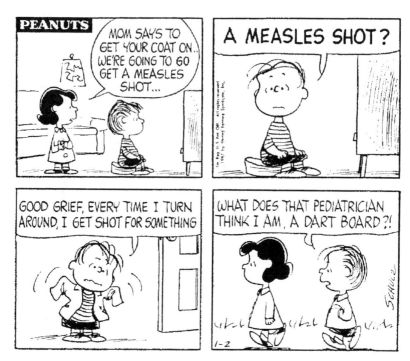

Figure 18. When the national measles eradication campaign kicked off in 1967, the cartoonist Charles Schulz devoted a week of the popular *Peanuts* comic strip to depicting Lucy and Linus's trip to the pediatrician to be vaccinated. Peanuts: © United Feature Syndicate, Inc. Reprinted with permission.

provided promotional materials, including posters, brochures, and children's coloring books, to cities around the country to assist them in their publicity.

As had been done during the anti-diphtheria campaign, New York City also attempted to reach parents more directly. Chief among these efforts was the "Immunization Reminder System" begun in January 1967. The system was a technologically more sophisticated version of a manual birth certificate follow-up program that the city had developed in the 1930s. A computer database generated reminder cards that were sent to the parents of the approximately 11,000 babies born each month in the city. The cards, printed in Spanish and English, were mailed ninety days after the child's birth and asked parents to indicate whether their children had received the recommended schedule of vaccines and to return the card to the health department.[53] Those who failed to return a card after one month were sent a second reminder card, and, if necessary,

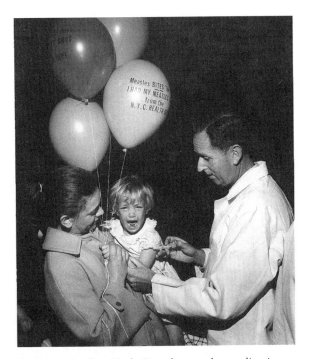

Figure 19. In New York City, the measles eradication effort, promoted with the slogan "Measles Bites the Dust," included health fairs featuring toys and games for the children attending. Courtesy New York City Municipal Archives.

a third. Reminder cards were also sent to parents one year after the child's birth to remind the parent about measles vaccination.

The federal war on poverty provided immunization programs around the country with both material assistance and conceptual support. Workers from government programs, including VISTA, the Job Corps, and Head Start, contributed efforts to measles vaccination programs in many cities.[54] As we saw in chapter 4, the 1961 "Babies and Breadwinners" anti-polio campaign had urged public health departments around the country to enlist the support of "neighborhood vaccination leaders" who might influence the decisions of their peers. In the years that followed, sociological research lent increasing credibility to the concept of the "indigenous nonprofessional," which became an important component of the federal Office of Economic Opportunity's Community Action Program.[55] Several vaccination programs around the country, working through neighborhood health centers funded by the OEO, recruited community members to serve as educators and canvassers urging their neighbors to get vaccinated.[56]

At the same time that the measles eradication campaign was launched in the United States, the most far-reaching of all eradication campaigns, the global effort to wipe out smallpox, was officially begun overseas. The program had been announced several years earlier, but it had made little progress because of an inadequate budget; the World Health Organization appropriated special funds to jump-start the effort, and the campaign officially kicked off at the beginning of 1967.[57] The launch overseas coincided with a debate at home over whether routine vaccination against smallpox should continue in the United States.

RISKS AND BENEFITS: THE CONSEQUENCES
OF SMALLPOX ERADICATION IN THE UNITED STATES

By the mid 1960s, the United States had been free from endemic smallpox for almost two decades—the last case had occurred in Texas in 1949— but health officials remained concerned about cases "imported" into the country through travel from overseas. Three physician inspectors checked all passengers arriving on international flights at Idlewild (later Kennedy) Airport, and although visitors to the United States from most other countries were required to present a certificate of vaccination, many of these documents were outdated or fraudulent.[58] The ongoing threat was vividly illustrated in the summer of 1962, when a fourteen-year-old boy flew into Idlewild Airport on a flight from Brazil, traveled into New York City in a taxi and spent several hours at Grand Central Terminal before taking a train to Montreal. After he was hospitalized in Canada and diagnosed with smallpox, New York City health officials launched an intensive hunt for anyone who might have come in contact with the youth and ultimately vaccinated more than ten thousand people.[59]

It was in response to incidents such as these, and surveys showing low levels of recent smallpox vaccination among adults, that the American Medical Association in 1963 undertook a publicity campaign urging people to update their protection.[60] In a strikingly short period of time, however, the prevailing medical and public health opinion would shift from a feeling that the nation was insufficiently vaccinated against smallpox to a belief that people should no longer undergo the procedure at all. This transformation occurred as a few physicians and public health experts began to question whether the harm from routine vaccination of infants and children outweighed the benefit.

Medical complications had, of course, been a central and contentious issue about the smallpox vaccine since the nineteenth century, and they had continued to occur even after the U.S. Public Health Service had been granted regulatory oversight of vaccine production in 1902. Reports from England and the Netherlands in the 1920s suggested the vaccine could trigger encephalitis, a sometimes fatal swelling of the brain, and that the risk was higher in school-age children than in infants.[61] In 1930, in response to anecdotal reports of central nervous system complications, the U.S. National Institute of Health undertook surveys to gauge the extent of the problem; the institute's director asked New York City Health Commissioner Shirley Wynne to be on the lookout for any such cases that might come to the attention of the department.[62] A. M. Stimson, medical director of the Public Health Service, argued in a 1930 letter to his superiors that vaccination should be limited to infants, because "complications, notably encephalitis, are very rare or absent during this period, while they are so frequent later on that it is doubtful if we should support compulsory vaccination at school ages."[63]

Beyond clinical anecdotes, however, there was little evidence of the extent of these problems, since reporting of complications to health authorities was neither legally mandated nor customary. In 1960, a Colorado pediatrician published a study in the journal *Pediatrics* documenting a variety of complications of vaccination that he had observed in young children.[64] The article raised an alarm that prompted more extensive investigations to determine the frequency of severe adverse events. In 1966, researchers from the Public Health Service, in the first systematic attempt to document the scope of the problem in the United States, determined that out of an estimated fourteen million smallpox vaccinations administered in a single year, there were more than four hundred severe reactions and seven deaths.[65] This new quantification framed the issue in stark terms: was the nation willing to accept a handful of fatalities every year in order to remain free of a disease that had become virtually nonexistent within its borders?

A key conclusion of the study was that, contrary to the earlier European findings, the frequency of complications overall was two to three times higher in infants under one year of age than in any other age group. In response, the federal Advisory Committee on Immunization Practices issued a recommendation in 1966 that a child's first vaccination be postponed to the second year of life. The committee was not ready, however, to abandon the practice altogether. The group's members noted that international air travel had increased substantially in recent years, and that because the condition was so rare in industrialized nations, physicians might not recognize an outbreak early enough to contain it. Continued universal vaccination thus "represents the only currently practicable approach for community protection in the United States."[66] Other experts agreed that the time for discontinuation had not yet arrived.[67]

But additional investigations, including a survey the following year that found a similar toll of some six hundred complications and nine deaths per year, made a stronger case that the nation's policies should at least be modified.[68] Because the risk of complications was known to be higher in people with certain biological conditions, especially eczema or other forms of dermatitis and immune suppression due to cancer or chemotherapy, many experts argued that more careful screening of potential vaccine recipients could reduce the toll. Others proposed increasing the investment in developing an improved vaccine that would produce fewer adverse reactions.[69] Some analysts suggested that a safer and more effective policy would be to limit vaccination only to those most likely to come in contact with an imported case of the disease: hospital and health care workers, emergency personnel, port and airline employees, and travelers to areas of the world where smallpox was still endemic.[70] One critic, after analyzing importations of smallpox into Europe over the previous twenty years, determined that the very limited spread of the disease in such incidents had been confined almost exclusively to health care workers caring for the initial cases. Given these data, smallpox could scarcely be considered a threat to the general population, the author concluded, noting wryly that "more people have recently died from space travel than from smallpox acquired outside a hospital."[71]

Underlying the arguments for more selective practices was a challenge to the assumption that routine childhood vaccination was doing anything to keep the country safe from smallpox. Given that the immunity conferred by vaccination waned after seven to ten years, and that rates of adult revaccination in the United States were low, the absence of the disease from the United States was attributable not to current vaccination practices, as proponents claimed, but rather to the dramatic decline of the disease worldwide.[72]

Disagreement about the most prudent course of action prevailed throughout the decade, even within the U.S. Public Health Service. At the end of 1969, the Advisory Committee on Immunization Practices reaffirmed its recommendation that universal vaccination of children should continue.[73] Just a month later, however, two employees at the CDC published a lengthy analysis in the *New England Journal of Medicine* in favor of abandoning the practice. Smallpox was increasingly confined to geographically and socially isolated areas of the globe, they argued, among people who were unlikely to travel by airplane. Any cases imported into the United States could be contained by "ring vaccination," in which limited numbers of people in an area where a case was found would be immunized in order to form a protective cordon of people that would halt the spread of the disease. Acknowledging that the decision to end vaccination carried risks of uncertain magnitude—including the possibility that the virus might be used in the future as a weapon of biologic warfare—the authors concluded: "We vaccinate against smallpox more because of the dramatic successes of the past than the needs of the present."[74]

At the heart of these debates lay the question of how to formulate policy in the face of scientific uncertainty. In this case, the situation was even more complex, because both the potential threat and the proposed remedy carried risks that were unknown and to some extent unknowable. Would ring vaccination be adequate to contain any future outbreak of smallpox? If routine vaccination were discontinued but then resumed at some point in the future because of a resurgence of the disease, what would be the consequences of having a large pool of never-vaccinated people? Would those receiving their first vaccination as adults be at increased risk of post-vaccinal encephalitis, the complication that most often resulted in death? Would discontinuation of one vaccine cast doubt in the public mind about the need for protection against other infectious diseases?

While increasing recognition of the dangers of vaccination catalyzed the growing sentiment against the practice, it was the rapid progress of the global eradication campaign that ultimately tipped the balance in favor of ending routine smallpox vaccination in the United States. When the effort had officially kicked off in 1967, thirty-three countries reported endemic smallpox. By 1970, that number had been reduced to fourteen, and by the middle of 1971, the disease was confined to only nine countries, all in west or central Africa or on the Indian subcontinent. Given the rapidly shrinking magnitude of risk from the disease, the dangers of the vaccine were no longer tolerable. In September 1971, the Advisory Committee on Immunization Practices issued a new position. "Today, nonselective vaccination against smallpox unnecessarily exposes a large segment of the United States public to the risk of complications resulting from vaccination—a risk greater than the probability of their contracting the disease," the committee declared. Health officials therefore "should consider the discontinuation of compulsory measures" to enforce the practice.[75] The following month the Committee on Infectious Disease of the American Academy of Pediatrics, the other influential advisory body on vaccination, passed a resolution unanimously supporting the ACIP's recommendation.[76] The era of routine smallpox vaccination in the United States was at an end.

While rank-and-file health care providers generally welcomed the new recommendation—an assistant commissioner in the New York State Health Department commented that "many physicians now consider the administration of smallpox vaccine to American children tantamount to malpractice"[77]—there were a few dissenting voices. Some city health commissioners, for example, remained concerned about the ability to contain an outbreak should a case arrive via one of the nation's international airports, while some private practitioners felt the recommendation was short-sighted.[78] But these were minority opinions. Cities and states around the country moved quickly to change smallpox vaccination laws, many of which had been on the books since the previous century.[79]

The abandonment of smallpox vaccination might have been a triumphant moment, validating the belief that infectious disease could be conquered and reaffirming the power of vaccination as a force for permanent good. But instead the decision came at a time of crisis for immunization programs around the country. The anti-measles effort had run aground amid recrimination and finger-pointing, federal financial support was no longer assured, and efforts to reach young children, especially those in poverty, were stalled. In stark contrast to the steady progress being made against smallpox, the goal of measles eradication seemed to be moving farther away than ever.

THE PERSISTENCE OF MEASLES

In 1968, the country recorded an all-time low of 22,000 cases of measles, compared to an average of 450,000 for the five years preceding the licensing of the vaccine. That year, CDC surveys showed that about half of children aged five to nine, and about 60 percent of those aged one to four, had received the vaccine.[80] But instead of a continuing downward trend in measles, and steady growth in the proportion of children vaccinated, as had been hoped and predicted, the opposite occurred. In 1969, the number of cases increased slightly. Cases in 1970 totaled forty-seven thousand, more than double the 1968 figure; in 1971, there were some seventy-five thousand cases, more than triple the number in 1968. At the same time, the CDC's surveys indicated that measles vaccination levels nationwide were stagnant.[81]

As had been the case with polio a decade earlier, the experience of poor neighborhoods in Chicago served as a harbinger of a new epidemiological pattern. In the winter of 1967–68, the city was struck by an outbreak concentrated among preschoolers on the south and west sides. "Spread of measles among pre-school children was particularly marked in high-rise, urban renewal dwellings where such children were found to congregate with common babysitters, at recreational facilities, and in other crowded situations," a report on the outbreak noted.[82] In February 1969, an outbreak in the South Bronx prompted the New York City Health Department to intensify efforts in clinics, run Spanish-language public service announcements on radio and television, and enlist the help of neighborhood charitable organizations.[83] But by spring, the outbreak had spread to high-poverty areas in Brooklyn. By the end of the year, New York had recorded more than twice as many cases as the previous year.[84] "None of us wants to repeat this year's measles outbreak and the dubious distinction New York City had, accounting for 25% of all reported cases in the country," a frustrated deputy commissioner wrote.[85]

This pattern soon became familiar. In 1969 and 1970, epidemics of measles occurred in almost every state in the country, heavily concentrated among the poor in inner-city and rural areas.[86] Cleveland, Chicago, and Baltimore all experienced outbreaks among African American and Latino children in central-city areas.[87] By the summer of 1969, with reported cases rising around the country, the AMA issued a pessimistic report declaring that eradication was "at a stand-still" because of outbreaks in "'hard-core' ghetto areas of the East."[88]

The leaders of the eradication campaign had been aware from the outset of the risk they took in announcing the imminent conquest of a problem so deeply embedded in the country's social fabric. Bruce Dull, who had read the eradication paper before the American Public Health Association in 1966, subsequently cautioned that the word "eradication" could be misleading because it suggested finality, when in fact an ongoing commitment to continuing immunization was needed.[89] Nevertheless, it seemed clear in hindsight that the architects of the eradication program had, like the leaders of the federal war on poverty, set themselves up for

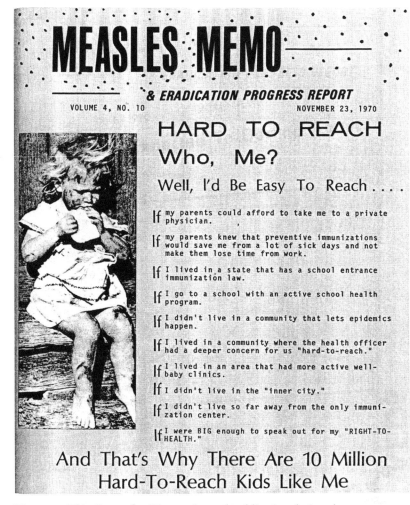

Figure 20. This Center for Disease Control publication designed to support frontline public health workers in the anti-measles campaign illustrated the factors that were perceived to be the greatest barriers to high immunization rates. The idea of "hard to reach" populations gained prominence during the 1960s, when the issue of infectious disease became increasingly identified with social crusades such as the federal war on poverty.

embarrassing failure. The most obvious proximate reason for the resurgence in the disease was that the four-point plan—especially routine vaccination of one-year-olds—had not been fulfilled. As the number of cases of measles continued to rise, a variety of explanations for the underlying reasons for the failure were proposed.

Some analyses of the failure questioned the epidemiological theory that underpinned the effort. The concept of herd immunity applied only to closed, randomly mixing populations, according to one critique, and a more complex model was needed to reflect the real-life situations of a national campaign. The question of what proportion of a population must be immunized in order to prevent epidemics was "not answerable in absolute terms"; factors such as the age, demographic, and geographic distribution of the population and the social habits that affected the mixing of group members all needed to be taken into account.[90] Another analysis claimed that the immunity needed for eradication "exists perhaps somewhere above the 90 percent level, if it exists at all."[91] Data emerging from measles control programs in West Africa suggested that either a mass campaign reaching 90 percent of children annually or an ongoing maintenance level of 75 percent of children—neither of which had been achieved in the United States—was necessary.[92]

A second framework for understanding the failure of the eradication effort was the idea of the "hard core" and the "hard to reach" that had emerged during the polio campaigns. Some of these analyses emphasized the difficulty of overcoming cultural differences related to race and ethnicity. Others drew on the concept of the "culture of poverty," popularized in academic and popular works such as Michael Harrington's influential 1962 book *The Other America*.[93] In this conceptualization, ethnic minorities and the poor had behaviors and beliefs fundamentally different from "mainstream" American society and were thus less accepting of vaccination. One review argued that the poor "take a rather cavalier attitude" toward illness, which accounted for their limited use of medical care: "if the lower and middle classes viewed illness with as great alarm as do the upper classes," the author contended, "their use of physicians would certainly rise."[94] A study of New York City's Washington Heights neighborhood found that Puerto Ricans were the "most divorced from the objectives and methods of modern medicine and public health"—a finding that explained, according to the author, "why Puerto Ricans, and to a lesser extent Negroes, constitute the core of the 'hard-to-reach' groups in public health and medical care."[95]

While these and other assessments implicitly characterized the "hard to reach" groups as dysfunctional, other analyses cast the failure to respond to public health appeals as a rational reaction to complex life situations. "Ghetto members lead crisis-ridden lives," asserted the authors of one article examining poor people's use of preventive health care. "Dealing with these crises creates a value system that gives highest priority to satisfaction of immediate needs. In this system, disease is a concern only when it is an emergency."[96] Vincent Guinee, who headed New York City's Bureau of Preventable Disease, echoed this view when he claimed, "When someone is struggling to get up the rent money, or the roof is falling in, a case of measles that may or may not happen just doesn't seem very real."[97] In this respect, the lack of severe complications of measles impeded the effort to eliminate the disease: it simply did not trigger the kind of anxiety that spurred people to action, like smallpox or polio. "Measles is still characterized as an uncomfortable but not very threatening interlude of childhood. Immunization is 'nice' but not critical," claimed a state health official in 1971. "The measles immunization program is *for* the people, but it is done *to* the people, not *with* the people, and certainly not as a response to a felt need *of* the people."[98] Reflecting several years later on assumptions behind the measles campaign, Alexander Langmuir, one of the campaign's chief architects, wrote:

> Intrinsic in my personal thinking was the mistaken belief that once measles was eliminated from a community its reintroduction and beginning spread would lead to a spontaneous community response to immunize all susceptibles in the immediate vicinity and thus promptly snuff out the disease. This community reaction I call "the typical smallpox reaction." In practice, this did not occur. Instead there was to me an amazing apathy on the part of both citizens and health authorities rather than alert "fire fighting."[99]

A third explanation for the failure of the anti-measles campaign centered on the inadequacies of the American health care system. In this view, rigid administrative procedures and impersonal service—not the characteristics of the "hard to reach"—lay behind the persistent low vaccination rates of some groups. "The traditional hours of a child health clinic, from 9 to 11 a.m. or from 2 to 4 p.m., may not meet the needs of a mother who works all day," noted a typical critique in a public health journal. "An immunization clinic on the downtown premises of the health department is difficult for a rural family to attend when traveling to it involves several bus transfers."[100] Such analyses were an indictment of immunization programs in general, not just those for measles. During efforts to control a diphtheria outbreak in Austin, Texas, waiting time in line was one to two hours, with many people forced to stand in the rain; clinics closed at the stated time regardless of how many people were waiting in line.[101] A review in Tennessee found that rigid and unfriendly administrative procedures led to failure to vaccinate even the children of highly motivated parents. "If children arrived on days that immunization clinics were not being held, they were refused vaccination even though they had traveled long distances or were in a high-risk group and it was unlikely that they would return at the specific time."[102]

Onerous bureaucratic structures made things difficult not only for low-income patients, but also for the health providers who had to work within the system. One physician contended:

> To have a child fully immunized in a county health station requires seven visits. The wait is long, and the service is impersonal. During the 1970–71 epidemic in New York City, the state Medicaid payment for measles immunization was $1.00 for a vaccine that cost the physician $1.69 to purchase. Physicians could receive a small free supply only if they went personally or sent a courier with a prescription containing the names of the patients they planned to vaccinate. This was obviously not a procedure designed to facilitate mass immunization.[103]

These harsh assessments from within the health care system dovetailed with a radical political critique by outsiders. Left-wing activist groups such as the Health Policy Advisory Center (HealthPAC), which published the widely cited polemic *The American Health Empire* in 1970, attacked the institutions of medicine as tools of capitalist power and profit-making that reflected and reinforced existing social inequities.[104] A frequent criticism in this vein was the long-standing failure of many physicians to cooperate with communitywide mass vaccination campaigns, instead vaccinating only those children in their own practices.[105] An incident that occurred at the start of the measles eradication campaign was emblematic. In San Francisco, a planned mass vaccination program was derailed when the city's Pediatric Society refused to support the provision of vaccination in community settings, insisting instead that all shots be given in visits to private physicians' offices. This action prompted Massachusetts Senator Edward Kennedy—who, as we shall see, had a special interest in measles control—to write to Surgeon General William Stewart seeking reassurance that the U.S. Public Health Service was taking all possible steps to enlist the cooperation of the medical profession in the eradication effort. The Public Health Service had no authority to compel any local medical society to give practical or rhetorical support to its programs, of course, and it conceded that, "In some instances, as was the case in San Francisco, the reluctance of the medical society to give support is enough to either delay or stop mass measles campaigns." But the service assured Kennedy that the CDC had secured the endorsement of major national medical groups, including the American Medical Association and the American Academy of Pediatrics, in the measles eradication effort.[106]

A final—and in the eyes of many analysts crucial—reason for the failure of the measles eradication campaign was the lack of a sustained financial commitment on the part of the federal government. By 1967, federal dollars constituted a major part of vaccination program budgets around the country. The CDC was supporting more than one hundred projects at the state, county, and city levels, serving some 84 percent of the U.S. population.[107] At this time, a political debate emerged about the appropriate way for the federal government to support the expenses of states. The Vaccination Assistance Act had embodied a "categorical funding" method, in which funds available to states were earmarked for specific needs. The incoming Nixon administration favored a block grant approach under which states were given lump sums, which they had wide latitude in determining how to spend. Laws passed in 1966 and 1967 changed the way the Public Health Service allocated money to states, and many categorical programs had been combined into block grants.[108] The Vaccination Assistance Act was not renewed when it expired in 1968, and money from the program ended in the middle of 1969. Funding for vaccination programs, which had been guaranteed through most of the 1960s, was folded into a new category of Public Health Service block grants called the "Partnership for Health" program. Many states, faced with a wide range of health issues they considered more pressing, chose to spend their money on programs other than immunization.[109]

Measles programs suffered most from the changeover, and the situation was worsened, ironically, by the arrival of a new vaccine against rubella (German measles), which was licensed in June 1969. Rubella is a relatively mild disease, but it was one that commanded special attention, because it most severely affected pregnant women and their newborns. In 1964, an epidemic in the United States resulted in some 20,000 children born with profound birth defects. The disease was known to occur in cycles of five to seven years, and a sense of urgency to forestall a potential epidemic was thus felt alongside the excitement that would normally greet the introduction of a new vaccine. The Department of Health, Education and Welfare made a special appropriation of almost $10 million for fiscal year 1969–70 for rubella immunization programs under a clause in the block grant program that allowed categorical earmarking for new and innovative programs. As a result, what federal funding there was for immunization was to be used exclusively to fight rubella. Although the timing of the two political developments was closely aligned, the block granting of federal vaccination funding was unrelated to the policy decision to support rubella. Nevertheless, many analysts characterized the sequence of events as federal bureaucrats taking money away from measles in order to give it to rubella.[110]

The decline in funding of routine vaccination affected other diseases besides measles. Following the mass community campaigns for the Sabin vaccine in the early 1960s, which had resulted in close to 90 percent of preschoolers being vaccinated, immunization rates against polio declined each year, to the point where only about 63 percent of children were protected in 1971.[111] At the end of the 1960s, diphtheria rates nationwide climbed to their highest level in years. To be sure, the numbers were nowhere near what they had been earlier in the century, when annual infectious disease deaths in every state had numbered in the hundreds or thousands. But even these very small numbers of cases seemed unacceptable in an era when the vaccines had been available for so long. The failure to control, much less eradicate, easily preventable conditions was an embarrassing comment on the inadequacy of the nation's health infrastructure.

Funding for immunization programs continued to be erratic for the next several years. In response to pressure from David Sencer, director of the CDC, about the rising incidence of childhood illnesses, Congress created a new discretionary grant-in-aid program (so-called "317" grants, named for the section in the enabling legislation) to help state and local governments fund vaccination programs.[112] The nationwide resurgence of measles prompted special federal allocations in 1971 and 1972. But in 1973, funds were cut to the lowest amount since the Vaccination Assistance Act had been passed in 1962.[113]

Regardless of the reason for the failure of the measles eradication effort—faulty epidemiologic theory, the entrenchment of infectious diseases within the "culture of poverty," the inadequacy of the nation's health care system, the lack of sustained federal financial commitment—it was clear in the early 1970s that officials at the CDC had experienced a stark reversal from the optimism of just a few years earlier. Rather than bringing measles eradication to a triumphant conclusion, health professionals nationwide found themselves fighting a rearguard action to shore up the basic protection against several diseases long thought to be under control. The anti-measles effort did, however, have a far-reaching effect on one key policy area that was widely viewed as a major step forward for public health: the enactment of state laws across the country requiring measles and other vaccinations prior to school entry.

"NO SHOTS, NO SCHOOL": THE RETURN OF COMPULSION

Through the middle decades of the century, a voluntaristic ethos prevailed with respect to vaccination. When the Salk vaccine was licensed, mandates were felt to be superfluous at best and philosophically objectionable at worst. The National Foundation's senior staff members believed that "vaccinations, like [charitable] giving, should be voluntary."[114] As health officials grew frustrated in the late 1950s with lagging public uptake of the vaccine, a few states considered using the law to increase coverage levels. The Indiana legislature, at the recommendation of the state health commissioner, opted for a voluntary system in which parents enrolling their children in school were required to furnish a written statement about whether or not the child had been immunized.[115] When a bill to make polio immunization compulsory was introduced in 1961 in South Carolina, the state medical society was split over the issue of compulsion. "Proponents of the action pointed out that voluntary immunization had been rather a fiasco," according to the state medical journal, while "die-hard defenders of the individual rights of man insisted that those who did not wish to be saved should not be forced to seek protection."[116] The bill failed to pass in the state legislature. In New Jersey, the state medical society passed a resolution supporting a legal requirement, but no bills made it through the legislature.[117]

In states that did implement mandates, the impetus sometimes came from legislators concerned about limiting fiscal burdens, rather than medical experts seeking the most effective way to fight the spread of disease. The text of a bill introduced in the New York state legislature in 1965 made this concern explicit:

> The typical polio cripple of the post-vaccine period is a child less than five years of age in an underprivileged family. It is unlikely that the family will ever be able to pay for the child's medical care and rehabilitation or that the child will be able to support himself when he grows up. Therefore these polio victims will cost thousands of tax and charity dollars in the years ahead.... [T]he large numbers of pre-school children who are unprotected against paralytic polio must be immunized and protected in their own self-interest as well as for the health and economic well-being of the community."[118]

In response to this bill, New York City Health Commissioner George James expressed his department's long-standing reservations about legal coercion. "[W]e do not like to legislate the things which can be obtained without legislation," James explained. Furthermore, he argued, school-age children were already well-protected—more than 95 percent in New York City had received either the Salk or Sabin vaccine—and thus the bill would simply divert attention away from the preschool child who was most at risk.[119] Governor Nelson Rockefeller vetoed the bill, citing James's argument. In response, legislators expanded the scope of the bill to include requirements for children entering day-care facilities, kindergartens, and preschool centers. Rockefeller signed the revised bill in August 1966, and it went into effect January 1 the following year. But New York was atypical. By the mid 1960s, only a handful of states had enacted a requirement for polio immunization prior to school entry.[120]

The measles eradication campaign radically transformed this legal landscape. Immunizing school-age children was one of the four programmatic pillars of the campaign (along with newborn vaccination, ongoing surveillance, and control of outbreaks) that the CDC had laid out in 1966. It is thus not surprising that laws mandating the vaccination of students were enlisted as a tool in achieving the goal. It was among kindergartners and first- and second-graders that the disease occurred most frequently, and CDC officials warned of allowing "an increasing pool of older susceptibles" to build up in the population.[121] In this context, many health officials began to rethink their long-standing opposition to vaccination laws.

An additional force behind the enactment of new laws was the Joseph P. Kennedy Foundation, a Washington D.C.-based charity concerned with mental retardation.[122] Measles-related encephalitis, which occurred in about one in one thousand cases of the disease, was a major cause of retardation, and the foundation took great interest in the licensing of measles vaccine. The organization had significant political connections—its president was Massachusetts Senator Edward Kennedy, and its executive vice president was Eunice Kennedy Shriver, sister of the senator and the former president and wife of Sargent Shriver, head of the federal Office of Economic Opportunity—and it encouraged legislators and health officials around the country to mount aggressive vaccination programs even before the eradication program had been officially announced.[123] In January 1968, the Kennedy Foundation sent letters, signed by Eunice Kennedy Shriver, to the governors and congressional delegations of numerous states urging them to enact laws requiring measles vaccination before entry into public schools. Appealing to the politicians' concerns for fiscal matters, each letter was tailored to the particular state and contained a projection, based on the most recent estimate of the state's current measles prevalence, of how many measles-related cases of mental retardation and deaths might be expected to occur in the coming year, and the total cost to the state in resulting medical and rehabilitative care.[124]

The data in the letters on each state's measles prevalence was supplied by James Bowes, a Kennedy Foundation consultant who worked for Pitman-Moore, a subdivision of the Dow Chemical Company, which manufactured measles vaccine. Bowes's potential conflict of interest in the matter—as a representative of a vaccine manufacturer, it was to his employer's advantage to magnify the extent of the measles problem—angered at least one state health officer who felt that the disease prevalence described in the letter was exaggerated. "I resent the inference that Massachusetts has in any way been dragging its feet on its Measles Immunization Program," wrote the state's head of communicable disease control in a letter to Bowes's superior at Pitman-Moore. "While Dr. Bowes perhaps did not write Mrs. Shriver's letter, he did supply the erroneous data on which the letter was based. I am sure that all State Health Departments will hold Pitman-Moore responsible for any unwarranted misrepresentations of their performance."[125]

Senator Jacob Javits passed on the letter he received from the foundation to New York State Health Commissioner Hollis Ingraham seeking comment. Ingraham's wary response echoed those of his predecessors who had opposed legal mandates for children on pragmatic grounds. "While commendable in intent, this approach must be regarded as something of a calculated risk," Ingraham replied, because it could lead parents to postpone the procedure until their children were of school age; health officials were having significant problems persuading people to immunize children against measles at one year of age.[126] Nevertheless, various bills on the subject were already wending their way through the state legislature, largely without the support or input of public health officials. The rationale for adding a measles requirement echoed concerns that had been expressed about polio: children who became sick with infectious disease cost a state money.[127] In 1968, with the measles eradication effort in full swing and the Kennedy Foundation making its push, Rockefeller signed a bill requiring measles vaccination, to take effect January 1, 1969.[128]

A "natural experiment" in 1970–71 provided empirical evidence for the effectiveness of school entry requirements and galvanized the growing national trend—promoted by some health officials with the slogan "no shots, no school"—for the enactment of laws. The city of Texarkana, which straddled the Texas-Arkansas state line, experienced a measles outbreak. Texas had no requirement for measles immunization before school entry; Arkansas did. The case rate among children in Bowie County, on the Texas side of the border, was twelve times higher than the case rate in Miller County, on the Arkansas side.[129]

The number of states with a school immunization requirement quickly grew. In 1968, just half the states had a law requiring one or more vaccinations prior to school entry; by 1974, forty states did.[130] The proportion of children aged five to nine who had received the measles vaccine climbed from about one-half in 1968 to about three-quarters in 1974. During the same period, the proportion of vaccinated children aged one to four remained constant (at around 60 percent).[131] Although the requirement for protection against measles provided the impetus for changing laws, many states took the opportunity to make sweeping updates, adding requirements for all, or most, other vaccine-preventable diseases. Many of the laws extended to include college students and daycare facilities. While exclusion from school was generally the penalty, some laws made it a misdemeanor for parents to violate the law or for school officials to fail to enforce it.[132] By 1981, all fifty states—with Idaho, Iowa, and Wyoming bringing up the rear—had made vaccination against most vaccine-preventable illnesses mandatory for school entry.[133]

It might seem ironic that the measles eradication campaign, undertaken amid the Great Society's spirit of community mobilization and empowerment, would leave as its most lasting legacy a nationwide network of compulsory regulations and laws. But proponents of school requirements, especially officials at the CDC, framed the laws in terms of their persuasive function, and characterized them as helpful prompts to action rather than tools of coercion. "[S]ome additional stimulus is often needed to provoke action on the part of a basically interested person who has many other concerns competing for attention," claimed Alan Hinman, one of the most vocal advocates of the enactment of school entry laws. In this view, the laws were essentially hortatory, serving as a "means of bringing to individuals' attention the continuing publicly perceived need for immunization."[134] This use of the law was thus consistent with a liberal vision of an activist state intervening to improve social welfare.

There were dissenting voices to the overall consensus about the appropriateness of using legal sanctions to boost immunization rates. "Adequate systems for health care delivery and education afford the best approaches to preventive medicine," wrote Samuel Katz, a prominent pediatrician and one of the developers of the first measles vaccine. "Laws are too apt at one extreme to afford a false sense of accomplishment or at the other extreme to impose a climate of conformity which stifles the intellectual and emotional impetus for change."[135]

Given the many controversies that had attended vaccination mandates in the nineteenth and early twentieth century, the swiftness with which legislators around the country placed new laws on the books in the 1960s and 1970s, and the failure of these actions to generate widespread or sustained public protest, are striking. The lack of contention was due largely to the fact that immunization had by this time achieved the status of an uncontroversial medical orthodoxy, and concerns about risk, which a decade later would surge to the forefront of public attention, were generally absent during this period. Although the decision to discontinue smallpox vaccination had cast unprecedented light on the potential risks of immunization, these deliberations had been confined to scientific circles and attracted little notice among the lay public. Moreover, a CDC survey in the late 1970s suggested that many people were not aware of their state's laws: about one-quarter of respondents said that their state did not require vaccination of children prior to school entry, even though virtually all Americans by this time lived in areas covered by such laws. More than nine out of ten respondents said that even if their state did not have such a law, they would have their child vaccinated anyway—an apparent vindication of Hinman's characterization of the laws as prompts.[136]

One immunization requirement did spark controversy: the mandate for protection against rubella. As we have seen, the licensing of the vaccine in 1969 was greeted with great excitement because another epidemic was thought to be imminent, based on a historic trend of the disease occurring in five- to seven-year cycles. City and state health departments across the country mounted extensive publicity campaigns to encourage use of the vaccine, and requirements were added to many state laws in the rush of legislation sparked by the anti-measles effort. But concerns were raised about the vaccine's safety and efficacy. It was known to cause joint pain, sometimes severe, in up to 10 percent of those who received it, prompting the CDC to issue a notice to all state epidemiologists and immunization project directors in August 1970 to be alert to potential problems and let parents know in advance of the likely side effect.[137]

More serious, at least two studies had raised doubts over the duration of protection the vaccine afforded, and some health experts worried about the long-term consequences of artificially replacing the permanent and certain immunity provided by natural infection with the less complete and long-lasting protection offered by the vaccine. The Nobel laureate John Enders, one of the country's most respected virologists, expressed concern in a *New England Journal of Medicine* commentary about the potential to create a generation of women of child-bearing age who might be vulnerable to the disease and suffer more severely from it than if they had contracted it naturally as children.[138] Enders was careful to emphasize that, on balance, he believed the current policy was beneficial and should continue, but the reporting of his concerns in the popular media raised doubts among parents, physicians, and lawmakers. Other medical experts were even more skeptical, claiming that no law should mandate the vaccine until the concerns about its efficacy and safety had been resolved through further research.[139]

But the most controversial aspect of universal rubella immunization was the fact that the children who received the shot did not themselves derive a significant benefit from it. Rubella was a very mild illness in youth that almost never caused serious or long-lasting complications; the disease was a threat only to pregnant women who might give birth to infants with congenital defects. Thus in contrast to all other immunization programs, in which the individuals who were vaccinated benefited along with the community, in the case of rubella, one segment of the population (youth) was being subjected to the intervention in order to protect another group (pregnant women). Vince Fulginiti, a leading immunization expert, questioned the ethics of this practice when he declared, with striking bluntness, that "women of childbearing age ... have the risk of congenital rubella among their fetuses; they should shoulder the risks associated with vaccine."[140] But this was a minority opinion. Because of the unknown effects the vaccine might have on a developing fetus, it was generally considered ethically unacceptable to run the risk of giving the vaccine to women of child-bearing years who might be pregnant and not know it.

Doubts about the use of the vaccine were further inflamed after a widely publicized report on a rubella epidemic in which several women in the town of Casper, Wyoming, contracted rubella even though a large majority of the town's children had received the vaccine. "It is apparent that in this community, the presence of an immune, prepubertal 'herd' was not effective in preventing community spread of rubella," a 1973 article on the epidemic concluded.[141] The Casper experience thus undermined the central epidemiological premise for universal rubella immunization of schoolchildren. An editorial accompanying the medical journal report declared that in light of the findings, compulsory rubella immunization laws should be repealed.[142]

In spite of the Casper study and the doubts it raised about the balance of risks and benefits, the epidemiological trend of rubella seemed to validate the continuing use of the vaccine. The feared national epidemic on the scale of the 1964 experience that had been forecast for the early 1970s never materialized; instead, cases of rubella declined over the decade. In 1977, the American Academy of Pediatrics took a formal position in favor of continuing the current rubella policy because of its apparent efficacy.[143] Laws requiring rubella immunization remained on the books, and although the controversy did not subside entirely, administration of the shot became increasingly routinized as part of the combined measles-mumps-rubella preparation licensed in 1971.

VACCINATION, RELIGION, AND THE COURTS

Although the new laws that swept the country in the 1960s and 1970s did not provoke the kind of high-profile political battles that had punctuated the era of smallpox, they did draw numerous court challenges. The focus of this litigation was the question of which children, if any, should be excused from school vaccination requirements. Unlike mandates in the nineteenth century, almost all of the new laws contained exemptions for children whose parents had religious scruples against the practice. These exceptions were included largely in response to the lobbying efforts of Christian Scientists.[144] Legislators in some states wrote their exemptions narrowly, out of concern that too liberal a policy would encourage parents to opt out. Some laws allowed exemptions only for members of "recognized" or "established" religious denominations whose tenets specifically proscribed vaccination (for all intents and purposes, Christian Science), while others allowed local education officials the discretion to waive the requirement as they saw fit. But limiting exemptions in this way left the laws on shaky constitutional ground. The specific bases of the legal challenges varied; so too did the outcomes of the suits.

Early salvos were fired in New York soon after the state adopted its requirement for polio vaccination in 1967. The law included, along with a medical exemption, a waiver for "children whose parent, parents or guardian are bona fide members of a recognized religious organization whose teachings are contrary to the practices herein." Legislators added the clause at the request of Christian Scientists.[145] The start of the 1967 school year brought four challenges to the new law. The backgrounds of the cases were similar. All the parents in question were chiropractors ("chiropractic ethics" held that introduction of foreign substances into the body was harmful); all practiced religions other than Christian Science; and all their cases were triggered when education officials charged the parents with neglect for their failure to protect their children against polio. None of their challenges to the new law was successful.

The argument of the plaintiff Thomas McCartney, a Roman Catholic, was typical of the four. He claimed that he held a "deep moral conviction" that vaccination was wrong, and that he should therefore be covered by the law's religious exemption. Roman Catholicism "does not have any proscriptions against inoculation," McCartney conceded, "but it does require that one follow his moral convictions."[146] If he had been a Christian Scientist, he argued, he would be allowed the exemption; the law thus interfered with his right to worship according to his conscience and favored one religious belief over others, in violation of the First and Fourteenth Amendment prohibitions against government establishment of religion. The other plaintiffs, two Catholics and a Methodist, made similar arguments. But the courts did not agree that "freedom of religion would be constitutionally prohibited or restrained by this statute," in the words of one of the judges on the family court. Furthermore, "the practice of one's religion must be exercised in the light of the general public welfare, and cannot conflict with the public welfare."[147] Citing *Jacobson v. Massachusetts* and other precedents, the judges in all four cases dismissed the parents' arguments.[148]

These legal actions were a source of chagrin for the state's education officials, who ended up in court because of their role in enforcing the vaccination law. A local school superintendent complained to Commissioner Ingraham that the "reports in the papers and the appearance in court made it appear that the school district was the aggressor, in fact, that the school district and its employees were the 'bad guys' for attempting to enforce the laws of the State."[149] The polio vaccination requirement "places school authorities in the position of being either policemen or theologians, neither of which we are especially well qualified for. The law should probably be changed, either to completely eliminate Subsection 8 [the exemption clause] or to clarify the instances of religious exemption."[150] At the beginning of 1968, the head of the state medical society urged Ingraham to issue a public clarification on the need for the law "to neutralize the statements of quacks in the press" and to assist principals and school board members who were having difficulties administering the requirement.[151]

In spite of the rebuffs to these initial challenges, another lawsuit in New York three years later—this time with a different legal strategy—brought success for the plaintiff. In December 1970, a school principal in the small town of Fabius, in central New York, ordered that the three children of William Maier be excluded from school because they lacked the required immunizations. Maier insisted that he followed the Christian Science tenet that "the sanctity of the human body cannot be violated by injection," even though he was "not a formal member of the Christian Science Church."[152] In a case he brought before a U.S. district court, Maier contended that the exemption clause violated the First Amendment prohibition against establishment of religion and the Fourteenth Amendment guarantee of equal protection. Although Maier's complaint was similar to the ones that had been brought by the four chiropractors—he too claimed he was entitled to an exemption because of his sincere religious beliefs—his legal aim differed. Whereas the earlier cases had sought to have the entire law declared unconstitutional, Maier challenged only the religious exemption clause, on the ground that it was underinclusive.

In this case, the court agreed with Maier's legal argument. The judges enjoined the school district from barring his children, but they abstained from deciding the case for procedural reasons and instructed Maier to seek redress in state court. The following year, Maier took his claim to the New York supreme court, which concurred with the opinion of the district court. "There does not appear to be any rational basis or legitimate purpose," the judge wrote, "in requiring a person to be a registered member of an organized church as opposed to one who can prove that he genuinely practices and lives his religious tenets in order to qualify for this religious exemption."[153] The judge declined to hold the clause unconstitutional, however; instead he granted an injunction that gave Maier the chance to prove the sincerity of his religious belief—that he was a "bona fide," if not formal, member of the church—in a trial.

In March 1971, one month after William Maier's first case was heard in U.S. district court, the Massachusetts supreme court took a strong stance against that state's religious exemption clause, which, like New York's, was limited to members of "a recognized church or religious denomination" whose tenets conflicted with vaccination. The case was brought by a Lowell resident, Beulah Dalli, who, although she practiced no organized religion, did not want her five-year-old daughter to be vaccinated because of the biblical command to "keep the body clean and acceptable to God." The court ruled that the statute violated the First and Fourteenth Amendments because it "extends preferred treatment" to members of certain religious groups who "enjoy the benefit of an exemption which is denied to other persons whose objections to vaccination are also grounded in religious belief."[154] In declaring the provision unconstitutional, the court left it to the legislature to determine whether the appropriate next step was to extend the exemption to other sincere religious beliefs or discard it altogether.

Other cases during the 1970s produced conflicting legal outcomes. In a law they placed on the books in 1971, New Hampshire legislators had decreed that "a child may be excused from immunization for religious reasons at the discretion of the local school board." Three years after the law was enacted, a U.S. district court judge threw out the provision, finding that it was "unconstitutionally vague" and violated the due process clause of the First Amendment.[155] The judges determined that the exemption clause could be severed from the rest of the law, leaving the mandate for vaccination intact—and the plaintiff, ironically, with no recourse for avoiding the requirement. Thus the judges concluded that "plaintiff may have won the battle, but lost the war."[156]

In a 1976 case, a three-judge panel on the U.S. district court in Kentucky disagreed with the decisions that had been reached in New York and Massachusetts. The exemption in that state was limited to members of "a nationally recognized and established church or religious denomination, the teachings of which are opposed to medical immunization against disease." Louis Kleid, a chiropractor in Fulton, Kentucky, argued that the state law violated the establishment clause of the First Amendment. The court found that the benefit conferred to religious groups opposed to vaccination was "at best, only an indirect, incidental and remote" one and therefore did not pose problems of establishment. Responding to the plaintiff's claim that the statute breached the wall between church and state, the judges replied tartly that "Kentucky legislators who enacted [the law] have not removed one stone nor even loosened any mortar from that constitutional wall."[157]

In the midst of these legal challenges, the potential epidemiological effects of religiously based refusal of vaccination were dramatically illustrated. In the fall of 1972, an outbreak of polio struck a Christian Scientist high school in Greenwich, Connecticut, resulting in eleven cases of paralytic disease among unvaccinated youth aged seven to eighteen.[158] It was the country's worst cluster of polio in many years—annual incidence of the disease had declined to near zero—and the episode starkly posed the question of whether safeguarding religious liberty was a more important societal goal than protecting the health of children. "I am deeply bothered," the head of a state health department wrote to the *New England Journal of Medicine*, "by the fact that disease-prevention measures of documented benefit can be withheld from children by their parents in the name of religious freedom, jeopardizing not only the health and lives of the children so denied but those of the community as well. The courts of this land have long since set precedent in the protection of children from the irresponsible acts of their parents."[159]

This comment was a reference to the landmark 1944 case of *Prince v. Massachusetts,* in which the U.S. Supreme Court had ruled that the religious beliefs of a Jehovah's Witness who sought to have her nine-year-old niece distribute tracts must be subordinate to the state's interest in proscribing child labor. In its famous formulation, the court had declared, "Parents may be free to become martyrs themselves. But it does not follow they are free, in identical circumstances, to make martyrs of their children."[160] In the context of exemptions from vaccination laws, many health authorities believed that withholding immunizations would, as had been the case in Connecticut, condemn children to the martyrdom of deadly illnesses.

The ruling in *Prince* had included a passage that buttressed the constitutional case that compulsory vaccination programs need not contain religious exemptions:

> Acting to guard the general interest in the youth's well-being, the state as *parens patriae* may restrict the parent's control by requiring school attendance, regulating or prohibiting child labor and in many other ways. Its authority is not nullified merely because the parent grounds his claim to control the child's course of conduct on religion or conscience. Thus, he cannot claim freedom from compulsory vaccination for the child more than for himself on religious grounds. The right to practice religion freely does not include liberty to expose the community or the child to communicable disease or the latter to ill health or death.[161]

It was thus clear that states were not *required* to grant religious exemptions. Less certain was whether they *could* do so, and with what restrictions on eligibility.[162]

By the mid 1970s, disagreement prevailed over several aspects of compulsory vaccination laws for students. Were they coercive or simply motivational? Should they cover all vaccinations or only those with an unequivocally favorable risk-benefit profile? To what extent should they excuse people who had religious scruples against the practice? But there was increasing agreement on one important point: that school mandates were in tension, if not irreconcilable, with the principle of informed consent, which assumed great significance during this period. As we shall see in chapter 6, the conflict between mandates and consent, along with a proliferation of lawsuits for vaccine-related injuries and an intensified focus on adverse events, created an unprecedented period of crisis for immunization programs around the country.

Consent, Compulsion, and Compensation

Vaccination Programs in Crisis

"Immunization policy has become a public concern, and society has declared its right to know and to participate in decision making," a prominent physician wrote in the *New England Journal of Medicine* in mid 1977. "It is the nature of immunization that its problems and hazards enter the daily lives of all people and attain a unique visibility as compared with other medical practices."[1] The "problems and hazards" had at this moment thrust vaccination policy under a spotlight. In the first three months of the year, some seventy health officials, researchers from academia and industry, and representatives of the lay public met in a series of federally sponsored working groups to conduct a thorough-going reassessment of some of the most fundamental aspects of policy. These committee members, like rank-and-file immunization providers around the country, confronted a thicket of legal, ethical, and political issues as they sought simultaneously to achieve high levels of coverage, provide accurate and useful information to the public about vaccine risks and benefits, administer school-based mandates in a way that respected parental autonomy, and maintain an adequate and stable supply of vaccines.

Several interrelated crises and trends fueled this intense scrutiny. The largest mass vaccination campaign in the country's history, an effort to protect against a feared epidemic of a deadly flu, had collapsed into a morass of legal claims and negative publicity. A series of tort actions against makers of the oral polio vaccine holding them liable for their failure to warn recipients of the small risk of vaccine-induced paralysis threatened to drive producers from the market and undermine supply. These lawsuits, along with the use of school mandates, sparked debates about whether the parents of vaccine recipients, like the parents of children receiving other clinical care, had a right to give informed consent, and whether those administering vaccines had a duty to warn about potential harms. All of these developments were situated within a broader social movement for patients' rights and a rejection of medical paternalism, in a political climate in which the judgment of government and scientific elites was met with increasing cynicism and mistrust.

This chapter examines events during the 1970s and 1980s, a period of both great success and unprecedented difficulty for vaccination programs. On the heels of the immunization work groups, Secretary of Health, Education and Welfare Joseph Califano announced a major new federal initiative in the spring of 1977 to boost the percentage of children fully protected. A dramatic increase in funding launched new rounds of publicity, which, in combination with a national push to enforce school entry requirements, succeeded in raising coverage levels among school-age youth. While the initiative was generally seen as a success, the issue of legal liability continued to hover ominously until the early 1980s, when a controversy erupted over the pertussis vaccine. Health officials clashed with parent activists who believed their children had suffered severe neurological damage from the vaccine. Their claims gave a powerful new force to the growing chorus of demands that the federal government take responsibility for compensating the few individuals inevitably harmed for the sake of ensuring society's protection from infectious disease.

INFORMED CONSENT, DUTY TO WARN, AND THE LIABILITY CRISIS

As the public health community was debating whether to end routine smallpox vaccination in the United States in the 1960s, another, more far-reaching controversy over vaccine risks and benefits unfolded. Unlike the decision-making about smallpox, which involved the deliberations of scientific advisory bodies and government bureaucracies, the new debates were conducted in a far more adversarial environment: the courtroom.

The success of polio control efforts gave rise to the controversy. Between 1969 and 1976, just 132 cases of paralytic polio were reported in the entire country. But fully one-third of these were thought to be caused by the vaccine itself, due to the phenomenon of reversion to virulence. The risk of vaccine-induced polio was estimated to be approximately one case of the disease for every 11 million people vaccinated.[2] The imminence of polio eradication thus posed the same ethical question that had arisen with smallpox: what level of risk from a vaccine was acceptable as a disease declined to vanishing levels? To this question was joined a new, corollary issue: what duties did those involved in immunization programs have to warn vaccine recipients of such risks?

Giving these questions special urgency was a string of court rulings against the makers of the polio vaccine. As we saw in chapter 1, the issue of legal liability for vaccine-related injury had first arisen in the late nineteenth century in cases of medical negligence or wrongful death brought against doctors. The first successful litigation against a manufacturer was in the case involving Cutter Laboratories for the ill-fated lots of its Salk vaccine that had killed or crippled hundreds of recipients in the spring of 1955. In 1960, a California appellate court had found for the plaintiffs in a case brought against Cutter by several recipients.[3] The decision in the case, *Gottsdanker v. Cutter,* held that the pharmaceutical company had not been negligent in its manufacturing, yet nevertheless was responsible for the harm the product had caused. The case was significant because it established the legal concept of product liability without fault.[4]

During the 1960s, makers of the Sabin oral vaccine also faced suits, but these differed in a crucial respect from the litigation arising from the Cutter incident. The Sabin vaccine was not a defective product—the potential to cause illness was an inherent property of the vaccine (though Sabin himself continued to question whether it was truly responsible for the rare cases of paralysis it was thought to cause).[5] Because the vaccine was considered in legal terms to be "unavoidably unsafe," the question arose of who, if anyone, had a duty to warn consumers of its tiny risk. Two court cases, one involving a mass vaccination campaign and the other arising from routine clinical practice, produced rulings that answered the question.

The first was the 1968 case of *Davis v. Wyeth.* The case originated when thirty-nine-year-old Glynn Richard Davis attended a mass vaccination clinic in West Yellowstone, Montana, in March 1963. Even though the surgeon general had issued a statement a year earlier that Sabin's live vaccine was not appropriate for adults over thirty because of the heightened risk of vaccine-induced paralysis in this age group, the Idaho Falls Medical Society, which was running the campaign, gave Davis the vaccine. One month later, he was diagnosed with paralytic polio, which was determined to be vaccine-induced. A three-judge panel on the ninth circuit court of appeals held that Wyeth Laboratories, the manufacturer, had a duty either to warn recipients of the small risk or be assured that the vaccine's purchaser—a medical society, public health department, or private physician—would give the warning.[6] One judge dissented from the opinion, claiming that the package insert that Wyeth included with each bottle of one hundred doses, which contained excerpts of the surgeon general's advisory, constituted sufficient warning.

The precedent established in *Davis* was extended from the context of a mass vaccination campaign to any clinical encounter in *Reyes v. Wyeth.* Eight-month-old Anita Reyes had been taken by her parents to a health department clinic in Mission, Texas, in 1970. Two weeks after being given a dose of the Sabin vaccine, she was hospitalized and diagnosed with paralytic polio. The nurse at the clinic who gave Anita Reyes the vaccine testified that she had not read the girl's parents the warning that Wyeth included as a package insert, and that it was not the policy of clinic staff to give such warnings to patients receiving vaccines. Anita Reyes's mother, the court held, could not assume the risk for her child, because no one had informed her of the danger inherent in the product. A federal district court in Texas awarded Reyes $200,000 in damages, a verdict that was upheld by a circuit court of appeals in 1974.[7] Citing the decision handed down six years earlier in *Davis,* the judges held that if the manufacturer could not warn the recipient directly, it would have to ensure that whoever gave it to the recipient would do so. Wyeth appealed to the U.S. Supreme Court, but the justices declined to hear the case.[8]

In amicus curiae briefs filed on behalf of Wyeth, both the American Academy of Pediatrics and the Conference of State and Territorial Epidemiologists protested that warning every recipient of a vaccine of the minuscule risk involved would unduly alarm the public and undermine the effectiveness of immunization programs—a position the court rejected as paternalistic: "[W]e believe that a warning advising a patron of a public health clinic of the relative risk of contracting polio from a 'wild' source against the slight chance of contracting it from the vaccine would not be terrifying or confusing."[9] In the court's view, "the right of the individual to choose and control what risk he will take" lay at the heart of the decision.

For many in the public health community, a bitter irony of the *Reyes* case was that, according to the best scientific assessments, Anita Reyes had almost certainly not contracted the disease from the vaccine. A polio outbreak was in progress in that region of south Texas at the time the child had been taken to the clinic. Several expert witnesses, including Neal Nathanson, the Johns Hopkins epidemiologist who had been one of the chief investigators of the Cutter incident, testified at the trial that the child's risk of contracting polio from someone in the community at the time she became ill was approximately one in 3,000, while her risk of contracting it from the vaccine was about one in 5.88 million.[10] Subsequent analyses of the *Reyes* verdict harshly criticized the court for ignoring powerful evidence that Wyeth's product was not responsible for the alleged harm; one report declared that the ruling in the case "signaled the unhinging of liability from causation, and made all previous experience meaningless in assessing the exposure of vaccine manufacturers."[11] Another legal expert noted, "It is difficult for the drug companies to defend in these cases, since they are trying to prove a negative—that is, that the drug did *not* cause the devastating injury and disability that was clearly sustained by the plaintiff from some cause."[12]

The rulings in *Davis, Reyes,* and a raft of other court cases in the 1960s and 1970s were alarming to public health authorities, and even more so to pharmaceutical companies, who saw them as opening the door to potentially ruinous legal costs. Drug makers contended that vaccines were relatively unprofitable compared to other biologic products, because profit margins were lower and patent protection was narrower.[13] Between 1962 and 1977, partly in response to the wave of litigation, half of the twelve companies producing vaccines withdrew from the market; in the case of several vaccines, including the live polio and measles vaccines, there was only one producer left by the late 1970s.[14]

The U.S. Department of Health, Education and Welfare was sufficiently concerned about both the legal and ethical implications of the risks of the live polio vaccine that it called upon the Institute of Medicine, a branch of the National Academy of Sciences that advised the government on health issues, to conduct a full reexamination of the nation's polio vaccination policy and revisit the relative advantages and disadvantages of the live and killed vaccines. Salk's inactivated vaccine had fallen into almost complete disuse by the late 1960s and was no longer produced nationally. But some experts argued that because of the fundamental shift in the balance of risks and benefits that the decline of polio had created, it was no longer appropriate for the country to rely solely on a vaccine that carried the risk, however minuscule, of causing paralysis. But because the inactivated vaccine was less effective at controlling the spread of polioviruses in the community, a switch back to using the Salk vaccine only, assuming approximately the same level of vaccination coverage that currently existed in the population, would put the country at risk of increased polio outbreaks. The committee therefore recommended a policy of continuing to use the live preparation as the principal vaccine, but offering the inactivated formula to people at heightened risk of vaccine-induced disease, including those with immune suppression and adults undergoing polio vaccination for the first time.[15]

The court rulings on the Sabin vaccine emerged from evolving legal concepts of tort liability that made it easier for consumers who were injured by defective products to recover damages from manufacturers.[16] The verdicts also reflected the erosion of the paternalistic ethos that had traditionally characterized relationships in the health care system. Drawing on the discourse of the civil rights movement, feminism, consumer activism, and other challenges to long-standing power hierarchies, a patients' rights movement arose during the 1960s and 1970s that demanded full participation in decisions involving medicine and bodily integrity.[17] At the same time, the stature of the medical profession, like that of many other social institutions, underwent a sharp erosion.[18] The revelation in 1972 of the U.S. Public Health Service's infamous Tuskegee syphilis study, and the exposé of hepatitis vaccine trials involving mentally retarded children at the Willowbrook State School in New York, which some considered ethically questionable, were just two of the most well-publicized examples of scientific experts being viewed as violating the public trust. In this climate, it was perhaps inevitable that vaccine manufacturers and health officials who managed immunization programs would become subject to the same demands for accountability. Thus by 1979, a representative of the National Consumers League could tell participants at a forum on immunization that "experts are not necessarily the best equipped to make judgments on acceptable public risks and benefits. Such judgments should be made by a broader-based group in which consumers must have significant participation."[19]

Both drawing on and contributing to these social changes was the popularization of informed consent. This ethical principal held that it was a basic right of all people to choose freely, based on full knowledge of potential risks and benefits, whether or not to undergo a medical procedure.[20] (Minors were generally considered to be incapable of giving informed consent; the consent of a parent or legal guardian was therefore needed on their behalf, although this varied by age and the type of procedure.)[21] Informed consent assumed great salience in health care during this period, becoming codified in ethical guidelines governing clinical medicine and biomedical research. But how the principle should be applied to vaccination was far from clear, especially since, as a result of the sweeping changes in legislation during the 1970s, most children were now legally required to receive several vaccines before they could attend school. LeRoy Walters, a prominent bioethicist, commented on the striking diversion of public health policy from the developments that were taking place in medicine:

> In the patient-physician relationship, we have seen an increasing emphasis on patient autonomy. Informed consent means that it is the patient who ultimately decides, on the basis of a fair presentation of the facts, what treatments shall be employed in the medical care context.... In the public health arena, the momentum during the 1970's has been in the opposite direction. Several state legislatures have passed new mandatory immunization laws, and old laws are being enforced with unaccustomed vigor.... In this public health context, there is little or no room for individual autonomy and informed consent.[22]

Alan Hinman of the Center for Disease Control, a leading proponent of school-based requirements, acknowledged that the use of legal mandates recast the very meaning of consent. "The concept of consent ... implies a free choice," he told participants at the annual immunization conference in 1978. "Sometimes, however, society decides to do things that may not necessarily include individual volition. Some of these include the military draft, income taxes, and school immunization laws. In these situations, the term 'consent' may be a misnomer. Nonetheless, I believe we can agree that the obligation to ensure an informed participant remains."[23]

The new focus on the inherent risks of vaccines and the proliferation of mandates for vaccination prior to school attendance gave rise to a growing chorus of demands that the federal government assume responsibility for vaccine-related injuries. As early as 1965, in the wake of the first lawsuits arising from the oral polio vaccine, the federal Advisory Committee on Immunization Practices had considered the desirability of a system through which vaccine manufacturers were freed from legal liability for non-negligent damages resulting from their products, and harmed individuals could receive publicly supported compensation. The committee predicted—correctly—that "the net cost of litigation and settlements resulting from the oral polio vaccine associated illnesses must necessarily be reflected in increased vaccine costs. Further, it would seem but a matter of time until lawsuits under the 'implied warranty' principle would be applied to other immunizing agents and in many additional states."[24] But it was not until a decade later, following the verdicts in *Davis* and *Reyes*, that calls for such a system grew widespread.

Typical was a commentary in 1975 in the journal *Pediatrics*, which asserted that the mandate of vaccination through school entry laws was placing the country on a "collision course" with its failure to adopt a coherent plan for dealing with vaccine-related injuries.[25] "Society— not the manufacturer, the physician, or the patient—should support those who suffer the adverse consequences of our laws," the author claimed. The Institute of Medicine committee that evaluated the policy on the live and inactivated polio vaccines had declared in its conclusions, "It is essential that liability for non-negligent losses sustained by persons with vaccine-associated ... cases of paralytic poliomyelitis be assumed by the federal government."[26] Proponents pointed out that several other countries had adopted some form of government compensation plan. West Germany had instituted the first such program in 1961, followed by France in 1964; in the 1970s, Japan, Switzerland, Denmark, New Zealand, Sweden, and the United Kingdom all adopted similar programs.[27]

These complex and interrelated ethical and legal issues—how risks and benefits should be balanced, whether and to what extent those responsible for immunization programs had a duty to warn participants, who should bear the liability for the small number of people inevitably harmed by vaccines—all crystallized over the course of 1976, when officials at the CDC had to deal with one of the most difficult crises in its history: forestalling a feared epidemic of swine flu.

SWINE FLU AND THE NATIONAL IMMUNIZATION WORK GROUPS

In January 1976, an army cadet at Fort Dix in New Jersey died of the flu. A culture of the virus revealed that the strain was closely related to the one that had caused the worldwide influenza pandemic in 1918 that had killed at least 20 million people. As alarmed officials at the CDC considered mounting a mass campaign to protect every American from the possible reemergence of the deadly strain, they were faced with an ethical dilemma. If they went ahead with the plan and the feared epidemic failed to materialize, some number of injuries, and possibly deaths, might result from needless use of the vaccine. If they failed to vaccinate preemptively and the epidemic occurred, thousands could die from the flu, and the CDC would be blamed for having failed to fulfill its duty. In April, David Sencer, the CDC's director, who had spearheaded the measles eradication effort a decade earlier, recommended that the program go forward, and President Gerald Ford announced it to the country.[28]

Problems plagued the enterprise from the beginning. Over the summer, the pharmaceutical companies making the vaccine announced that their insurers were refusing to provide them with coverage because of liability concerns in light of the recent verdict in *Reyes;* only after the U.S. Congress passed a bill authorizing the federal government to assume liability was the program able to move ahead. Prominent scientists and researchers attacked the program as unnecessary and dangerous, recommending instead that the vaccine be stockpiled for quick deployment only if the feared epidemic actually began to occur. The informed consent forms that Congress, as a condition of the government's assuming liability for the program, had required the CDC to develop to warn recipients of potential side effects were criticized as confusing and even misleading by some experts, including members of the National Commission for the Protection of Human Subjects.[29] Just days after the program began its late start in October, three people with cardiac conditions died shortly after receiving the vaccine, prompting nine states to suspend their programs. The deaths, though ultimately judged to have been coincidental, inflamed doubts about safety that were exacerbated by persistent negative coverage in the media. In a survey in New York City in mid November, more than half the respondents said they had not been vaccinated and did not intend to be, citing as reasons that the vaccine was unnecessary, that they were afraid of it, or that their physician had recommended against it.[30]

Then, in late November, reports came in to the CDC of people who had recently been vaccinated being stricken with Guillain-Barré Syndrome (GBS), a rare, sometimes life-threatening neurological disorder that can cause paralysis. By the middle of the next month, more than fifty cases of GBS had been reported in ten states; the majority of cases had received the vaccine within the previous month. On December 16, 1976, the program was suspended, never to resume. Some 40 million people had received the vaccine. Although this was the largest number of people ever vaccinated in a single mass campaign, it was less than one-fifth of the national target population.

The handling of the swine flu program was widely viewed as a debacle for all concerned.[31] In February 1977, incoming Secretary of Health, Education, and Welfare Joseph Califano fired Sencer; ostensibly the reason was that the new secretary wanted to select his own staff, but Sencer's handling of the swine flu program was widely believed to be the reason for the dismissal.[32] Many critics of the program claimed that the CDC's handling of it had served to undermine already shaky trust in the public health system and vaccination in particular, and that the program had diverted scarce resources from routine immunization programs that were of greater value.[33] Commenting in early 1977, Califano said it was "undeniable that the swine flu program has affected the public's perception of influenza immunization and immunization generally. People were confused by the disagreements between experts and by the difficulties that beset the program once it was under way."[34]

The extent to which the negative publicity generated by the swine flu debacle hurt immunization rates for other diseases is uncertain. A survey a year later commissioned by the CDC to gauge national attitudes and, in particular, to determine whether there had been a change in people's intentions to be vaccinated or have their children vaccinated suggested that, for the most part, people distinguished between the swine flu vaccine and those for other illnesses. Approximately 90 percent of respondents felt that vaccinations in general were either "very safe" or "moderately safe"; when asked about those that were unsafe, people singled out the swine flu vaccine. In general, the survey concluded, "behavior and beliefs about Influenza vaccines are different from behavior and beliefs about vaccines for other diseases." But the survey also found there was "a general lethargy and feelings of 'it can't happen here' and 'it can't happen to me or my children.'... People's theoretical beliefs about immunization in general and actual personal practices are two very different things."[35]

The most significant legacy of the swine flu affair, then, was not its impact on public acceptance of vaccination. Rather, the episode forced to the top of the policy agenda the issues of informed consent and liability for vaccine-related injuries that had been percolating for the previous decade. Over a four-month period in late 1976 and early 1977, in the wake of the aborted swine flu program, the Department of Health, Education and Welfare convened a series of working groups made up of academics, health officials, and representatives of vaccine manufacturers and consumer groups, who prepared recommendations on key policy areas, including financing and supply, public education, liability, and informed consent.[36]

Perhaps most challenging were the deliberations of the committee on informed consent, chaired by the bioethicist LeRoy Walters. In light of the international consensus that had emerged about the rights of bodily integrity in medical contexts, were mandatory vaccination laws ethically tenable? Could a parent faced with the exclusion of a child from school be considered to have freely consented? The committee concluded that there were several essential differences between immunization and other medical procedures that made it uncertain whether the model of informed consent that prevailed in biomedical research and the clinical encounter was applicable. Because of the high numbers of people involved in mass vaccination programs, opportunities for interaction between the participant and the health care provider were limited. Because immunization was sponsored by the government on behalf of society, individuals were under special obligations to participate. The risks of receiving a vaccination were much lower than the risks associated with most types of medical procedures where informed consent was customary.[37]

The committee members agreed that voluntary programs were preferable to mandatory ones, and that compulsion for adults should be invoked only in cases of urgent health threats. But the devil was in the details, of course, and members were unable to agree on a precise wording for a policy that would cover the varied situations in which compulsion might be invoked. The committee split evenly between two very similarly phrased position statements that differed subtly in the emphasis they gave to questions of autonomy and public participation in decision-making.[38] In its final report, the committee recommended the establishment of a national council that would formulate "clear, publicly announced criteria" for determining whether immunization programs for particular diseases should be mandatory or voluntary.[39]

The difficulty of achieving consensus on the issue was further illustrated by the numerous dissenting and supplementary opinions filed by committee members as appendices to the official report. Four members of the panel stated that the final recommendations did not go far enough in stressing that compulsory vaccination was acceptable only in cases where the unvaccinated posed an imminent danger of spreading disease to others. Implicitly invoking the "harm principle" of the utilitarian philosopher John Stuart Mill, the four asserted that people should not be forced to be vaccinated simply for their own good.[40] This same group also objected that the committee's final proposal for a national advisory council on vaccine policy did not stipulate that a majority of members be representatives of the lay public.[41] Quite different was the perspective of a state health commissioner on the committee, who objected to the very idea of a national council. Given the constitutional delegation of health authority to the states, and the extensive network of laws already in place, she claimed in a dissenting opinion that creating such a council would represent a "presumptuous" intrusion on states' rights.[42]

In the wake of the swine flu affair and the meetings of the immunization work groups, disagreement prevailed over who should be responsible for warning consumers about vaccine risks, how these warnings should be conveyed, and what information they should contain. Documents detailed enough to provide legal protection for pharmaceutical companies were not the most useful to consumers. In response to the liability verdicts against them, makers of the oral polio vaccine had developed information forms that the Institute of Medicine described as "lengthy, complicated and defensively written documents for protecting manufacturers, rather than conveying usable information to those vaccinated."[43] Nevertheless, HEW's general counsel determined that an informational form to be signed by recipients was the most appropriate way for the federal government to deal with the issue, and in 1977, the CDC developed a series of forms that would be included with all federally supplied vaccine administered in public settings. Each form described the disease in question, the estimated effectiveness of the vaccine, the number of doses needed, possible side effects of the vaccine, and contraindications.

Striking a balance between providing legal protection and educating the public proved difficult, however. In pilot testing, between one-fifth and one-third of those given a vaccine stated that they had not read the entire form, and around 10 percent did not understand what they had read; as many as one in four could not answer basic questions about the information on the form after they had read it.[44] The forms also received mixed reviews from health officials and legislators when the CDC submitted them for comment. After reviewing one of the forms with legal counsel, Donald Lyman, head of disease control for New York State, wrote to the CDC that the forms were "unnecessary, burdensome and of no legal status in a jurisdiction such as New York with mandatory immunization laws."[45] Echoing the concerns expressed in the amicus briefs in *Reyes,* other health officials objected to the fact that the proposed information forms were framed as "warnings" of possible risks.

IMPORTANT INFORMATION
ABOUT MEASLES AND MEASLES VACCINE
Please read this carefully

ME 12/1/77

WHAT IS MEASLES? Measles is the most serious of the common childhood diseases. Usually it causes a rash, high fever, cough, runny nose, and watery eyes lasting 1 to 2 weeks. Sometimes it is more serious. It causes an ear infection or pneumonia in nearly 1 out of 10 children who get it. One child out of every 1,000 who get measles has an inflammation of the brain (encephalitis). This can lead to convulsions, deafness, or mental retardation. One child in every 10,000 who get measles dies from it. Measles can also cause a pregnant woman to have a miscarriage or possibly a deformed baby.

Before measles vaccine shots were available there were hundreds of thousands of cases each year. Nearly all children got measles by the time they were 15. Now, because of the wide use of measles vaccine, a child's risk of getting measles is much lower. However, if children stop getting vaccinated, the risk of getting measles will go right back up again.

MEASLES VACCINE: Immunization with measles vaccine is one of the best ways to prevent measles. The vaccine is given by injection and is very effective. In over 90% of people, one shot will give protection, probably for life. Since protection may not be quite as good if the shot is given very early in life, measles shots should be given at 15 months of age or older. Measles vaccine can be given along with rubella (German measles) and mumps vaccine.

POSSIBLE SIDE EFFECTS FROM THE VACCINE: About 1 out of every 5 children will get a rash or slight fever 1 or 2 weeks after the shot. Although experts are not sure, it seems that about 1 out of a million children who get the shot may have a more serious reaction such as inflammation of the brain (encephalitis).

WARNING — SOME PERSONS SHOULD *NOT* TAKE MEASLES VACCINE WITHOUT CHECKING WITH A DOCTOR:

- Those who are sick right now with something more serious than a cold.
- Those with allergies to eggs or an antibiotic called neomycin.
- Those with cancer or leukemia or lymphoma.
- Those with diseases which lower the body's resistance to infection.
- Those taking drugs that lower the body's resistance to infection, such as cortisone.

PREGNANCY: Measles vaccine experts do not know if measles vaccine can cause special problems for pregnant women or their unborn babies. However, doctors usually avoid giving any drugs or vaccines to pregnant women unless there is a specific need. To be safe, pregnant women should not get the shot. A woman who gets the shot should wait 3 months before getting pregnant.

QUESTIONS: If you have any questions about measles or measles vaccination, please ask us now or call your doctor or health department before you sign this form.

REACTIONS: If the person who received the vaccine gets sick and visits a doctor, hospital, or clinic in the 4 weeks after vaccination, please report it to:

PLEASE KEEP THIS PART OF THE INFORMATION SHEET FOR YOUR RECORDS

I have read the information on this form about measles and measles vaccine. I have had a chance to ask questions which were answered to my satisfaction. I believe I understand the benefits and risks of measles vaccine and request that it be given to me or to the person named below for whom I am authorized to make this request. ME 12/1/77

INFORMATION ON PERSON TO RECEIVE VACCINE			FOR CLINIC USE
Name (Please Print)	Birthdate	Age	Clinic Ident.
Address	County		Date Vaccinated
State, ZIP			Manufacturer and Lot No.
X			Site of injection
Signature of person to receive vaccine or person authorized to make the request		Date	

Figure 21. In response to the concerns about liability that the litigation over the oral polio vaccine and the swine flu program had raised, the Center for Disease Control developed a series of information forms in 1977 for parents that described both the risks of the vaccine and the disease it prevented. These were not true "consent" forms, since most children were now required by law to be vaccinated before they could attend school, but they were designed to fulfill the ethical duty to warn consumers about vaccine risks.

"If the word 'warn' is used, with its connotation of danger, the safety of vaccines could be seriously questioned by parents who must provide consent for their children's immunizations," wrote the Massachusetts director of communicable disease control. "There is almost universal antipathy and hostility on the part of state and territorial epidemiologists, as well as private physicians, on [sic] the suggested Risk Benefit Forms we have previewed."[46] Others took the essentially paternalistic position that parents could not be relied upon to make appropriate judgments. "It is unreasonable and unfair to burden parents fully with the responsibility of decisions for or against immunization, based on descriptions of benefits and hazards," the medical director of the New Haven Health Department said. "From observing 10,000 people signing consent forms before flu immunizations, it appears that less than 3 percent read the forms and fewer understand it. This is a cumbersome time consuming and useless ritual."[47]

As an attempt to reconcile the legal and ethical mandates of informed consent and the duty to warn with the practical realities of the clinical encounter, the CDC's forms were a compromise that satisfied no one. They were nevertheless required for use with all publicly administered vaccines beginning in early 1978. The broader issue of compensating those few people who suffered harm from vaccines remained stalled amid seemingly intractable political disagreements over how such a system might function. It would take a new crisis in vaccine safety to propel the various parties to this debate toward a solution. Meanwhile, the U.S. Public Health Service was eager to recover from the public relations debacle of the swine flu program and reinvigorate a system that was widely seen as foundering. The necessary political will—and funding—for such a recommitment was soon to come from the new presidential administration.

Betty Bumpers, the wife of the Arkansas senator and former governor Dale Bumpers, had championed the cause of childhood vaccination when she had been the state's first lady. Bumpers was a friend of Roslyn Carter, and when President Jimmy Carter took office at the beginning of 1977, Betty Bumpers convinced Roslyn Carter that the issue should be elevated to the top of the nation's health priorities. The Carters requested that HEW Secretary Joseph Califano move ahead with a national program.[48] In April 1977, just a few months after Carter had taken office, Califano announced the Childhood Immunization Initiative.

Having been burned by the failure to eradicate measles a decade before, CDC leaders no longer framed their objectives in terms of disease reduction. Instead, the goal, for the first time, would be the achievement of a target level of fully immunized children. The initiative set an eighteen-month timeline for boosting the percentage of children fully protected by recommended vaccines to 90 percent by October 1978. Federal funding increased dramatically, rising from about $5 million under the final year of the Ford administration to $17 million in 1977 during the first year of the Childhood Immunization Initiative, and $23 million in 1978.[49]

The central pillar of the initiative was a national push to enforce the school immunization mandates that had been passed during the previous decade.[50] Placing a law on the books was one thing, health officials had quickly discovered, but verifying the immunization status of all children in a school—much less dealing with students who faced exclusion because they were delinquent in their shots—was another matter altogether. Giving teeth to the laws would require confronting thorny questions about how to balance two desirable social goals: controlling infectious disease and providing universal public education.

"NO SHOTS, NO SCHOOL": COMPULSION AND ITS DISCONTENTS

Conflict over the enforcement of school vaccination requirements was as old as the laws themselves. Ensuring that all students had the mandated protection entailed cooperation at the state and local levels between health and education administrators, who had differing missions, priorities, and political constituencies. In the 1920s, as we saw in chapter 2, New York's smallpox law for students was a dead letter in much of the state because school boards were unwilling or unable to enforce it. Parents who were hostile or indifferent to vaccination openly flouted the law, while local health officials fumed that school authorities—who saw smallpox as a very remote threat that did not warrant disrupting classes—did little to ensure compliance. By the 1970s, when school laws became universal in the United States, enforcement had grown more complicated. Vaccines against seven diseases, not one, were now required, and schools thus had to keep track of more student records than ever, with scant resources to do so. Parents were in general supportive of vaccination, as the CDC's survey following the swine flu episode had shown, but they were often uncertain which vaccines a child had received. If the documentation had been lost or mislaid, many schools admitted the child anyway. The result was the persistence of diseases that, like smallpox in the 1920s, were readily preventable.

Especially problematic was measles, the most contagious of childhood infections.

States found that they had to take aggressive actions to ensure that school laws were enforced. Tennessee had enacted a law covering all recommended immunizations in 1967, but it was not until 1973 that any of the state's counties were fully compliant with the law. Cooperation was achieved only after the state health department leaned heavily on schools, threatening to expel unprotected children and bring civil actions against noncompliant principals.[51] Missouri's law had gone largely ignored for years until the health department adopted what one official called a "no more Mr. Nice Guy" approach—gaining the backing of the state attorney general to pursue legal action against schools where unvaccinated children were found to be attending.[52] In New York, lax enforcement was especially prevalent in middle schools, which viewed the law as a concern of the elementary grades, and in which there were repeated outbreaks of measles among teenagers in the mid 1970s.[53] In the fall of 1976, the state health department, increasingly exasperated that control of measles should prove to be so elusive more than a decade after effective vaccines had become available, for the first time took a hard-line stance and insisted on enforcing the exclusion of all unvaccinated students from any school where a case of measles had occurred. "Excuses, excuses," a health department doctor wrote in a testy note to a local school health officer:

> Physicians and public health personnel last year continually blamed the outbreaks on everything but poor immunization status. "The vaccine didn't work." "The parents thought the child got measles vaccine in 1971; it was really rubella vaccine." "No parents keep good records." "They don't speak English." "Private physicians should protect their patients." "The county has no authority to intervene in an outbreak."... Our point of view is simple. You as the school health official are either satisfied the child is protected or you have him vaccinated.[54]

The record was especially bad in Nassau County on Long Island, which had been, according to the state health department, "consistently timid in its approach to control."[55] The standoff between health and education officials came to a head in the town of Oceanside in the spring of 1978, when a fifteen-year-old boy attending Boardman junior high school was diagnosed with measles. Health authorities met with the school superintendent, who was accompanied—in a reflection of the litigious climate surrounding immunization—by the school district's insurance agent and its attorneys. The insurers and lawyers advised the superintendent against taking any action to exclude unvaccinated pupils and rejected the proposal that vaccinations be given on site at the school unless there was a "hold harmless" agreement covering any liabilities or costs of the program. Fed up with what he viewed as procedural stonewalling, State Health Commissioner Robert Whalen obtained a court order barring ninety unvaccinated students from school.[56]

Less than two weeks later, a similar standoff developed in a district on Long Island. School officials there refused to go along with the state's immunization program until the county government agreed to indemnify them against all possible claims that might result from vaccine-related injuries. In May, Whalen once again obtained a court order against the board of education, superintendent of schools, and a school principal in the district demanding that they enforce the exclusion of unvaccinated students or face civil and criminal penalties.[57]

Skirmishes such as these and the belief that the promise of vaccination mandates for students remained unfulfilled provided the rationale for the focus on schools in the 1977 initiative. The CDC coordinated a massive drive to help states audit millions of student immunization records. One of the main barriers at the outset of the effort was uncertainty about whether immunization files held by schools were protected under federal law that guarded against the release of student records. That potential barrier was removed in 1978 when the federal Office of Education issued a ruling that immunization documents need not be accorded confidential status. In the wake of the decision, state health departments around the country, with the encouragement and assistance of the CDC, reviewed the school immunization records for some 28 million students. At the same time, HEW Secretary Califano wrote to the governors of all forty-five states that had mandatory school vaccination laws asking that they be enforced to the fullest extent possible. Califano also encouraged those states where the legal language was not "sufficiently comprehensive" to strengthen their laws and close any loopholes that allowed children to remain unvaccinated.[58]

The legal, political, and ethical issues around school mandates were nowhere more apparent than in the New York City school system, the nation's largest. The 1977 immunization initiative set in motion a series of confrontations over the responsibility for determining which students were vaccinated and what should be done about those who were not.

The health department had for several decades offered immunizations as part of its program of school-based clinical services. But in the

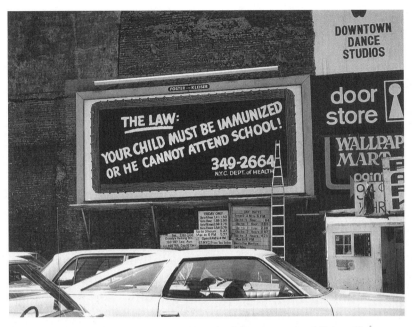

Figure 22. In 1978, New York City launched an intensive publicity effort to educate parents about the "no shots, no school" policy. Cities around the country in the late 1970s ran into numerous logistical problems with enforcing their school vaccination requirements. Courtesy New York City Municipal Archives.

wake of the CDC's introduction of mandated information forms—which required the parent or legal guardian to give consent for each shot a child received—it was forced to abandon its long-standing practice: "it would be impractical," health officials determined, "to attempt to continue school based immunization programs because of the unlikelihood of obtaining multiple informed consents."[59] Instead, the department would operate special walk-in clinics around the city where parents could bring children to get their shots before it was time to start classes. At the same time, an aggressive advertising campaign, including billboards, flyers, and mailings, was launched to educate parents about the "no shots, no school" policy. The magnitude of the problem facing the city was revealed when an audit of the city's schools found widespread failure to keep records of students' immunization status. At one school, less than half of the pupils had the required documents on file, and the education official responsible for the records was fired.[60]

Over the next two years, the city's health and education bureaucracies remained locked in a stalemate over implementing the "no shots, no school" policy. In the fall of 1978, only a few students were excluded from classes.[61] When the health department audited several schools' records the following autumn, it found that thousands of children were being allowed to attend classes though they were not in compliance with the law.[62] School principals, whose work revolved around keeping students *in* class, were reluctant to keep them out; furthermore, keeping track of students' immunization records "places demands on schools ... which are already burdened with a great many priorities," the chancellor explained in a letter to the health commissioner.[63] Health officials, for their part, saw the schools' lack of cooperation in stark terms: it was failure to observe a law that was sensible and straightforward. Continued outbreaks of measles—evidence that unvaccinated students were still in class—led the health commissioner to seek the advice of legal council to determine his options for forcing recalcitrant principals to comply with the law and exclude unprotected pupils. (State law allowed civil penalties of up to $500 to be levied against the noncompliant principals.)[64]

Finally, in the fall of 1980, after two years of pressure from the city council president and the health department, school officials adopted a get-tough stance toward those students—estimated to be almost one-fourth of the city's 930,000 K-12 students—who lacked proof of the required protection.[65] Repeated notices in multiple languages were sent home to parents, and announcements were made over school loudspeakers. As an emergency measure, health department officials agreed to hold on-site clinics at selected schools with especially low rates of vaccination (though they later discovered, to their dismay, that some principals ended up signing students' consent forms, or allowing them to sign their own forms, in order to expedite the process).[66] In spite of the extra efforts, some 28,000 youths—about 3 percent of the student population—were barred from classes in November 1980. The board of education received "average daily attendance" reimbursement from the state based on its student census, and the absences cost the city thousands of dollars per day.[67] By the end of the 1980–81 school year, the health department had summoned the principals of eleven schools (one public, three parochial, and three private) before its administrative tribunal to face fines for not cooperating with the effort.[68]

In the fall of 1981, when mass exclusions were once again enforced, the strategy began to attract public criticism. "Why are we punishing the kids?" an op-ed columnist in the *New York Times* asked. "Once a child misses a few classes, then a few days, the slide toward permanent absence often becomes irreversible."[69] Even some health experts questioned the wisdom of controlling contagion at the expense of children's education. A former New York City health commissioner termed the exclusions "a latter-day version of outdated public-health police action."[70] But officials with the American Academy of Pediatrics rose to the defense of the city's actions. Concerns about forcing students into truancy were overblown, they contended, noting that just 1 percent of students remained excluded because of vaccination status as of November 1981, while an average of 16 percent of students were absent on any given school day.[71]

While New York City was notable for the magnitude of the problem and the amount of friction between health and education administrators, the situation there was not unique. Many American cities, including Los Angeles, Detroit, and Cincinnati, saw thousands of students barred from schoolhouses during the late 1970s.[72] These mass actions were the most visible side effect of the nationwide emphasis on schools as a site of vaccine promotion. A less high-profile, though equally significant, consequence was continued litigation over exemptions from school laws. As we saw in chapter 5, the enactment of the laws had provoked a flurry of suits from the mid 1960s to the mid 1970s by plaintiffs who were denied an exemption. In the wake of the 1977 immunization initiative, legal challenges continued, on varied constitutional bases.

In Mississippi and Maryland, exemption clauses were severed from school vaccination laws after courts found them unconstitutional. Mississippi granted a waiver only for children of parents "whose religious teachings require reliance on prayer or spiritual means of healing." In a 1979 case, the state supreme court agreed with the claim of Charles Brown, a chiropractor, that the exemption violated the equal protection provision of the Fourteenth Amendment because it discriminated against the large majority of parents who had no religious convictions against the practice.[73] In Maryland, a parent could opt out of vaccination if it conflicted with "the tenets and practice of a recognized church or religious denomination of which he is an adherent or member." In the decade following the addition of the exemption clause in 1972, waivers had been granted to members of only two groups: the Christian Science church and the Worldwide Church of God. Irving Davis, who objected to vaccination because of "personal religious views," was charged by school authorities with violating the state's mandatory education law for keeping his eight-year-old son out of school rather than consent to vaccination. Davis went to court, arguing that the statute violated the First Amendment's establishment clause. The court agreed that the exemption "contravenes the principle of government neutrality regarding different religious beliefs" and severed the provision from the rest of the law.[74]

In Ohio, however, a less restrictive law withstood judicial challenge. The exemption in that state was available to any "parent or guardian who objects to the immunization for good cause, including religious convictions." The chiropractor Stanley Hanzel made three constitutional arguments against the provision. He claimed it infringed on his right to privacy (this right did not exist in the Constitution, of course, but the U.S. Supreme Court had recently recognized a limited right to privacy in the context of certain personal decisions such as the use of contraception); that it contravened due process, because it authorized "local school officials to burden a fundamental right without providing guidelines for the officials' exercise of their authority"; and that it breached the equal protection clause, because school officials could deny a claim grounded in "chiropractic ethics" while granting exemptions to "similarly situated individuals" whose objections were religious. A U.S. district court in Ohio rejected all three of these arguments and left the law intact.[75]

One of the most interesting series of events occurred in New York State, where some of the first legal challenges against a religious exemption had been launched. In 1972, the state supreme court had found that the law posed problems with establishment of religion, but the judges had stopped short of declaring the exemption clause unconstitutional. In the fall of 1987, two families in the Long Island town of Northport brought suit against the school district after they were denied exemptions. Both couples, Alan and Claudia Sherr and Louis and Valerie Levy, challenged the law on the same ground that had been the basis of the 1972 case of *Maier v. Besser*: that the law's religious exemption discriminated against those whose faith did not explicitly proscribe vaccination. Citing the rulings that had been handed down in various states over the previous two decades, a U.S. district court judge held that New York's law violated the establishment and free exercise clauses of the First Amendment; instead of limiting the exemption to "bona fide members of a recognized religious organization," the state was obligated under the constitution to extend it to anyone who held sincere religious beliefs. "The primary effect of [the] limiting clause is manifestly the inhibiting of the religious practices of those individuals who oppose vaccination of their children on religious grounds but are not actually members of a religious organization that the state recognizes," the judge declared. Thus the statute was "blatantly discriminatory."[76]

As a result of the court's ruling, New York legislators were forced to revise the statute. No longer would an exemption be contingent on the petitioner belonging to a particular religious organization; instead, any sincerely held religious belief would be sufficient. Under the revised law, education officials had to assess individually each parental request for an exemption in order to determine whether or not the belief was founded in sincere religious convictions as opposed to secular ethical principles.[77] The cases of the two Northport families, the Sherrs and the Levys, provided a preview of the types of judgments that would henceforth be necessary. Although the legal actions of the two families had been consolidated before the court because they raised the same constitutional questions, the plaintiffs had quite different backgrounds and belief systems. Under cross-examination, Alan Paul Sherr, a chiropractor, admitted that he had joined what the judge called a "mail order church"—the "Missionary Temple At Large, Universal Religious Brotherhood, Inc.," based in Sarasota, Florida—in order to qualify for an exemption. Although Sherr had claimed that he opposed on religious grounds any "intrusion" into the body, he admitted on the stand that he had taken his son to a dentist to have cavities filled, that he had had the boy's leg x-rayed when it was thought to be broken, and that the boy had been circumcised. The judge determined that the Sherrs' objections to vaccination stemmed from "chiropractic ethics, not from any religiously inspired source" and thus denied the couple's claim to an exemption.[78] Louis Levy, on the other hand, spoke thoughtfully on the stand about the tenets of bodily integrity that governed his practices and "greatly impressed the court with the seriousness with which he ha[d] contemplated the foundations of his religious beliefs and their implications for his family's daily life."[79] The court therefore granted the Levys an exemption.

By the mid 1980s, immunization rates among school-age youth had risen substantially. The CDC's push to ensure enforcement of school mandates was bolstered by the results of a 1981 study demonstrating that states with comprehensive and strictly enforced school entry laws had significantly lower measles incidence than those that did not.[80] The improved compliance with the laws came at a cost. Education for some youth was temporarily disrupted if they could not provide proof of their protection; some parents opposed to vaccination were denied the right to make decisions about an aspect of their children's health care. Most health officials, politicians, and jurists considered these acceptable trade-offs in order to control infectious disease. But the confrontations in schoolrooms and courtrooms over the implementation of the laws were eclipsed during this period by a series of events that raised even more difficult questions about risks, benefits, and the costs of immunization.

PERTUSSIS, PARENTS, AND THE PATH TO A FEDERAL COMPENSATION SYSTEM

In early 1978, as the Childhood Immunization Initiative was in full swing, the state health commissioner of New Jersey, in a letter to the president of the Association of State and Territorial Health Officials, warned of "the devastating effect of the overhanging cloud of liability" on vaccination programs. Her comments reflected growing dissatisfaction among frontline immunization providers with what was widely perceived as the U.S. Public Health Service's dilatory handling of the urgent problems caused by tort claims against vaccine manufacturers. The CDC's information forms were seen as a Band-Aid, at best. "Until the liability issue is resolved through a different mechanism than the torts procedures now employed," she wrote, "production, supply, public information and education, consent and effective immunization status will all lag."[81]

The American Academy of Pediatrics had taken the lead in pushing the passage of legislation to create an indemnification and compensation system similar to those that existed in several other countries. Because immunizations were being required for school entry in the service of the public good, the AAP declared in a 1977 policy statement, society had an obligation to compensate those few who were injured in the course of complying with the laws. In 1981, the AAP issued a detailed outline of the specific elements that such a system should contain.[82] Meanwhile, some states began to take steps to address the problem. In 1977, California established a state-run compensation system to reimburse the medical and rehabilitative expenses of anyone who suffered a severe reaction from one of the vaccines mandated by state law (by the end of 1980, however, only one claim had been filed under the program).[83]

Those wary of the federal government's assuming liability pointed to the indemnification program that Congress had enacted in the summer of 1976 to enable the swine flu campaign to move ahead. In the wake of the campaign's collapse, almost four thousand injury claims seeking some $3.5 billion in damages were filed against the government. Close to two-thirds of these were ultimately denied or withdrawn. Most of the claims, according to a report commissioned by Congress, "were trivial at best, mischievous at worst, and ... a great deal of time and money has been wasted on distinguishing potentially valid claims from frivolous ones."[84] Even accounting for the large portion of claims that were dismissed, the federal government paid out some $20 million in the five years following the program.[85] These results did not bode well for an even more comprehensive system that would cover some or all routinely recommended vaccines.

In 1980, the U.S. House of Representatives asked the Congressional Office of Technology Assessment to prepare a report examining the possibility of creating a federal compensation program for vaccine-related injuries. The report laid out a host of complicated questions that would have to be answered. What should the program cover—all vaccines or only those legally mandated? What types of injuries should be compensated? Should compensation differ based on severity? What types of expenses should be compensated? Should there be a cap on awards? How should such a system be funded? Should the system provide an exclusive remedy or should tort claims through traditional legal channels still be permitted? And perhaps the most contentious question: How was a causal connection between a vaccination and an adverse event to be reliably established?[86] Because of the complexity of the issues, and the reluctance of the Reagan administration to involve the federal government in a new regulatory role, attempts to create a national system remained stalled in the early 1980s. But much as concerns over the risks of the polio and swine flu vaccines had sparked the initial calls for a compensation program, a new safety controversy—this time, over the vaccine for pertussis, or whooping cough—propelled the issue forward.

As we saw in chapter 3, the pertussis vaccine had a somewhat checkered history. In 1947, a pair of New York City physicians published a case report suggesting that fatal neurological complications might in rare instances result from the vaccine. "Despite this report, the risks of not immunizing against whooping cough are vastly greater than the risks of immunizing," the two authors concluded. "We can best summarize our belief in the safety of the pertussis vaccine by remarking that the authors' own children have been inoculated."[87] Over the next several years, scattered reports about severe side effects appeared in the medical literature but, as had been the case with injuries resulting from the smallpox vaccine, lack of systematic surveillance made it impossible to determine the frequency of these occurrences. The pertussis antigen had been implicated in a lawsuit involving Parke, Davis & Co.'s ill-fated product Quadrigen, which combined vaccines against diphtheria, pertussis, tetanus, and polio. Quadrigen was introduced in 1959 and pulled from the market three years later after reports of severe reactions, and in 1969, a federal judge ruled that the pertussis component had been responsible for an infant's brain damage.[88]

Nevertheless, use of the pertussis vaccine, typically given as one component of the combined diphtheria-pertussis-tetanus (DPT) preparation, continued to be widespread and uncontroversial. The vaccine became known for causing mild and transient reactions, including prolonged periods of fussiness and crying, and soreness and redness at the site of injection. But the incidence of more severe or long-lasting consequences remained unknown.

In 1974, however, an article in the British medical journal *Archives of Disease in Childhood* described thirty-six children who had experienced severe neurologic complications within two weeks of receiving the vaccine, including convulsions, prolonged unconsciousness, and partial paralysis; two children had died.[89] Widespread press coverage of the findings in Great Britain inflamed public fear. A prominent physician at the University of Glasgow, Gordon Stewart, became a highly visible spokesperson against pertussis vaccination, writing several articles and letters to the editors of scientific journals in Britain and the United States, appearing on British television, and appearing with the activist Association of Parents of Vaccine-Damaged Children.[90] Stewart claimed that the risk of a child suffering severe and possibly permanent brain damage from the vaccine far exceeded the risk of dying from, or even contracting, pertussis.[91] Amid a flood of negative press coverage, public uptake of the vaccine plummeted in the United Kingdom from about 80 percent in 1974 to about 30 percent in 1978.[92] At the end of 1977, and continuing through 1979, an epidemic of pertussis swept through the country, with some 100,000 cases of the disease reported and more than thirty deaths.[93] The controversy in the United Kingdom was followed by a similar (though less dramatic) sequence of events in Sweden and Japan as acceptance of the DPT shot fell in the wake of bad publicity.

Physicians and public health experts in the United States were troubled by the British findings but concluded that the risks of the vaccine were outweighed by the benefit of its ability to prevent pertussis. There was broad agreement, however, that research leading to the development of a safer vaccine was needed, as was better tracking of adverse events.[94] In the wake of the events in Great Britain, the CDC responded in 1978 to calls for better monitoring of vaccine adverse events by establishing a system through which the parents of children who received publicly funded vaccines were given the number of a hotline to call to report any illness occurring within four weeks of vaccination.[95] Because of the system's reliance on parental reporting, without medical verification, some of the reports were vague and incomplete.[96] The system suffered from underreporting because parents either did not keep the form or did not associate an adverse event with the vaccination, as well as from overreporting of some conditions that were subsequently judged to be unrelated to the vaccination. (In a revealing sign of the times, the CDC also established a system in the late 1970s to track the amount of litigation related to vaccine adverse events.)[97]

In spite of the new concern about the pertussis vaccine among health professionals, the controversies abroad attracted scant attention from the general public in the United States until 1982. In April of that year, a television station in Washington, D.C., aired a one-hour documentary titled "DPT: Vaccine Roulette," which featured dramatic personal testimony by numerous parents who believed the pertussis component of the DPT shot had caused severe and in many cases permanent neurological damage to their children. Portions of this were subsequently broadcast nationally on the NBC morning program *Today*, and it was also aired by several NBC affiliates around the country. In the weeks that followed, pediatricians around the country reported being inundated by calls from frightened parents.[98] The program drew widespread condemnation from the medical and public health community for what was viewed as a sensationalistic and unbalanced picture that overplayed the risks of side effects while barely mentioning the severe and more frequent consequences of the disease itself. The CDC's director, William Foege, labeled it "journalistic malpractice," while a UCLA physician whose research on the frequency of adverse events following the DPT shot had been cited in the program termed it "totally distorted."[99]

After the show aired, several parents in the Washington area who believed their own children had suffered harm from the DPT shot called the television station to see if any local groups were doing anything about the events described in the program. The station took their names and phone numbers, and the parents got in touch with each other. Eventually they formed an organization called Dissatisfied Parents Together (DPT), taking as their acronym the name of the vaccine which was the target of their activism.[100] The creation of Dissatisfied Parents Together added a highly vocal new constituency to the already broad array of groups pressing for action on the issues of liability and compensation. The group was made up largely of well-educated, middle-class parents and was led by a lawyer who had formerly worked for the federal government, and their actions jump-started the languishing efforts to move the issue forward in the political arena.[101]

A month after "Vaccine Roulette" aired, Senator Paula Hawkins (R-Fla.), devoted a hearing originally scheduled to discuss funding for immunization programs to considering instead the newly prominent charges of vaccination dangers. "It would be tragic," Hawkins declared in opening the session, "if efforts to eliminate or control communicable disease were to become hampered because the public's confidence was so eroded as to cause frightened segments of the population to oppose and reject vaccines."[102] The bulk of the hearings were concerned with the evidence as to whether and to what extent the pertussis component of the DPT vaccine caused neurological damage in children who received it. In addition to testimony from health officials, the committee heard from numerous parents who believed their children to have been harmed by the shot. In the wake of these hearings, Hawkins indicated that she might sponsor legislation creating a national compensation program if a plan were developed jointly by Dissatisfied Parents Together and the American Academy of Pediatrics.[103]

The concerns about the safety of the DPT shot quickly ballooned into a full-blown crisis with legal and economic dimensions that went beyond what had occurred with the oral polio vaccine, which had until then been the source of most vaccine-related legal activity. Lawyers began to run advertisements on television and in print media offering to represent the claims of parents who believed their children had suffered neurological damage from the DPT vaccine. The number of legal actions related to the vaccine across the country skyrocketed, rising from just two suits in 1978 to more than two hundred fifty annually by 1986.[104] A rise in the price of vaccines paralleled the trend in court cases. Between 1981 and 1986, the price of a dose of the DPT vaccine rose from about $.10 to about $3; although this was the most extreme increase, all other recommended childhood vaccines also rose in price.[105]

Pharmaceutical companies defended these increases as a necessary adaptation to the newly litigious climate—Lederle Laboratories contended that its potential liability for DPT injury lawsuits exceeded two hundred times its annual sales from the product—but skeptical parent groups questioned whether the pursuit of profits was the true motive and accused the firms of "crying 'liability crisis' all the way to the bank."[106]

The situation reached a critical juncture in the second half of 1984, when two of the five manufacturers of the DPT vaccine announced they were pulling out of the market and a third withdrew a planned shipment because of quality control problems. The CDC was forced in December to notify physicians around the country that there might be a national shortage of the vaccine and recommended that the fourth and fifth doses of the shot be delayed pending stabilization of the supply. After tense negotiations between the pharmaceuticals and the federal government, the makers committed to continuing production.[107] The publicity surrounding these events drew widespread attention to the precariousness of the nation's vaccination system and the problems it faced, and intensified calls for a federal response. A *New York Times* editorial claimed that vaccination was "a triumph of preventive medicine ... marred by a cruel injustice"—society's failure to provide for individuals harmed for the sake of community protection—and urged Congress to pass legislation based on the proposal that had been drafted by Dissatisfied Parents Together and the American Academy of Pediatrics.[108]

It was in the midst of the legal and political battles over liability that *DPT: A Shot in the Dark* was published. The book was co-authored by Harris Coulter, a historian who had written on medical dissidents of the nineteenth century, and Barbara Loe Fisher, one of the co-founders of Dissatisfied Parents Together.[109] Fisher's son Chris suffered from learning disabilities and attention deficit disorder, which Fisher believed were caused by the DPT shot he had received at age two and a half. The book was dedicated to the daughter of Dissatisfied Parents Together co-founder Jeffrey Schwartz; Julie Schwartz had suffered a grand mal seizure within hours of her first DPT shot when she was six months old and regularly suffered severe convulsions until her death two years later. The book interspersed a narrative about the dangerous history of the pertussis vaccine with dramatic vignettes of loving parents who fought against an unfeeling medical establishment after their children suffered severe and often permanent damage from the shot. While some reviewers found the book's claims misleading or tendentious, it served as a modern-day manifesto for those who questioned the vaccination orthodoxy.[110]

With its numerous personal histories of damaged youth, *A Shot in the Dark* was a direct descendent of the self-published 1914 tract in which James Loyster had collected photographs and anecdotes about people who had been killed by smallpox vaccination. But unlike those who had challenged the medical orthodoxies of the Progressive Era, Dissatisfied Parents Together emphatically rejected the label of "anti-vaccination." The group's members did not question the basic principles of immunization; instead, they advocated more research into the potential dangers of vaccines, increased transparency of medical decision-making, and greater commitment on the part of government and industry to ensuring safety. In contrast to the adversarial stance that earlier activists had taken toward members of the scientific establishment, DPT collaborated with the American Academy of Pediatrics on drafting the provisions of the legislation that was introduced. At a congressional hearing, Jeffrey Schwartz stressed that his group was not anti-vaccination, and characterized as "a false choice" the idea that society had to either accept the continued use of a vaccine suspected of causing neurological damage or face renewed epidemics of pertussis.[111]

Because of the wide range of parties with stakes in the outcome of the legislation, it faced a circuitous and difficult journey on its way to enactment. In late 1983, the American Medical Association convened an ad hoc committee made up of representatives from leading doctors' groups and pharmaceutical companies, which the following year issued a set of recommended components of a national system.[112] Nearly identical bills were introduced in both the House and Senate in 1984. President Ronald Reagan opposed the system called for in the legislation because it would be financed by a new excise tax on vaccines and would be administered through the judiciary rather than the executive branch; some administration figures also feared the system would become a model for other programs to provide government relief for people who claimed to have been injured by hazards such as Agent Orange or radiation from nuclear power plants.[113] The administration put forward a proposal that rejected the idea of a federally sponsored program and called instead for reforms in tort law.[114]

Of the many vexing issues, perhaps the most contentious was whether the new system would provide an exclusive remedy for those who claimed a vaccine-related injury or whether tort suits would still be allowed. Both the House and the Senate versions of the bill permitted suits against manufacturers. Because the compensation would be funded through an excise tax on vaccines, pharmaceutical companies claimed that to continue to allow tort claims would subject them to "double jeopardy."[115] But Dissatisfied Parents Together, along with other parent advocacy groups that had been formed in response to the pertussis controversy, staunchly opposed any move to limit plaintiffs' access to the legal system, arguing that disallowing punitive damages would remove a necessary incentive for pharmaceutical companies to improve the safety of their products.[116]

It was not until mid 1986 that a compromise version of the legislation acceptable to all parties could be hammered out. "I recognize that the bill I have introduced is probably not the first choice of most parties to this controversy," said Henry Waxman, the California Democrat who sponsored the House legislation, during the final negotiations on the terms of the bill. "Manufacturers would undoubtedly prefer greater insulation from liability. Parents of injured children would certainly prefer larger compensation and fewer restrictions on court activity. The Reagan administration would, I am sure, prefer legislation that spends no money."[117] In spite of these divisions, the idea of a compensation system had broad bipartisan congressional support, and legislation was ultimately passed in October 1986 on the last day of the Ninety-ninth Congress. It was part of an omnibus budget measure that, in a compromise to gain the support of vaccine manufacturers and the Reagan administration, allowed pharmaceutical companies to export drugs that were not approved in the United States to countries where they had been approved. The following month, in spite of "serious reservations," Reagan signed the National Childhood Vaccine Injury Act of 1986 (NCVIA) into law.[118]

The NCVIA's centerpiece was the National Vaccine Injury Compensation Program, which provided reimbursement for a wide range of medical and rehabilitative care for those injured by any vaccine designated by the CDC for "routine administration to children." Allowable expenses included loss of earnings, attorney's fees, and up to $250,000 for pain and suffering. In the event of a death that was judged to be vaccine-related, a lump sum of $250,000 was automatically awarded. The system allowed no punitive damages against manufacturers or anyone involved in administering vaccines unless there was evidence of gross negligence. All claims were reviewed by a "special master" in the U.S. court of federal claims; in order to streamline the process for plaintiffs, normal rules of evidence and other legal procedures were relaxed.

Although the system did not provide the exclusive remedy that pharmaceutical companies had sought, petitioners could file a claim in a civil court only if they had first gone through the special master and had rejected that decision or had their claim denied.[119]

The key to the compensation program was a "vaccine injury table," which set forth the various adverse events and conditions that were eligible. For each vaccine, the table listed the conditions with which, according to the best scientific evidence, they were plausibly associated, along with the time limit within which the event had to occur in order for it to be considered vaccine-related. The purpose of establishing a standard list was to remove from the claims process the need to prove causation, which was the most contentious issue from the standpoint of both law and epidemiology. Instead, if an event appeared on the vaccine injury table, it was presumptively compensable, provided it had occurred within the specified time. Parents could also file for compensation for events not listed in the table, but in those cases they bore the burden of proving that the condition was caused by a vaccine.[120]

In addition to the compensation program, the NCVIA included several measures related to improving the safety of vaccines. Satisfying one of the key goals of parent activists who had complained that no one knew how often DPT and other vaccines sickened or killed children, the act mandated, for the first time, that all physicians report adverse events following vaccination along with the vaccine's manufacturer and lot number. The Vaccine Adverse Event Reporting System (VAERS), administered jointly by the CDC and the Food and Drug Administration, became operational in 1990.[121]

The act also mandated that the Institute of Medicine, which had earlier evaluated policy on polio vaccination, conduct a series of studies examining the safety of all the vaccines covered under the compensation program. In 1991, the IOM issued its report on the two vaccines that had been most debated, those against pertussis and rubella. The report considered a wide range of evidence, including biological studies in humans and animals, epidemiological investigations, case reports, and biological plausibility. In examining the suspected relationships between the two vaccines and the more than twenty adverse events they were suspected of causing, the committee conceded that there were many gaps in knowledge and insufficient evidence to reach conclusions. The committee did determine, however, that there was sufficient evidence to declare a causal relationship, in rare instances, between pertussis vaccine and anaphylaxis and protracted, inconsolable crying, and between rubella vaccine and acute arthritis.[122] Three years later the IOM published its second summary, a review of the seven other vaccines routinely recommended for children (diphtheria, tetanus, polio, measles, mumps, *Haemophilus influenzae* type B, and hepatitis B). Once again illustrating the difficulty of establishing causation, there was inadequate evidence in about two-thirds of the relationships examined to definitively accept or reject a causal link.[123]

Perhaps the most striking aspect of the protracted and often bitter debates over vaccine injuries and liability during the 1980s was how little effect they had on immunization rates nationwide. Nothing comparable to the sequence of events that had occurred in Great Britain, where outbreaks of pertussis had followed closely on the heels of a dramatic drop in vaccine use, occurred in the United States. Coverage rates among infants in the United States lagged behind those of most European countries but, as we shall see in chapter 7, the causes were rooted in economic and structural barriers rather than in active opposition to vaccines. Nevertheless, the open challenges to the judgment and integrity of public health and medical experts that emerged during the pertussis controversy set the stage for an even more far-ranging critique of vaccination programs in the 1990s.

Expansion and Backlash

Vaccination at the Turn
of the Twenty-First Century

The scientists and parent activists who testified in the summer of 1999 at a packed congressional hearing on the topic of "Balancing Personal Choice and Public Safety" offered starkly differing views of the risks and benefits of vaccination. In counterpoint to health professionals emphasizing the potential dangers of preventable contagions, a House of Representatives committee heard emotionally wrenching personal stories from parents who believed that their children had been harmed or killed by one or more vaccines. Dan Burton (R-Ind.), who convened the hearing—and who believed that a vaccine had caused his grandson's autism—suggested that the increasing number of recommended shots for children represented "a good intention gone too far."[1] The hearings illustrated the challenges in maintaining public confidence in an era when vaccine-preventable illness had declined to negligible levels and the risks of immunization had come to seem more threatening.

At the turn of the twenty-first century, vaccination programs around the country confronted the limits imposed by their own success. For the first time, coverage rates among infants under two climbed to levels comparable to what had been attained for school-age youth. A major federal funding program enacted in 1993 gave a new influx of money to providers serving children of low-income families, while an effort to improve clinical efficiency by building a national network of computerized databases containing children's immunization records was under way, with broad private and public sector funding and support.

At the same time, however, a growing chorus of individuals and groups publicly challenged the safety of vaccines and, with increasing bitterness, questioned the integrity of health officials and pharmaceutical companies. Reminiscent of the diversity of vaccination dissidents during the Progressive Era, the modern generation of activists encompassed a range of political and philosophical views but was united in its antagonism to compulsion. The most vocal segment was made up of parent groups who rejected the risk-benefit calculations that had long been used to justify routine immunization. These activists insisted that vaccines carried greater dangers than health experts were willing to acknowledge; as proof, they offered the experiences of their own children. Amid a flood of negative publicity and Internet-based activism, the crisis in public confidence grew serious enough that by 2001 an analysis in the journal *Pediatrics* could declare that "the broad cultural consensus that has enabled the United States' universal childhood immunization programs of the past 50 years shows signs of eroding."[2]

The emergence of the most vocal anti-vaccination movement in almost a century created a sense of historical déjà vu that was intensified in the wake of the terrorist attacks of September 11, 2001. As the nation confronted the possibility that smallpox might be used as a biological weapon, scientists, politicians, and the public grappled with issues not seen since the nineteenth century, when isolation, quarantine, and the limits of the police powers were the defining features of vaccination policy. These debates underscored the extent to which fundamental features of civic and political culture, as much as scientific evidence, shaped decision-making around vaccination.

VACCINES FOR CHILDREN

By the late 1980s, the effect of laws requiring immunization before children could attend school was clear: at least 90 percent of those aged five to nine had the recommended protection. But infants under two—the age by which children were supposed to have received the majority of their shots—lagged far behind. Nationwide, less than half had received the full course of recommended vaccines, and in many of the nation's largest cities, a scant one-third of preschoolers were up to date with all the recommended immunizations.[3] From 1989 to 1991, a dramatic resurgence of disease forced this disparity in rates to the top of the political agenda. The worst measles outbreaks in over a decade swept across the country. The cases, heavily concentrated in low-income inner-city areas in Chicago, Houston, and Los Angeles, occurred mostly in children under five years old, who were disproportionately African American and Latino. In addition to highlighting the need for more efforts to reach the youngest children, the epidemic provided yet another example of the socioeconomic gradient that had long characterized immunization coverage.

The preponderance of disease among very young children prompted some public health experts to consider ways to extend the use of compulsion to preschoolers. No legal or practical mechanism comparable to school entry mandates, which had been successful with the "captive population" of students, existed for reaching the younger age bracket. In light of the concentration among the poor, some officials at the Department of Health and Human Services suggested that an effective way of targeting the problem would be to require children to be vaccinated as a condition of their parents' receiving public benefits such as Medicaid or Aid to Families with Dependent Children (AFDC).[4] This type of compulsion—the threatened denial of a benefit to which one would otherwise be entitled—could be considered ethically acceptable in the case of school mandates because it affected children of all socioeconomic backgrounds equally. But denying welfare benefits represented coercion of the disadvantaged and, in the eyes of critics, carried unseemly overtones of victim-blaming. The very rationale for such a policy raised ethically troubling questions of fairness and justice.

Tying the receipt of public benefits to completed immunization was not a new idea. During the national debates over reforming welfare in 1971, New York State had floated a proposal under which parents receiving payments from the state's Department of Social Services would have their allowances reduced but could "earn back" payments by engaging in various socially desirable behaviors, including ensuring that their children had received all their recommended vaccinations.[5] The idea was swiftly shot down as regressive and punitive. New York City mayor John Lindsay called the program "a step back into the dark era of the 19th century Poor Laws," while a Columbia professor of social work called the idea "morally repugnant" and argued that it "reflects a contempt for relief recipients as though they cannot be expected to care properly for their children except under duress."[6] By the 1990s, efforts to control the conditions of welfare had grown more politically acceptable, and at least two states, Georgia and Maryland, instituted programs denying AFDC benefits to parents whose children were inadequately immunized. Acknowledging that such targeted coercion was "arguably unfair," a researcher who evaluated Georgia's program nevertheless defended it. "It is both a public health obligation to encourage low-income parents to have their children immunized for these diseases and a benefit to these families and to the public as a whole."[7]

The debates over these programs hinged on vexing old questions: Why did some children—especially those in low-income families—remain unvaccinated? Did the responsibility lie with individual parents or with the health care delivery system—and thus, by extension, with society as a whole? The pendulum of opinion had swung between these two positions over the course of the century, and in the early 1990s, societal explanations were increasingly favored. Programs that attempted, through incentives or sanctions, to manipulate individual behavior were overshadowed by ambitious efforts to rethink the way the nation provided for its children's health.

In response to the measles epidemics, the National Vaccine Advisory Committee (NVAC), the policy-making body that had been established under the terms of the 1986 injury compensation act, issued a set of recommendations for improving coverage rates. The committee's report, while noting the need for better education and promotion to parents, focused primarily on reducing barriers of cost, access, and availability.[8] Known as the "Measles White Paper," the report reflected the growing consensus that if immunization rates were to improve, the health care system, not parental attitudes and behaviors, needed to change. "Though it is tempting for health care providers to attribute low immunization uptake to consumer apathy," noted a typical analysis in a public health journal, "much evidence points to correctable deficiencies of the health care system."[9]

The "system" for childhood immunizations during this period was in fact a disconnected patchwork of venues and payment mechanisms. About half of all children received their shots in the private sector and half in public facilities, including city or county health departments, community clinics, or public hospitals. Federal funds, administered by several different agencies, including the Centers for Disease Control, paid for about half of the public sector vaccines, with states and local governments making up the remainder.[10] State Medicaid programs varied widely in their reimbursement rates, but in many states, they did not even cover the physician's cost of the vaccine. Most private health insurance plans did not cover routine immunization; as a result, many parents who had a regular pediatrician were forced to take their children to a public clinic when it was time for shots. By 1990, the cost in the private sector of fully immunizing a child through the age of eighteen, including the vaccine and the doctor's fee, could run as high as $300, often paid out of pocket.[11] The rising cost was due partly to an expansion in the schedule of recommended vaccines; two new vaccines, requiring a total of seven shots, were added in the early 1990s, along with an additional measles booster. This proliferation of shots would have an important impact on public perceptions of vaccine safety as the decade progressed. But its most immediate effect was to price the full course of immunizations out of the reach of many parents.

The dissatisfaction with a fragmented system that seemed designed to thwart rather than facilitate timely and complete immunization was just one element of a much larger sense of crisis about how the nation's medical services were delivered and paid for. Concern about the growing number of people without health insurance helped propel Bill Clinton to the presidency in 1992; at the time of Clinton's election, polls showed that an overwhelming majority of Americans believed there was a health care crisis in the country.[12] Clinton's first major domestic initiative upon taking office was national health care reform (an effort that eventually came to grief in a miasma of partisan rancor and interest-group lobbying).[13] As planning for the reform effort got under way in the first weeks of the new presidency, the administration sent Congress a plan to allocate $1 billion to purchase and distribute vaccine free to providers. Hillary Rodham Clinton and incoming Secretary of Health and Human Services Donna Shalala had served on the board of the advocacy group the Children's Defense Fund, which had taken up the issue of immunization in the 1980s. The initiative was explicitly designed to stem the flow of children from private to public sector facilities.[14]

The question of why children remained unvaccinated was a central point of contention at congressional hearings on the proposal. Some skeptical legislators questioned whether inability to pay was the true cause of the nation's low immunization rates among preschoolers. Senator Nancy Kassebaum, a moderate Republican, contended that the president's initiative "misdiagnoses the causes of the problems and prescribes a remedy that is likely to be ineffective and perhaps wasteful."[15] Kassebaum instead laid the blame for poor coverage levels on lack of parental education, overburdened public health clinics, and the failure of private physicians to accept Medicaid because of low reimbursement rates. Especially problematic to Kassebaum and others in Congress was that under the plan, all children, even those of the well-to-do, would receive free vaccines. Secretary Shalala defended the proposal by arguing that to structure the plan otherwise would require means testing, and that full immunization was "a basic right" for all children.[16]

A wide range of health and child welfare groups, including the Children's Defense Fund, the American Academy of Pediatrics, and the Association of State and Territorial Health Officials, lined up in favor of the bill. Because the plan would involve the government negotiating a "reasonable price" for bulk purchase and distribution, vaccine manufacturers uniformly opposed it. Notably absent from debates were the parent activists who had played a prominent role in the enactment of the National Childhood Vaccine Injury Act in 1986. Dissatisfied Parents Together was at a low point in funding and morale and was devoting its limited resources to advocating for parents as the compensation system worked through a huge backlog of cases.[17] No groups opposed to vaccination testified before Congress against the initiative (though a letter from a Wisconsin-based parents' group was entered into the record in opposition to the bill).[18] Nevertheless, more than one member of Congress reported hearing from constituents concerned that a plan for universal distribution would lead to universal mandates. Senator Ron Wyden (D-Ore.), for example, said that the telephones in his office "rang off the hook" with parents wanting assurances that the legislation would not entail compulsory vaccination for all children.[19]

In August 1993, with the Clintons' ambitious plan for national health insurance foundering, Congress passed a scaled-back version of the immunization initiative. It was no longer a universal purchase program. Instead, the legislation established the "Vaccines for Children" program, which provided federal funding to buy vaccines from manufacturers and distribute them free to health care providers in the public and private sectors who served children eligible for Medicaid, those who lacked insurance, and Native American children.[20] Perhaps the most significant feature of the legislation was that for the first time, federal funding could be used to cover costs directly related to administering immunizations, such as the salaries of physicians, nurses, and other clinic personnel. Previous federal allocations, such as those under the 1962 Vaccination Assistance Act, had been limited to ancillary activities such as surveillance and promotion.[21] Although most child health advocates applauded the new measure for removing financial hurdles, some were concerned that a new categorical funding program might not be in the best long-term interests of vulnerable children, who lacked a wide range of preventive services. "Separate financing and delivery systems for immunizations could dilute and fragment the provision of these services to underinsured and uninsured children," warned an editorial in the *New England Journal of Medicine*.[22]

COUNTING ALL KIDS

The 1989–1991 measles outbreaks, besides drawing attention to the costs of vaccines, catalyzed efforts to reduce fragmentation in their delivery. Many children received their shots in multiple clinical settings from providers who had no way of knowing which immunizations had already been given and which were still needed. As the schedule became more complex, parents were increasingly uncertain whether or not their children had received all the recommended vaccines and tended to over-estimate the extent of their children's coverage.[23] One component of the Clinton initiative (removed from the final version) was a national computer tracking system that would help ensure that health care providers had access to the immunization history of all the children they saw.

The dream of using computers to enhance immunization efforts dated to the 1960s. "To picture an ideal situation, perhaps in the rather distant future," the CDC's director James Goddard had predicted in 1965, "the capabilities of electronic computers for storing and retrieving information could greatly facilitate our immunization programs. Computers could be used to store information with regard to the immunization given each individual, automatically print out a listing of those due repeat or booster immunizations, and manipulate data to compute the preventive effects of immunization."[24] The Vaccination Assistance Act of 1962 had included funding for cities and states to set up "reminder and recall" systems that could automatically generate letters or phone calls to parents around the time that children were due for their shots. In the 1980s, the CDC had piloted office-based systems running on desktop computers in several state and local health departments that could provide clinicians with a listing of which vaccines children in their practices needed.[25] But because of the variability of financial support for immunization activities over the years, few of these programs were sustained.

In the wake of the measles epidemic, the idea of computer registries gained new currency. At the National Immunization Conference in 1991, Kay Johnson, a youth health advocate who had worked with the Children's Defense Fund and the March of Dimes and had helped draft the "Measles White Paper," called for the creation of a national database to track the immunization status of all children from birth.[26]

Most immunization proponents, however, favored the development of
state or regional registries rather than a single national system, on the
grounds that they would be more technologically feasible and politically palatable. In particular, there were fears that a federally controlled
database with records on the nation's entire birth cohort would be seen
as unacceptably intrusive.

Even the task of establishing smaller-scale registries presented significant obstacles. The up-front expenses of computer hardware and soft-
ware were substantial, especially for cash-strapped public sector health
facilities. Senior managers at the Robert Wood Johnson Foundation, one
of the largest health-related philanthropies in the country, began discussions with CDC officials to determine how the charitable sector could
augment federal financial support for the development of registries, and
in 1991, they established the "All Kids Count" program with the goal of
fostering the development of registries nationwide. The following year, the
foundation awarded twenty-three planning grants, and in 1993, it funded
a dozen grantees, mostly city or county health departments, for four-year
periods to develop fully operational registries containing the records of
all the children within a defined area (city, county, region, or state). The
foundation devoted some $9 million to the program in its initial round
of funding, while a coalition of five other foundations with an interest in
health care funded an additional nine projects.[27]

By the time the Clinton administration submitted its ambitious immunization initiative to Congress in early 1993, many states and localities
were thus already developing their own registries, which was one reason
the creation of a national database was dropped from the final version
of the legislation. Some health officials in states that had their own registries told Congress that a single national system, in addition to being
technologically unrealistic, would lack the flexibility to meet varying
local and regional needs.[28] Although plans for the national database
were set aside, the Clinton initiative did provide substantial funding,
administered through the CDC, for registry development.[29]

Beyond technological hurdles, a key difficulty in building registries
was gaining the cooperation of private sector providers. Whatever benefits the systems might promise, an additional layer of administrative
procedures was a hard sell to busy pediatric practices already overburdened with paperwork related to insurance coverage through managed
care and other third-party payers. Although time- and labor-intensive
outreach by registry employees making personal visits to doctors' offices
was the most common way of persuading providers to participate, legal

means were used as well. In 1994, Mississippi became the first state to require by law that all physicians report immunizations to a statewide registry, a step soon taken by many other states.[30]

In 1998, the Robert Wood Johnson Foundation funded a second round of sixteen grantees, eight of which had been among the first group of All Kids Count programs. The areas covered under the grants included nine states, two counties, two multiple county regions, and three large urban areas (New York City, Philadelphia, and Baltimore); together they served approximately one-fifth of the nation's annual birth cohort.[31] In 1999, more than two hundred fifty health departments were developing some form of immunization registry (though most of these were only partly functional).[32]

The development of immunization registries took place amid a groundswell of public concern about the confidentiality of electronic information, especially health data.[33] Registries typically contained information such as address, parental marital and employment status, and sometimes family income, making the agreement of civil liberties groups and privacy rights organizations crucial in establishing them.[34] In order to head off public opposition on the basis of privacy concerns, the CDC held a series of focus groups around the country in the fall of 1998 to identify concerns that parents might have about the systems. Most parents in the groups supported the idea of registries, generally viewing them as a helpful public service rather than as an invasion of privacy, and few respondents indicated that they would not wish to participate. But many expressed concerns about who would have access to the information, with health insurance companies being the object of particular mistrust. Most of those interviewed felt it would be inappropriate for all children to be automatically included in the registry, and that laws should require the explicit written consent of parents to include their information.[35] Nevertheless, about half of the registries operating at the time linked automatically to birth certificate registries.[36]

Immunization status was not generally considered to be a sensitive or potentially stigmatizing piece of information, unlike some data that were collected by city and state health departments, and the creation of registries did not provoke the kind of widespread opposition that had met other types of epidemiologic surveillance, most notably attempts to mandate reporting by name of people with HIV infection. But efforts to monitor the immunization status of children electronically did draw the ire of those who questioned the value and safety of vaccines. At a 1998 public meeting on immunization registries held by the CDC,

Barbara Loe Fisher, one of the co-founders of Dissatisfied Parents Together, invoked the specter of Big Brother in denouncing the databases as a "violation of privacy and civil liberties" that "could be used to discriminate against and economically or socially punish loving, conscientious parents and their children if they do not conform with every government recommended health care policy."[37] Fisher called upon all registries to require written parental consent before a child could be included. Her strong stance reflected more than just the prevailing concern about medical privacy. It exemplified the heightened scrutiny, and often hostility, that efforts to increase vaccination rates were generating by the end of the decade.

VACCINATION "UNDER SIEGE"

Although the controversy over the DPT vaccine in the 1980s focused public attention on the potential harms of vaccines, it did not immediately give rise to the type of widespread and sustained resistance that had characterized battles over vaccination earlier in the century. But during the 1990s, a series of high-profile incidents and a proliferation of theories about the untoward effects of one or more vaccines galvanized a growing number of activists who brought new challenges to the judgment of scientists, public health officials, and pharmaceutical companies. The debates unfolded in the popular media, congressional hearings, academic journals, and, increasingly, on the Internet.

The backlash was in part a by-product of the success of vaccine research and development that had brought new products to market. In 1990, a vaccine against *Haemophilus influenzae* type B, one of the most common childhood infections and a leading cause of bacterial meningitis, was introduced; it was given in a series of either three or four doses. In 1991, three doses of a vaccine against hepatitis B were added to the schedule, the first given just hours after birth. Also around this time, a second dose of the measles-mumps-rubella preparation was recommended to provide additional protection. By 2000, two more vaccines, against chicken pox and pneumococcal disease, were universally recommended. Depending on which combination vaccines were used, a typical child received a total of eleven vaccines in a possible twenty injections by two years of age.

As early as 1993, after the *Haemophilus influenza* B and hepatitis B shots had been added to the recommended schedule, some clinicians began to worry about the pain and discomfort from the increasing number of injections infants were receiving—what was sometimes described as the "pediatric pincushion phenomenon."[38] (Somewhat surprisingly, one survey found that physicians were more concerned than parents about children receiving multiple injections in a single office visit.)[39] Some physicians worried that the increasing use of combined vaccines would make it more difficult, when adverse events occurred, to determine which, if any, of the antigens was responsible.[40] A more serious concern was that somehow receiving so many injections might prove to be "too much" for an infant's immune system. Experts in immunology insisted that such fears had no scientific basis; since the human immune system was theoretically capable of responding to more than 10 million antigens, there was little possibility that even a dramatically expanded vaccine schedule risked "overwhelming" or "using up" a child's immune capabilities.[41] Moreover, because of the discontinuation of the smallpox vaccine and the reformulation of the pertussis vaccine to an acellular formula, the number of antigens to which children were exposed through immunization had actually decreased in the previous four decades, from more than 3,000 to about 130.[42] But as the number of recommended vaccines for children grew during the 1990s, theories began to surface that too many immunizations were responsible, directly or indirectly, for a variety of child health problems including allergies, asthma, sudden infant death syndrome, and juvenile diabetes.[43]

The preoccupation with vaccine safety grew also out of a climate in which the ubiquity of risk in modern industrial society had emerged as a central concern—even obsession—of American politics, law, and popular culture.[44] In areas as diverse as nuclear power plants and AIDS, the assessment, quantification, regulation, and communication of risks dominated civic discourse in the last decades of the twentieth century, giving rise to a large body of analysis of what types of risks are deemed acceptable or unacceptable and how people can best be reassured under conditions of uncertainty. Psychologists identified several heuristics and biases that affected people's judgments about risk. The degree of concern a given risk aroused was not solely, or even primarily, based on a rational calculation of empirical features such as likelihood and severity, but was in addition influenced by a wide range of psychological and cultural factors. To vaccination supporters, this literature suggested that the classic approaches to vaccine promotion of previous eras—appeals to parental obligation or civic duty, warnings of the threat of infectious disease—were inadequate tools in the new climate of fear and concern. Clinicians and health officials began to draw explicitly on analyses that had emerged in other domains, such as the regulation of environmental hazards, to engage directly with the perceptions of vaccine risks.[45]

According to these models, several features of vaccine-induced injuries served to magnify concern about them. They primarily affected children; they were man-made, rather than naturally occurring; and they were involuntary, because of school entry mandates. In a signal of the seriousness with which vaccine proponents viewed the threat to public trust that the theories of vaccine-related harm might create, the Institute of Medicine (IOM), the branch of the National Academy of Sciences that had issued earlier reports on vaccine adverse events, held an all-day workshop in 1996 on risk communication and vaccines at which public health officials, pharmaceutical representatives, child health advocates, and parent activists concerned about safety discussed the growing perceptions of risk and the ways in which the public and private sectors should respond, both substantively and discursively.[46]

More than any other health concern, it was autism that propelled vaccine safety into the public spotlight. An umbrella term for a spectrum of developmental disorders characterized by severe limitations in social interaction and communication, autism began to draw attention in the media due to anecdotal reports of increasing prevalence. In early 1998, the British medical journal *The Lancet* featured an article by a team of British physicians describing a group of twelve children in their practice with severe intestinal abnormalities and autism, which, they hypothesized, might be associated with the children's having received the measles-mumps-rubella (MMR) injection years earlier.[47] At a press conference called by the hospital to publicize the findings, the lead researcher, Andrew Wakefield, declared that the MMR vaccine should be withdrawn (a position not held by his co-investigators in the study).[48] Wakefield's willingness to draw sweeping conclusions from relatively scant data, and what was viewed as unseemly grandstanding in his public statements, drew stinging criticism from public health officials in the United Kingdom.[49] The article reporting the team's findings was accompanied by a skeptical editorial pointing out numerous methodological limitations in the investigation: the conclusion was based on case reports with no control data; the temporal association between the vaccination and the onset of autistic symptoms was based solely on parental recall.[50] But the hypothesis quickly took on a life of its own. In Britain the MMR shot (or "jab," as injections are known in the United Kingdom) became the subject of negative press coverage, and acceptance rates began to decline.[51]

In the United States, concern about autism surged the following year when the California Department of Developmental Services issued a highly publicized report showing an increase in autism in the state of almost 300 percent between the years 1987 and 1999. The figures set off alarms among parent groups and politicians and prompted the *Los Angeles Times* to declare that "an epidemic of autism" was raging in the state.[52] Critics of that report and a follow-up study issued in 2002 cited numerous methodological weaknesses and sources of potential bias in the figures, and disagreement remained over whether the rise in rates was real or an artifact of expanded diagnostic criteria and increased awareness.[53] But parent activists seized on the data and the suspected link that Wakefield and his colleagues had identified in *The Lancet,* and calls for investigations into the suspected MMR-autism connection grew widespread.

As these concerns were drawing media attention, another vaccine dispute emerged from the U.S. military. In December 1997, U.S. Defense Secretary William Cohen announced a plan to vaccinate all 2.4 million members of the military against anthrax, a highly lethal bacterial infection. It was the first time that the military had attempted to immunize all active and reserve members against a potential biological weapon, and reflected a growing concern that countries hostile to the United States were developing a variety of agents that could be used for chemical warfare.[54] The vaccine—administered in six injections over the course of eighteen months—was known to cause minor side effects such as pain and swelling at the injection site, headache, and fever, but rumors soon began to circulate among service members that it could cause sterility and paralysis. Many soldiers refused the shots and, in so doing, faced a variety of disciplinary actions, including court-martial. The resistance was fueled in part by widespread mistrust of the military's past responses to soldiers' health problems, including its failure to be forthcoming about issues such as Agent Orange and Gulf War Syndrome.[55] By early 2000, some three hundred fifty service members had refused the shots, and an unknown number had left the service rather than be forced to undergo them. The problems with morale and refusal attracted the attention of some members of Congress, who called on the Pentagon to suspend the program in light of concerns about the vaccine's safety and efficacy.[56]

The confluence of concerns about the safety of vaccines led to a remarkable series of hearings beginning in May 1999 before the House of Representatives Committee on Government Reform. The committee chair and leading congressional critic was Indiana Republican Dan Burton, whose granddaughter had been hospitalized after receiving her hepatitis B vaccine, and whose grandson had autism, which Burton believed was the result of the measles-mumps-rubella shot the child had received.

First to come under the congressional microscope was the hepatitis B vaccine and the hypothesis that it was causally linked to multiple sclerosis and sudden infant death syndrome. This theory had been at the center of a protracted legal battle in France, where the program of routine childhood immunization against hepatitis B was thrown into turmoil after tribunals ruled in favor of plaintiffs who claimed that the vaccine had caused their multiple sclerosis. The French government appealed the decisions, and in 1999, a higher court overturned the verdicts and appointed a panel of medical experts to investigate the link.[57] The animus against the vaccine among critics in the United States was rooted not only in concerns about its safety but in the fact that it protected against a blood-borne disease spread primarily by sexual contact and injection drug use (though transmission also occurred perinatally and among children in day-care facilities). Some congressional testimony barely concealed a distaste for those most at risk of the illness. "Almost every newborn baby is now greeted on its entry into the world by a vaccine injection against a sexually transmitted disease because they couldn't get the junkies, prostitutes, homosexuals, and promiscuous heterosexuals to take the vaccine," charged one parent activist who believed the vaccine had caused the death of his infant daughter.[58] In what would become a leitmotif running throughout the Burton hearings, critics charged that the expansion of the schedule of recommended vaccines during the 1990s was a profit-making conspiracy among pharmaceutical companies, scientists, and government bureaucrats; in the words of one parent, "a program to vaccinate newborns [against hepatitis B] is of no worth to anyone except those who sell vaccines."[59]

In the summer of 1999, in the midst of this intensive political scrutiny, another controversy that had been brewing came to a head. Thimerosal, a preservative that contained trace amounts of ethylmercury, was used in some multidose vaccines to prevent contamination once the vial had been opened. Inquiry into thimerosal had begun when the U.S. Food and Drug Administration (FDA) asked vaccine manufacturers to provide information about the amount of mercury contained in their products. Because vaccines were available in different formulations, some multidose and others single dose, and could be given at different ages during infancy, there was variability in the amount of mercury from thimerosal that any given infant might receive; a child who received all of the vaccines that contained thimerosal according to a certain schedule could theoretically be exposed to an amount of mercury during the first six months of life that exceeded the threshold set by the Environmental Protection Agency for mercury exposure. The clinical significance of exceeding this limit was unknown.[60]

Concerned about the imminent release by the FDA of manufacturers' thimerosal data and the potential for further damage to public confidence, a group of the nation's leading vaccine researchers and representatives of medical and public health organizations hastily convened a meeting in June 1999 to determine the best course of action. Participants were sharply divided over the significance of the findings and the most prudent course of action. Options ranged from recommending immediate cessation of all vaccines containing the preservative to advising no change in the current schedule but urging manufacturers to eliminate the chemical from vaccines as soon as possible. Looming large over the debate was the widespread criticism to which the immunization system had recently been subject, resulting in deliberations that were, according to a subsequent analysis, "a process under siege."[61]

This was the backdrop against which the U.S. Public Health Service and the American Academy of Pediatrics issued a joint statement on July 7, 1999, calling for the removal of thimerosal from childhood vaccines. The statement noted the trade-off between risks and benefits entailed in the recommendation: "The large risks of not vaccinating children far outweigh the unknown and probably much smaller risk, if any, of cumulative exposure to thimerosal-containing vaccines over the first six months of life." Nevertheless, the statement declared that "because any potential risk is of concern," such vaccines should be removed as soon as possible.[62] The statement further recommended that the dose typically given at birth against hepatitis B, one of the vaccines that contained the preservative, be delayed, unless the mother was known to be a carrier of the virus.

Many scientists and health care providers sharply criticized the statement for elevating a theoretical risk over an actual one. The available data did not warrant the shift in policy, they contended, and the sudden nature of the recommendation with relatively limited study left pediatricians and other clinicians confused.[63] There were widespread reports that infants born to mothers with hepatitis B were not getting the birth dose as a result of their providers misunderstanding the guidelines, and that the change in the one vaccine disrupted the overall schedule, resulting in infants missing other vaccinations as well.[64] The American Academy of Pediatrics subsequently issued statements attempting to clarify its position and emphasizing the importance of continuing to use thimerosal-containing vaccines during the transition period as they were being phased out, so that children would not be unnecessarily put at risk of diseases that the vaccines were able to prevent.[65]

Just one week after the announcement about thimerosal, the nation's immunization system got another black eye when the CDC released data on fifteen cases of intussusception, a potentially fatal intestinal blockage, in children who had received a rotavirus vaccine that had been introduced just a year earlier. Rotavirus is one of the most common viral infections in children and a leading cause of severe dehydrating diarrhea, responsible for some 50,000 hospitalizations and as many as forty deaths each year in the United States.[66] In the wake of the reports, the manufacturer of the vaccine suspended distribution and three months later withdrew the product from the market entirely. A flurry of negative press coverage and worried calls to the CDC's immunization hotline followed.[67] Although skeptics seized on the episode as further evidence of the dangers of vaccines, immunization proponents contended that the sequence of events in fact demonstrated the effectiveness of the government's system for monitoring safety.[68] A handful of cases of intussusception in vaccine recipients had been reported during clinical trials, but the difference in the rate from those receiving the placebo was not statistically significant, and the cases did not prevent the product from being licensed. After reviewing data from the trials, both the Food and Drug Administration and the Advisory Committee on Immunization Practices recommended continued monitoring of the suspected side effect after the licensing of the vaccine. Clinicians were alerted to the possibility of the complication in a package insert, and extra efforts were made to ensure that occurrences were reported to the Vaccine Adverse Events Reporting System.[69]

The ongoing scrutiny of vaccination programs—the House Committee on Government Reform held seven hearings in 1999 and 2000—prompted the U.S. Public Health Service to ask the IOM to convene a special standing committee to review immunization safety. The committee's two dozen members, representing a variety of scientific specialties related to immunization, were charged with conducting comprehensive reviews of all available evidence on any suspected safety concerns, assessing the strength of the evidence for and against the suspected hazard, and making policy recommendations. Members of the committee were carefully screened to ensure that no accusations of conflict of interest could be made.[70] Over the course of the next three years, the committee investigated and issued reports on the hypothesized connections between vaccination and sudden infant death syndrome, multiple sclerosis, immune dysfunction, and autism. In some cases, the group found insufficient scientific evidence to either support or refute a given theory of harm, but for the most part, it determined that the overall body of evidence weighed against the suspected causal links.[71]

As these reports were being issued in 2001–2003, the fundamental inability of scientific inquiry to prove (or disprove) a negative—to demonstrate conclusively the absence of the suspected causal connections—was a source of continual frustration for vaccine critics. The first report issued by the Institute of Medicine on pertussis and rubella vaccines in 1991 had sounded a cautionary note about the limits of science. "[T]he concept of 'proof' in its common-sense meaning," the report noted, "is not strictly applicable to scientific observations. Even when scientists conclude that an experiment demonstrates ('proves') causation, they know there is a small, statistically definable probability that the conclusion is incorrect."

Differing views of what science could accomplish and what constituted proof were starkly evident in an exchange at a congressional hearing in April 2001, just after the IOM committee had released its report on the suspected connection between the measles-mumps-rubella vaccine and autism. In carefully measured scientific language, the report had declared that the majority of evidence pointed to a rejection of the hypothesized link:

> [T]he committee concludes that the evidence favors rejection of a causal relationship at the population level between MMR vaccine and autism spectrum disorders (ASD).... However, the committee notes that its conclusion does not exclude the possibility that MMR vaccine could contribute to ASD in a small number of cases, because the epidemiological evidence lacks the precision to assess rare occurrences of a response to MMR vaccine leading to ASD and the proposed biological models linking MMR to ASD, although far from established, are nevertheless not disproved.[72]

When Representative Dan Burton questioned Marie McCormick, the Harvard researcher who chaired the committee, about the wording of the conclusion, their exchange encapsulated not only the differences between lay and scientific thinking but also the adversarial relations between members of the scientific establishment and those who doubted the safety of vaccines.

> Mr. Burton. Let me read this to you again, "although far from established, are nevertheless not disproved." So what you are saying is that the causal link is not disproved. Is that right?
>
> Dr. McCormick. No, we are saying it is not established.
>
> Mr. Burton. But you are saying that it is not disproved.
>
> Dr. McCormick. It is not established, either.
>
> Mr. Burton. So you do not know, do you? Can you say categorically, 100 percent, that the MMR vaccine is not a contributing factor to autism? Can you say that?
>
> Dr. McCormick. No, because we said in rare cases—
>
> Mr. Burton. That is the point. You put out a report to the people of this country saying that it does not cause autism, there is no causal link, and then you have an out in the back of the thing. You cannot tell me, the committee chairman, under oath, that there is no causal link because you just do not know, do you?
>
> Dr. McCormick. Because in part we were not provided the evidence—
>
> Mr. Burton. Do you know?
>
> Dr. McCormick. I do not know.
>
> Mr. Burton. Then why did you say so in the report?
>
> Dr. McCormick. Because the bulk of the evidence—
>
> Mr. Burton. Because the bulk of the evidence? But you do not know. You just said that.
>
> Dr. McCormick. In fact, most of the reports I saw indicated that.
>
> Mr. Burton. Do you know what it is like to have an autistic child?
>
> Dr. McCormick. I do.
>
> Mr. Burton. You have an autistic child?
>
> Dr. McCormick. No. My brother has two.
>
> Mr. Burton. Your brother has two?
>
> Dr. McCormick. Yes.
>
> Mr. Burton. Then you know what he goes through?
>
> Dr. McCormick. Yes.
>
> Mr. Burton. Do you know how many kids are getting autism? Every 3 hours in California, there is a new child with autism. It used to be every 6 hours. You used to have 1 out of every 10,000 kids who were autistic. We do not know all the answers. We do not know if the mercury, the thimerosal in the vaccinations are causing autism. You do not know for sure whether the MMR vaccine is causing autism.

Dr. McCormick. I know it is not causing most of the cases of autism.

Mr. Burton. But the point is, if you are the one that it does cause—if your
      child is the one that does get it and we find out there is a causal link,
      isn't that awful? Isn't that awful?[73]

In a further illustration of the subtleties of communicating risk to the
public, the IOM in 2002 decided to avoid using the term "biologically
plausible" in its reports on vaccine safety because of concerns that most
people did not fully understand the term's meaning and mistook it to be
synonymous with "possible" or even "probable."[74]

SCIENCE IN A DEMOCRACY, REDUX

The involvement of parent activists in the debates over vaccine safety
reflected broad social changes that emerged in the 1960s, especially the
environmental and feminist movements. As we saw in chapter 6, a more
open, democratic, and often adversarial atmosphere began to prevail
with respect to the interpretation of science and its use in public policy;
deference to medical expertise and other elite knowledge was replaced
with skepticism and even hostility. During the 1980s, challenges to the
paternalistic authority of the scientific and medical establishment grew
more prominent as lay activists opened previously closed decision-
making processes and were increasingly able to shape research and
policy agendas. Communities with elevated rates of cancer fought to
prove that toxic pollutants in their environment were responsible and
rejected the analyses of epidemiologists who argued that alleged
"clusters" of illness could not be statistically proven.[75] Gay activists
with HIV and AIDS lobbied successfully for changes in clinical trial
design and the approval process for experimental drugs and thereby
effected fundamental transformations in the relationship between
researchers and communities affected by illness.[76]

The growing influence of knowledgeable and politically astute advocacy groups who mobilized around health issues made possible a far-
reaching critique of vaccination programs. The parent activists who
believed that their children had suffered harm from vaccines engaged in
highly technical debates about biological mechanisms and the strengths
and weaknesses of epidemiological data and forged alliances with dissident scientists who brought the credibility of academic degrees and
appointments.[77] The political dynamic of the vaccination battles in the
1990s bore striking similarities to the debates over the safety and efficacy of smallpox vaccination during the Progressive Era and the 1920s.

At issue in both eras was the legitimacy of public participation in determining the meaning and implications of scientific inquiry.

Although some public health officials persisted in using the label "anti-vaccination" to describe the widespread if loosely organized movement that questioned the safety of vaccines, activists themselves insisted they were "vaccine safety advocates" seeking to counter the pervasive pro-vaccine bias that made the scientific establishment unwilling or unable to give credence to theories of harm. In a reflection of this orientation, Dissatisfied Parents Together, the group that had been formed in the wake of the pertussis controversy of the early 1980s, changed its name in the 1990s to the National Vaccine Information Center (NVIC). The NVIC's president, Barbara Loe Fisher, emerged as the most visible spokesperson of this new perspective. When the *Journal of the American Medical Association* published an article on "anti-vaccination" web sites, Fisher shot back with a column on the NVIC site that labeled the *JAMA* authors "anti-science." "What exactly is their definition of 'antivaccination?'" Fisher asked. "Is it ... those challenging 'the safety and effectiveness of recommended vaccines'? If that is the definition of anti-vaccine, we can label these authors anti-science for suggesting that challenging and testing existing knowledge in science can be abolished in favor of protecting the status quo."[78]

As much as activists adopted the discourse of science to press their case, a sharp epistemological divide remained over the place of anecdotal evidence in scientific inquiry. In the view of many parents, the experiences of their own children constituted a form of proof superior to what population-level data could provide. In 2002, the NVIC's national conference featured a group of workshops titled "Anecdotal Evidence Shows the Way," which highlighted the importance of individual case reports in bringing attention to problems too rare to be detected through the standard methods of epidemiological research.[79] In a similar spirit, Representative Dan Burton declared in a congressional hearing in June 2002, "Parents have been our best investigators."[80] A corollary of this outlook was the rejection of the risk-benefit calculations that had long been used to justify routine immunization. This view was captured most succinctly in a motto frequently repeated by parent activists: "When it happens to your child, the risks are 100 percent."[81]

One important factor in the spread of dissenting views of vaccination during the 1990s was the explosive growth of the Internet, which served as a force for laicizing knowledge, especially related to medicine and health care. By 2002, dozens of web sites were challenging the orthodox

view of vaccination and on-line message boards provided a forum for
sharing dissident opinions.[82] As a result, parents seeking to inform themselves by searching on-line, in addition to encountering pro-vaccine
material from official sources such as the CDC and the AAP, were
increasingly likely to find sites that cast vaccines in a negative light,
showing dramatic vignettes and photos of damaged children and char-
acterizing the medical establishment as a conspiracy of greedy pharmaceuticals and corrupt health bureaucrats. "I just typed in the word
'vaccines' and everything that popped up was antivaccine material,"
one mother told *Consumer Reports* of her experience using an Internet
search engine.[83] One analysis suggested that it was the growth of the
Internet that caused the uproar about the possible link between the
MMR vaccine and autism to spread to the United States much more
quickly than the DPT controversy had two decades earlier.[84]

Although parents who believed their children had suffered vaccine-
related harm were in the vanguard of the modern wave of activism,
opposition to immunization encompassed a range of attitudes and beliefs
related to health and healing. In rural areas of Northern California, for
example, large communities made up of what one reporter described as
"artists and writers, urban refugees and back-to-the-land folks" devoted
to "natural" and holistic healing spurned vaccination as part of an overall philosophy of bodily integrity.[85] Residents of Boulder, Colorado,
where alternative healing methods enjoyed great popularity, had high
rates of exemptions from the state's vaccination law.[86] As had been the
case earlier in the century, alternative healers such as chiropractors represented an important constituency among those resistant to vaccination. A survey of chiropractors in the United States found that one-third
of respondents felt that vaccination caused more illness than it prevented, and that contracting an infectious disease was safer than undergoing vaccination.[87] Some chiropractic guides to child health contained
strong statements against vaccination.[88] The official positions on vaccination adopted by both the International Chiropractors Association
and the American Chiropractors Association stressed the inherent risks
of the practice and the importance of individuals' rights to freedom of
choice in health care.[89]

Other critics of the vaccination system were motivated by antipathy
toward the use of coercion and what they viewed as an overweening
government bureaucracy attempting to dictate choices about health that
should be left to individuals. Conservative doyenne Phyllis Schlafly
called compulsory vaccination "un-American."[90] The Association of

American Physicians and Surgeons, a libertarian doctors' group, opposed all mandates for vaccination on the ground that such requirements overrode parental choice and represented an intrusion by the state into the doctor-patient relationship.[91] The extent to which an anti-statist political ideology dovetailed with dissident views about health and healing was illustrated by the quotation that appeared on the opening page of the National Vaccine Information Center web site: "If the State can tag, track down and force citizens against their will to be injected with biologicals of unknown toxicity today, there will be no limit on what individual freedoms the State can take away in the name of the greater good tomorrow."[92]

For those who objected to compulsion, laws requiring vaccination prior to school enrollment were anathema. Many Internet sites prominently featured calls to repeal mandates for students; at a site called "Vaccination Liberation," based in Idaho, readers could download all fifty states' forms for exempting children from legally required vaccines.[93] Although many states tightened their laws during the 1990s to make it more difficult to obtain a religious or philosophical exemption, at the end of the decade, this trend reversed.[94] In 2003, at least twelve state legislatures considered laws that would make school entry requirements less restrictive or add a philosophical exemption.[95] (Fifteen states had laws that allowed exemption based on philosophical or personal beliefs in addition to religion.)[96]

As a result, some health officials grew increasingly concerned that permissive opt-out clauses had the potential to undermine the high levels of coverage that had been achieved in school-age youth. There was no uniform procedure across the country for obtaining an exemption, and in many states it was far easier to decline—simply signing a form provided by the school district was often sufficient—than it was to have the child vaccinated.[97] Indeed, a survey in Washington State found that more than half of schools were encouraging parents to sign an exemption request simply to expedite the process of enrollment.[98] Some individual school districts allowed parents to opt out on the basis of philosophical objections even though their state laws did not authorize such exemptions.[99]

The increasing public demand for more liberal exemptions led some health professionals to call for a more robust and open discussion of compulsory laws that gave full credit to the varying viewpoints involved. "Just as war is too important to be left to the generals, so immunization mandates are too important to leave to public health authorities,"

Edgar Marcuse, a professor and former member of the Advisory Committee on Immunization Practices, asserted. "We must explore how better to involve the public in the issue of mandates as policy is formulated. If we do not, ultimately the issue of mandates will wind up in our state legislatures. A legislature has too little time to understand these complex issues and is subject to influence by articulate, well-organized groups with a particular axe to grind."[100]

As the steady drumbeat of negative coverage continued on the Internet and in the media, many health officials grew concerned about a massive public turn against vaccines. Suspected dangers garnered prominent and often sensational media attention, with reports in magazines such as *Time* and *Newsweek* and on the popular television news programs *60 Minutes* and *20/20*. Even stories that refuted theories of harm— "Vaccine Did Not Kill Teen," ran one newspaper headline—helped perpetuate a subtle yet increasingly pervasive association between immunization and danger in the popular imagination.[101] Strikingly, a nationwide survey of attitudes in 1999 revealed much that gave public health and medical officials cause for confidence: the vast majority of respondents agreed that immunization was extremely important in keeping children healthy and viewed most routinely given shots as safe and effective. Of concern, however, was the finding that about a quarter of respondents believed that children received more shots than were good for them, and that too many vaccinations could weaken a child's immune system.[102] Another survey among a predominately African American and Latino population in an inner-city neighborhood found similar levels of concern.[103] In the spring of 2000, more than two-thirds of surveyed physicians reported a "substantial increase" in the number of parents expressing concerns about vaccine safety in the previous year.[104]

Although most immunization controversy at the turn of the new century surrounded children, the issue of vaccinating the general adult population suddenly and dramatically reemerged in the aftermath of the terrorist attacks of September 11, 2001. As the country prepared for the possibility that smallpox might be used as a biological weapon, health officials, politicians, and the public confronted questions that had largely receded from view over the previous one hundred years: how best to gain the cooperation of the public in a health emergency, and what curtailment of freedom of movement and property rights might be necessary to protect the community from a potentially catastrophic threat.

THE "DARK WINTER" OF OUR DISCONTENT: THE RETURN OF SMALLPOX VACCINATION

Fear that smallpox might be used as a potential biological weapon began to emerge in the mid 1990s. Stocks of smallpox virus had been retained in laboratories at the CDC in Atlanta and in Moscow since the World Health Organization had officially declared the global eradication of the disease in 1980, but after the fall of the Soviet Union, it was widely believed that supplies of the virus had fallen into the hands of countries hostile to the United States and were being cultivated, along with other lethal biological agents, in an unknown number of chemical weapons laboratories around the world.[105] Fear of biological weapons prompted the U.S. military's program to vaccinate soldiers against anthrax and led in the summer of 2001 to "Dark Winter," a simulated exercise in emergency planning sponsored by the Johns Hopkins Center for Civilian Biodefense Strategies.

In an enactment of what was deliberately designed to be a "worst-case scenario," participants gathered over the course of three days at a midwestern conference facility to simulate the policy and planning decisions that would have to be made in the event of three simultaneous attacks with smallpox on shopping malls in Oklahoma City, Philadelphia, and Atlanta. The purpose of the exercise was to identify areas of weaknesses in the nation's emergency preparedness systems and to galvanize efforts to ensure better protection. As envisioned in the scenario, thirteen days after the initial attack, the nation's limited supply of smallpox vaccine had been depleted, panic and civil unrest were spreading, international borders had been closed, and food shortages were growing; by the end of the scenario, some three million Americans had been stricken with the disease and a million had died.[106]

A second effort, independent of Dark Winter but similar in spirit, was also in progress in mid 2001 and would strongly influence the debates about renewed smallpox vaccination. One of the many policy initiatives that the increasing concern over potential bioterrorism sparked in the late 1990s was an effort to ensure that the fifty states' health laws were adequate to meet the threat posed by new chemical or biological weapons. Central to this concern was uncertainty about whether the patchwork of state-level public health laws around the country, many of which had not been updated in decades, provided for the emergency measures that might be needed. The CDC, in collaboration with several other professional organizations, spearheaded the drafting of a model law that would serve as a template to help states increase the adequacy of their legal infrastructure to deal with catastrophic events that threatened public health.[107]

The drafting of the Model State Emergency Health Powers Act (MSEHPA) was already in progress before September 11, 2001, but it assumed sudden and dramatic relevance when it was released for public comment a month after the terrorist attacks. Under the model act's provisions, those who refused to comply with compulsory vaccination orders could be charged with a misdemeanor and subjected to immediate quarantine or isolation.[108] Some legislators moved quickly to incorporate its recommendations into their state's laws, but the act also drew fire from across the ideological spectrum, uniting in opposition activists from the political Left with libertarians on the Right, all of whom argued that it contained insufficient protection for civil liberties.

One of the act's most incisive critics was George Annas, a prominent professor of health law. While Annas conceded that the 1905 case of *Jacobson v. Massachusetts* provided a constitutional basis for many of the compulsory measures proposed in the model act, he doubted whether that seminal opinion remained a tenable foundation for modern health law in light of subsequent jurisprudence on questions of civil liberties and due process:

> Today, almost 100 years after *Jacobson*, both medicine and constitutional law are radically different. We now take constitutional rights much more seriously, including the right of a competent adult to refuse any medical treatment, even life-saving treatment. Of course, we would still permit public health officials to quarantine persons with a serious communicable disease, but only if they could not or would not accept treatment and thus put others at risk for exposure.... This model act seems to have been drafted for a different age; it is more appropriate for the United States of the 19th century than for the United States of the 21st century.[109]

In the view of Annas and other critics, securing public trust through open discussion of the risks and benefits of emergency measures—not legal sanctions—was the cornerstone of an ethical and effective public health policy.

The authors of the act, a team of health law experts led by Lawrence Gostin at the Center for Law and the Public's Health at Georgetown University, defended their work and insisted that the act contained adequate safeguards for civil liberties. In their view, securing voluntary public cooperation in an emergency was paramount, but the failure to recognize that legal force might be necessary in some cases was unrealistic and dangerous.[110] After three months of public comment, a revised draft of the act was released in late December 2001. Although broad police powers remained, some of the most controversial provisions for restrictions on personal liberty had been moderated with new procedures for due process.[111]

The federal response to the threat of smallpox in the months after September 11 thus unfolded amid bitter partisan debates about persuasion and compulsion and the permissible scope of government action. In the immediate aftermath of the attacks, the nation seemed woefully unprepared to meet potential biological threats. Only about eight million doses of aging smallpox vaccine existed, a supply that could be rapidly depleted in the event of a widespread outbreak, as the Dark Winter scenario had demonstrated. In October, as the nation confronted frightening scenarios in the popular media, the federal government announced plans to stockpile 300 million doses of smallpox vaccine, enough to vaccinate everyone in the country.[112] In provisional guidelines issued in late November 2001 for local and state health departments, the CDC called for ring vaccination rather than efforts to provide protection for the entire population. Although the CDC's plan gave priority to the least restrictive measures for controlling the spread of the disease, it warned that large-scale compulsory measures, including placing entire cities under quarantine and interrupting regional transportation, might be necessary in the event of a deliberate smallpox attack.[113]

Throughout 2002, disagreement prevailed about whether the vaccine should be made available to the general public as a preemptive measure. Because of the HIV epidemic, the increasing frequency of organ transplantation and cancer chemotherapy, and the rise in the rate of eczema, the number of people for whom vaccination was medically contraindicated was far greater than it had been in the 1960s.[114] Based on the studies that had been conducted at that time on the frequency of adverse events associated with the vaccine, it was reasonable to predict that vaccinating large segments of the civilian population would result in a handful of deaths and dozens, if not hundreds, of reactions serious enough to require hospitalization. But some contended that waiting to begin vaccinating until after an attack occurred could be disastrous. "[T]he logistical complexity of administering millions of vaccine doses in a crisis is daunting," warned William Bicknell, a former commissioner of health for Massachusetts and the most vocal proponent of voluntary mass vaccination. Bicknell argued that ring vaccination, while an effective tool for controlling small, localized outbreaks, would be useless in the face of the deliberate, simultaneous spread of smallpox in multiple locations. "An epidemic is highly likely to outrun the vaccinators," he predicted. "Effective enforcement of quarantine is also difficult. Official reassurances followed by further uncontrolled outbreaks could provoke panic, flouting of authority, and even the breakdown of medical and public health services."[115] Citing the dire outcome of the Dark Winter exercise, Bicknell insisted that the only prudent course of action was mass vaccination under circumstances in which it could be offered in a calm and orderly manner, with medical contraindications more carefully assessed, and post-injection complications monitored.

A position similar to Bicknell's was taken by libertarian groups such as the Cato Institute think tank and the Association of American Physicians and Surgeons (AAPS), both of which advocated making the vaccine available to the general public, with full disclosure of its risks.[116] This position was ideological rather than epidemiological: it was unacceptably paternalistic, both groups argued, for the government to deny a preventive desired by the some segments of the population. In position papers on the issue, however, neither group addressed the potentially more difficult question of what should be done in the event that an outbreak occurred and people refused to be vaccinated. This question was an especially delicate one for the AAPS, which had a long record of vociferous opposition to compulsory health laws and was forced to issue a statement, in the wake of its endorsement of widespread civilian vaccination, that it "has not wavered in its position AGAINST vaccine mandates."[117]

In deciding whether the most prudent course was to vaccinate preemptively or withhold action until the feared epidemic actually materialized, a looming unknown was how rapidly smallpox might spread in the event of a deliberate attack. The transmissibility of infectious diseases is described by the epidemiological parameter R_0, or reproductive rate, the number of secondary cases produced for every primary case in a susceptible population.[118] Measles, for example, has an R_0 of ten; each infected person on average infects ten others. The Dark Winter simulation had posited a smallpox R_0 of ten, an assumption that many public health experts—including some who had participated in the global smallpox eradication effort in the 1970s—challenged as unrealistic and exaggerated; most epidemiologists put the number at around two or three.[119] A variety of other analyses that used mathematical modeling to estimate the total number of illnesses and deaths likely to result from an attack arrived at radically different scenarios. Because so many of the parameters of such models remained either highly variable or unpredictable, including the method of introduction and spread, the models yielded very different outcomes, which pointed to varying policy recommendations.[120]

In mid 2002, the federal Advisory Committee on Immunization Practices recommended that approximately 15,000 health care workers and emergency responders be vaccinated, but in September, the committee came out in support of a more ambitious plan to vaccinate approximately 500,000 health care workers. The group remained strongly opposed, however, to the idea of making the vaccine available to the general public, on the grounds that this might lead to harms unjustified by the level of the threat.[121]

A nationwide poll conducted during the last three months of 2002 revealed widespread ignorance and misconception about both smallpox and the vaccine. A large majority of respondents believed, incorrectly, that there was an effective treatment for smallpox that could prevent death or serious effects even after a person developed symptoms, and that cases of smallpox had occurred somewhere in the world within the previous five years. Almost half of those who said they had been vaccinated against smallpox thought—again, erroneously—that their immunity to the disease would still be in force. About two-thirds favored a plan to make the vaccine available to the general public on a voluntary basis, and a similar percentage said that they themselves would choose vaccination if it were offered. But while three-quarters said they would want to be vaccinated if their own physician and most other physicians were vaccinated, only one-fifth said they would be willing if most doctors refused vaccination.[122]

It was thus against a backdrop of confusion among the public, sharp disagreements among health professionals, bioterrorism experts, and politicians about risks, benefits, and precautionary action, and the buildup to an increasingly likely war with Iraq that President George W. Bush announced a comprehensive plan to protect the nation from smallpox in mid December 2002. While admitting that his administration had "no information that a smallpox attack is imminent," Bush outlined an ambitious three-phase plan.[123] In the first phase, about half a million health care workers and emergency personnel were to be vaccinated within thirty days. Thereupon a broader effort would commence, targeting some 10 million health care workers. Finally, in late spring or early summer, the vaccine would be made available to any adult for whom it was not medically contraindicated.

Mixed reactions greeted the announcement. A *New York Times* editorial called the plan "a sensible approach" and said that it was right for the government to eventually make the vaccine available to "well-informed citizens ... if they want it."[124] Both the American Medical Association and the American Public Health Association offered cautious support but called for the government to assess the program carefully as it moved forward.[125] Others were concerned, however, that moving so far beyond the pool of half a million emergency responders to target ten million health care workers would incur substantial risks without a clear benefit. In recommending such a large-scale operation, the administration had, in an unprecedented move, overruled the advice of the federal Advisory Committee on Immunization Practices. Sources close to the decision-making indicated that the more far-reaching plan was being pushed by Vice President Dick Cheney and officials at the Department of Defense, over the objections of health experts in the CDC and outside of government.[126]

Former CDC director William Foege was among many who publicly criticized the scope of the plan. Foege's years of experience on the front lines of the global smallpox eradication program in the 1970s gave him special credibility on this issue, which he drew upon when he argued in a *Washington Post* op-ed column that ring vaccination, not blanketing the general population, was the wisest course of action. Ring vaccination had been effective, he wrote,

> even in a place like India, with its high population density, millions on trains at any one time and many people without actual addresses. For anyone not involved in that effort, ring vaccination seemed—and probably still seems—counterintuitive. But in India we went from the highest incidence of smallpox recorded in decades in May 1974 to zero in May 1975.... Compare this with the record of mass vaccination programs, which had been tried in India for more than 150 years without success. The key to fighting smallpox proved to be not background immunity but diligence in finding and vaccinating every possible contact of every patient.[127]

To the Bush plan's critics, the most egregious aspect of it was not so much the scope of the effort but the fact that the administration, citing national security, refused to release what it knew about the likelihood of smallpox being used as a biological weapon, thus making it impossible to weigh the program's risks and benefits. "It may come as a surprise to some that we don't make health policy in this country based on portentous warnings from behind closed doors," Linda Rosenstock, dean of the school of public health at the University of California, Los Angeles, and a former official in the Clinton administration, declared. "There is actually a science to calculating risk. Making such sweeping decisions as President Bush has done on smallpox vaccination—keeping the public and experts in the dark—is simply indefensible."[128]

These public expressions of skepticism were echoed throughout the health care rank and file. Hundreds of hospitals, nurses' associations, and unions representing health care workers and municipal employees came out against the plan, in large part because the government had not adequately addressed the issue of liability for vaccine-related injuries. Hospitals were worried about recently vaccinated health care workers transmitting vaccinia (the disease that could result from smallpox vaccination) to their patients, and their insurers indicated that vaccine-related losses would not be covered by workers' compensation programs.[129] Even those fully supportive of increased bioterrorism preparedness were concerned that the focus on smallpox vaccination was overshadowing other efforts, such as enhanced research and surveillance that would enable the country to respond to threats of anthrax, plague, botulism, and a variety of livestock diseases that could also be used. The feeling was widespread that the government was pushing a program fraught with known risks and unknown benefits, at the inevitable expense of other, more routine programs whose value was well proved; cash-strapped state health departments were forced to redirect money and personnel from core functions in order to administer an effort that many believed was of little value.[130]

Because of the administration's failure to win the support of frontline health care providers around the country, the program never met the goal laid out in phase one, much less progressed to the second or third stages. Out of the half a million health care workers targeted to receive the vaccine in the first phase, less than ten percent—approximately 40,000 people nationwide—were vaccinated. The coverage was neither uniform nor distributed in areas thought to be the most likely targets of a smallpox attack; more than half of the people who had been vaccinated were in just six states: Texas, Florida, Tennessee, Ohio, Minnesota, and Nebraska.[131] Ten months after it had been announced, officials at the CDC indicated quietly that the smallpox vaccination plan had "ceased" and been folded into larger bioterrorism response efforts.[132]

The administration's inability to make a compelling case for the public health necessity of the Bush smallpox vaccination effort proved in the end to be its fatal weakness. Although this might be read as an indication that scientific evidence plays a decisive role in successful public health policy-making, a more apt lesson to draw pertains to the unpredictable effects that the sociopolitical context may have on acceptance of vaccination. Although fear of disease has served as a powerful motivation to be vaccinated, it did not in this case trump other, more pressing concerns that emerged upon a weighing by the targeted populations of the risks and benefits that were thought to be involved.

VACCINATION IN THE TWENTY-FIRST CENTURY: THE OLD AND THE NEW

Vaccination policies and practices in the United States at the turn of the twenty-first century had by many measures achieved remarkable success. Perhaps the most striking achievement, in view of the extended and often acrimonious debates over safety, were record high levels of public acceptance for routine childhood immunization. Coverage among children under age three stood at an all-time high in 2004, with levels above 90 percent for most vaccines.[133] These rates suggested the efficacy of the broad systemic efforts undertaken in the 1990s to improve access and delivery. Disparities in full immunization persisted among children of different racial and ethnic backgrounds, but the gaps in levels of coverage between white children and African American or Latino children were smaller than those for most other health indicators.[134] Even as the controversy about the alleged connection between measles vaccine and autism crested between 1998 and 2003, and public acceptance of the MMR shot plummeted in the United Kingdom, rates of coverage for the vaccine increased slightly in the United States.[135]

Why the debates over safety had not caused greater public rejection of vaccines in this country remained a matter of speculation.[136] What was clear was that the relationship between vaccine critics and the public health establishment had become increasingly adversarial. Activists who believed that vaccines caused health problems such as autism leveled charges of corruption and bias against immunization proponents. There was an inherent conflict of interest, critics argued, in the fact that the CDC's National Immunization Program was responsible both for promoting the use of vaccines and ensuring their safety.[137] It was in response to such criticisms that the CDC announced in February 2005 that it would separate its vaccine advocacy and safety monitoring functions.[138]

By this point, the evidence against a connection between vaccines and autism had grown stronger. A raft of studies published in 2003 and 2004, conducted in Sweden, Denmark, the United Kingdom, and the United States, using a variety of epidemiological methods, all found no evidence of an association between autism and either the MMR vaccine or vaccines containing the preservative thimerosal. In response to the new evidence, the Institute of Medicine's immunization safety review panel, which had examined both hypothesized links in previous reports, reconvened to conduct an updated evaluation. In May 2004, the committee released a new report that reasserted the conclusion of its earlier reviews: that the evidence "favors rejection" of both causal relationships.[139]

The report's language bore the imprint of the controversies from which it had emerged. Acknowledging "the anger of some families toward the federal government (particularly the CDC and FDA), vaccine manufacturers, the field of epidemiology, and traditional biomedical research," the committee went out of its way to emphasize that autism was a grave problem that imposed enormous burdens on those affected. But the group insisted that "available funding for autism research [should] be channeled to the most promising areas"—which did not include vaccines.[140] Advocacy organizations for parents of autistic children were not reassured, however. The Coalition for SafeMinds (Sensible Action for Ending Mercury-Induced Neurological Disorders), one of the most vocal parent advocacy groups, slammed the IOM report as "flawed science" that was tainted by "pervasive conflicts of interest."[141]

Meanwhile, the disputes over the research of Andrew Wakefield, whose study in *The Lancet* had ignited much of the concern about autism, took an unexpected turn. In early 2004, the journal disclosed allegations of ethical improprieties that had been made against the investigators, including that, at the time the study had been conducted, Wakefield was also gathering evidence for a potential lawsuit by several parents who suspected that their children's autism was vaccine-related.[142] In the wake of the accusation of conflict of interest, ten of the original thirteen scientists who had participated in the research retracted their support for the conclusion about the MMR-autism connection.[143]

While debates over safety raged on, the other most contentious area of policy, the use of legal compulsion in schools, remained in dispute in courtrooms and statehouses around the United States. Although no court rulings suggested that either the century-old affirmation of compulsory laws in *Jacobson* or the 1922 *Zucht* decision validating school entry requirements was on the verge of being struck down, controversy continued to swirl around the acceptable scope of exemptions. In 2001, several Arkansas families sued the state after being denied exemption from the requirement for schoolchildren to be vaccinated against hepatitis B. The following summer a U.S. district court in Arkansas declared that the religious exemption, which was limited to practitioners of a "recognized church or religious denomination," was unconstitutional, arguing that the provision "clearly runs afoul" of the free exercise and establishment clauses of the First Amendment and the due process clause of the Fourteenth Amendment.[144] In so ruling, the court concurred with the decision handed down in New York in the 1987 case of *Sherr v. Northport* that had resulted in that state's rewriting its law. After the exemption clause, which was severable from the rest of the law, was thrown out, Arkansas joined Mississippi and West Virginia as the only states lacking either a religious or philosophical exemption. In response, Arkansas legislators in 2003 rewrote the law to allow parents with philosophical objections to opt out.[145]

The issues of risk and compulsion had the potential to undermine the success of the immunization system. So too did structural issues related to supply and financing. The production of vaccines remained concentrated among only a handful of pharmaceutical companies, and the possibility of shortages or interruptions in availability was an ongoing threat. Some new vaccines, including the heptavalent preparation against invasive pneumococcal disease introduced in 2000, were far more expensive than older products, raising questions about cost-benefit ratios and the continuing viability of public- and private-sector funding streams.[146]

The history of vaccination in the twentieth century cannot be viewed as a teleological narrative in which scientific advances produced a steady stream of increasingly sophisticated vaccines, leading to ever-greater levels of infectious disease control. It is clear that whatever new vaccines might emerge in the coming years, a volatile mix of social, political, and legal factors will shape the deployment of those innovations. Declaring in 2004 that "the easy work in vaccine-preventable diseases has been done," three officials with the Institute of Medicine, which had devoted so much study to vaccination over the previous two decades, laid out the challenges for the future:

> How many more vaccinations will parents, physicians and nurses, and insurance providers tolerate? Is the goal to develop vaccines for every infectious disease or only for serious diseases? How serious should a disease be to warrant a vaccination program? Who is to judge the seriousness of a disease? At some point, this health promotion and disease prevention strategy could wear out its welcome with the population

at large. It has already done so with some segment of society. The United States lacks a comprehensive scientific and policy approach to explore fully the ramification of the increasing number of vaccines that will soon be available.[147]

Vaccination policy underwent numerous transformations over the course of the twentieth century, reflecting shifts in popular perceptions of contagious disease and iatrogenic risk, evolving legal and constitutional ideas of bodily integrity, changes in the structure and priorities of the nation's health care system, and, of course, developments in science and technology that produced new vaccines. At the same time, however, fundamental questions have persisted. How should individual liberty be balanced against the need to protect the common welfare? How should authorities act in the face of incomplete or inconsistent scientific information, and how should the public be involved in these decisions? What are the best ways to secure the cooperation of the public in reducing the incidence of disease? Are some or all public health measures inherently, and necessarily, paternalistic? The ways that these questions have been answered by parties to these debates—scientists, physicians, public health officials, parents, legislators, jurists, and activists of all ideological persuasions—have reflected not only their assessment of the value of vaccination but also their views about personal choice and freedom in matters of health and the appropriate role of the state in shaping the decisions of individuals.

Notes

INTRODUCTION

1. Charles Hoppe to Shirley Wynne, January 23, 1931, NYCDOH, box 141375, folder: Vaccination.

2. Shirley Wynne to Charles Hoppe, January 29, 1931; and I. Robert Wolf to Shirley Wynne, April 24, 1931, NYCDOH, box 141375, folder: Vaccination.

3. Paul E. M. Fine and Jacqueline A. Clarkson, "Individual versus Public Priorities in the Determination of Optimal Vaccination Policies," *American Journal of Epidemiology* 124 (1986): 1012–1020; 1013.

4. Douglas S. Diekema and Edgar K. Marcuse, "Ethical Issues in the Vaccination of Children," in G. R. Burgios and J. D. Lantos, eds., *Primum Non Nocere Today* (Amsterdam: Elsevier, 1998); Paul Menzel, "Non-Compliance: Fair or Free-Riding," *Health Care Analysis* 3 (1995): 113–115; Tim Dare, "Mass Immunisation Programmes: Some Philosophical Issues," *Bioethics* 12 (1998): 125–149.

5. Garrett Hardin, "The Tragedy of the Commons," *Science* 162 (1968): 1243–1248; 1247.

6. John Stuart Mill, *On Liberty* (1859; Indianapolis: Bobbs Merrill, 1956), 100.

7. Ross D. Silverman and Thomas May, "Private Choice versus Public Health: Religion, Morality, and Childhood Vaccination Law," *Margins* 1 (2001): 505–521. For a contrasting view, however, see Dare, "Mass Immunisation Programmes."

8. The literature on risk and its meanings is voluminous. The topic has been approached from numerous disciplinary perspectives. Among many notable works, see Ulrich Beck, *The Risk Society: Towards a New Modernity* (London: Sage, 1992); Mary Douglas, *Risk and Blame: Essays in Cultural Theory* (New York: Routledge, 1992); National Research Council, *Improving*

Risk Communication (Washington, D.C.: National Academies Press, 1989); Daniel Kahneman, Paul Slovic, and Amos Tversky, *Judgment under Uncertainty: Heuristics and Biases* (Cambridge: Cambridge University Press, 1982); Cass Sunstein, *Risk and Reason: Safety, Law and the Environment* (Cambridge: Cambridge University Press, 2002); and Allan M. Brandt, "Blow Some My Way: Passive Smoking, Risk, and American Culture," *Clio Medica* 46 (1998): 164–187.

9. Joseph A. Bell, "Current Status of Immunization Procedures: Pertussis," *American Journal of Public Health* 38 (1948): 478–480; 480.

10. Henry M. Gelfand, "Vaccination: An Acceptable Risk?" *Science* 195 (1977): 728–729; 728.

11. Cheyney C. Ryan, "The Normative Concept of Coercion," *Mind*, n.s., 89 (1980): 481–498; Gerald B. Dworkin, "Compulsion and Moral Concepts," *Ethics* 78 (1968): 227–233; Ronald Dworkin, *Taking Rights Seriously* (Cambridge, Mass.: Harvard University Press, 1977); Willard Gaylin and Bruce Jennings, *The Perversion of Autonomy: The Proper Uses of Coercion and Constraints in a Liberal Society* (New York: Free Press, 1996).

12. Ronald Bayer and Amy Fairchild, "The Genesis of Public Health Ethics," *Bioethics* 18 (2004): 473–492.

13. Vaccination News web site, www.vaccinationnews.com (accessed January 12, 2004).

14. Ann Bostrom, "Vaccine Risk Communication: Lessons from Risk Perception, Decision Making and Environmental Risk Communication Research," *Risk: Health, Safety, and the Environment* 8 (1997): 183–200.

15. On inoculation in the colonial period, see Elizabeth A. Fenn, *Pox Americana: The Great Smallpox Epidemic of 1775–82* (New York: Hill & Wang, 2001).

16. Donald Hopkins, *Princes and Peasants: Smallpox in History* (Chicago: University of Chicago Press, 1983), 268.

17. Pedro Jose Salicrup, "Smallpox and the Value of Vaccination as a Preventive," *New York Medical Journal* (1893): 605–610.

18. "Anti-Vaccinism," *Boston Medical and Surgical Journal* 130, no. 14 (1894): 346–347.

19. William W. Welch, "A Statistical Record of Five Thousand Cases of Small-Pox," *New York Medical Journal* 59 (1894): 326–330.

20. "The Question of Vaccination," *New York Daily Tribune*, September 2, 1896, 6; *New York Times*, March 13, 1897, 8.

21. Patricia Cline Cohen, *A Calculating People: The Spread of Numeracy in Early America* (Chicago: University of Chicago Press, 1982).

22. "Opposed to Vaccination," *New York Times*, June 6, 1895, 8.

23. Jay Frank Schamberg, "What Vaccination Has Really Done," in *Both Sides of the Vaccination Question* (Philadelphia: Anti-Vaccination League of America, 1911).

24. Theodore M. Porter, *Trust in Numbers: The Pursuit of Objectivity in Science and Public Life* (Princeton, N.J.: Princeton University Press, 1995).

25. Mark A. Miller, Alan R. Hinman, "Economic Analyses of Vaccine Policies," in Stanley A. Plotkin and Walter A. Orenstein, eds., *Vaccines*, 4th ed. (Philadelphia: Elsevier, 2004).

26. Chris Feudtner and Edgar K. Marcuse, "Ethics and Immunization Policy: Promoting Dialogue to Sustain Consensus," *Pediatrics* 107 (2001): 1158–1164.

27. Cyrus Edson, *A Plea for Compulsory Vaccination in Defence of Assembly Bill No. 474, Entitled "An Act Regulating Vaccination in the State of New York"* (New York: Trow's Printing and Bookbinding, 1889), 7.

28. David T. Karzon, "Immunization on Public Trial," *New England Journal of Medicine* 297 (1977): 275–277; 276.

29. Nadja Durbach, *Bodily Matters: The Anti-Vaccination Movement in England, 1853–1907* (Durham: Duke University Press, 2005). See also Dorothy Porter and Roy Porter, "The Politics of Prevention: Anti-Vaccinationism and Public Health in Nineteenth-Century England," *Medical History* 32 (1988): 231–252; and Roy MacLeod, "Law, Medicine and Public Opinion: The Resistance to Compulsory Health Legislation, 1870–1907," *Public Law* (1967): 106–128.

30. Martin Kaufman, "The American Anti-Vaccinationists and Their Arguments," *Bulletin of the History of Medicine* 41 (1967): 463–478; 465.

31. "Vaccination and Revaccination," *Boston Medical and Surgical Journal* 130, no 1 (1894): 21–22.

32. William Fowler, "Principal Provisions of Smallpox Vaccination Laws and Regulations in the United States," *Public Health Reports* 56, no. 5 (1941): 167–173; Charles L. Jackson, "State Laws on Compulsory Immunization in the United States," *Public Health Reports* 84, no. 9 (1969): 787–795.

33. John Duffy, "School Vaccination: The Precursor to School Medical Inspection," *Journal of the History of Medicine and Allied Sciences* 3 (1978): 344–355.

34. Kaufman, "American Anti-Vaccinationists and Their Arguments," 464.

35. Jackson also makes this point in "State Laws on Compulsory Immunization," 787.

36. *Hazen v. Strong*, 2 Vt. 427 (1830).

37. James A. Tobey, *Public Health Law: A Manual for Sanitarians* (Baltimore: Williams & Wilkins, 1926), 89–98; William Fowler, "Smallpox Vaccination Laws, Regulations, and Court Decisions," *Public Health Reports*, suppl. 60 (1927): 1–21.

38. Lawrence O. Gostin, *Public Health Law: Power, Duty, Restraint* (Berkeley: University of California Press, 2000); on the police powers, see 47–51.

39. Matthias Nicoll, "The Age of Public Health," *New York State Journal of Medicine* 27 (1927): 114–116; 116.

40. Ibid., 114.

41. New York State Health Department, Spot # 2, March 1, 1978, NYSDOH, series 13307–82, box 8, folder: Immunizations (1977–78).

42. *Achieving Public Response* (Atlanta: Communicable Disease Center, 1963), 1, NARA, RG 90, box 334062, folder: Achieving Public Response to Immunization Programs.

43. See, e.g., Janna Merrick, "Spiritual Healing, Sick Kids, and the Law: Inequities in the American Health Care System," *American Journal of Law and Medicine* 29 (2003): 269–299; and Rita Swan, "On Statutes Depriving a Class of Children to Rights to Medical Care: Can This Discrimination Be Litigated?" *Quinnipiac Health Law Journal* 2 (1999): 73–95.

44. Ross D. Silverman, "No More Kidding Around: Restructuring Non-Medical Childhood Immunization Exemptions to Ensure Public Health Protection," *Annals of Health Law* 12 (2003): 277–294.

45. P. Bradley, "Should Childhood Immunisation Be Compulsory?" *Journal of Medical Ethics* 25 (1999): 330–334; 334.

46. "Outbreak of Measles among Christian Science Students—Missouri and Illinois, 1994," *Morbidity and Mortality Weekly Report* 43 (1994): 463–465; Daniel R. Feiken, David C. Lezotte, R. F. Hamman, et al., "Individual and Community Risks of Measles and Pertussis Associated with Personal Exemptions to Immunization," *Journal of the American Medical Association* 284 (2000): 3145–3150.

1. BETWEEN PERSUASION AND COMPULSION

1. "The Value of Revaccination," *New York Daily Tribune*, January 4, 1902, 10.

2. *Annual Report of the Board of Health of the Health Department of the City of New York for the Year Ending December 31, 1894* (New York: Martin Brown, 1895), 45.

3. *Annual Report of the Board of Health of the City of Brooklyn for the Year 1886* (Brooklyn, 1887), 37.

4. See, e.g., F. G. Attwood, "Vaccination," *New York Medical Journal* 70 (1899): 803–804; "Proceedings of Societies," *Brooklyn Medical Journal* 15 (1901): 712–715.

5. Frank S. Fielder, "What Constitutes Efficient Vaccination?" *New York State Journal of Medicine* 2 (1902): 107.

6. *Annual Report of the Board of Health of the City of Brooklyn for the Year 1888* (Brooklyn, 1889), 45.

7. *Annual Report of the Board of Health of the City of Brooklyn for the Year 1887* (Brooklyn, 1888), 12.

8. The first permanent municipal health department was founded in New York City in 1866 and the first state board was created in Massachusetts in 1869. On the growth in the authority of health departments and scientific medicine during this period, see, e.g., Elizabeth Fee and Evelynn M. Hammonds, "Science, Politics and the Art of Persuasion: Promoting the New Scientific Medicine in New York City," in David Rosner, ed., *Hives of Sickness: Public Health and Epidemics in New York City* (New Brunswick, N.J.: Rutgers University Press, 1995); Stanley K. Schultz and Clay McShane, "To Engineer the Metropolis: Sewers, Sanitation, and City Planning in Late-Nineteenth-Century America," *Journal of American History* 65, no. 2 (1978): 389–411; and Barbara Gutmann Rosenkrantz, *Public Health and the State: Changing Views in Massachusetts, 1842–1936* (Cambridge, Mass.: Harvard University Press, 1972).

9. Rosenkrantz, *Public Health and the State*, 65–67; Judith Walzer Leavitt, *The Healthiest City: Milwaukee and the Politics of Health Reform* (Princeton, N.J.: Princeton University Press, 1982), 8–9 and passim.

10. F. A. Jewett, "Smallpox in Brooklyn," *Brooklyn Medical Journal* 8 (1894): 290–292. On German immigrants' mistrust of the health department, see also *Annual Report of the Board of Health of the City of Brooklyn for the Year 1888* (Brooklyn, 1889), 11, 45.

11. Claudia Huerkamp, "The History of Smallpox Vaccination in Germany: A First Step in the Medicalization of the General Public," *Journal of Contemporary History* 20 (1985): 617–635. On the resistance of German immigrants to health department authority in Milwaukee, see Leavitt, *Healthiest City*, 80–83 and passim.

12. Cited in Donald Hopkins, *Princes and Peasants: Smallpox in History* (Chicago: University of Chicago Press, 1983), 282.

13. "The News of Brooklyn," *New York Tribune*, April 6, 1902, II-10.

14. *Annual Report of the Board of Health of the City of Brooklyn for the Year 1894* (Brooklyn, 1895), 18, 87.

15. Exhibit C, Rules for Vaccinators, March 20, 1984, *In re Smith*, New York State Supreme Court Cases and Briefs, vol. 4269, Appellate Division 1896–1911, 68–69.

16. "No Vaccination for Him," *New York Sun*, March 23, 1894, 1.

17. "Quarantined Family Escapes," *New York Times*, March 23, 1894, 9.

18. "The McAuleys Vaccinated," *Brooklyn Daily Eagle*, March 26, 1894, 1. The *Times* and *Eagle* spellings of the family's last name are discrepant.

19. Cited in *In re Smith*, 146 N.Y. 68 (1895).

20. "Bungling Health Board Doctors," *Brooklyn Daily Eagle*, April 8, 1894, 3. The department of health did not record how many houses were placed under quarantine during the outbreak, so it is impossible to determine precisely how widespread the practice was, but it seems to have been uncommon relative to the number of vaccinations administered.

21. "Smallpox Precautions," *Brooklyn Daily Eagle*, March 30, 1894, 7. The validity of this complaint is uncertain. The city did contract with private physicians to serve as vaccinators during epidemics, but it is unclear from health department records whether they were paid a flat or per capita salary.

22. "Vaccination Is Safe," *Brooklyn Daily Eagle*, March 26, 1894, 5. See also "Smallpox Precautions," ibid., March 21, 1894, 12.

23. Edwin G. Burrows and Mike Wallace, *Gotham: A History of New York City to 1898* (New York: Oxford University Press, 1999), 1227–1228; David Rosner, *A Once Charitable Enterprise: Hospitals and Health Care in Brooklyn and New York, 1885–1915* (Princeton, N.J.: Princeton University Press, 1982), 24.

24. *Annual Report of the Board of Health of the City of Brooklyn for the Year 1894* (Brooklyn, 1895), 12.

25. Exhibit A, *Smith v. Emery*, New York State Supreme Court Cases and Briefs, vol. 4269, Appellate Division, 1896–1911, 48.

26. "Proceedings of Societies," *Brooklyn Medical Journal* 8 (1894): 643.

27. Cited in *Brooklyn Medical Journal* 8 (1894): 576.

28. "Physicians Fighting Hard," *New York Times,* March 29, 1894, 9. See also "Brooklyn's Small-Pox Outbreak," *New York Sun,* March 29, 1894, 1.

29. "Great Increase in Smallpox," *New York Times,* March 27, 1894, 9. Newspaper accounts during the outbreak do not specify mass vaccination at all-female workplaces, but there is no reason to believe that the health department systematically neglected them. Indeed, health department annual reports frequently express concern over the work of seamstresses and laundresses because of the danger posed by infected clothes and bedding.

30. "Vaccinators Start a Riot," *New York Sun,* April 19, 1894, 1.

31. *Annual Report of the Board of Health of the City of Brooklyn for the Year 1894* (Brooklyn, 1895), 178.

32. Leavitt, *Healthiest City,* 76–121.

33. "Preparing to Stamp Out Smallpox," *New York Times,* April 24, 1894, 9.

34. "Chicago's Small-Pox Scourge," *New York Sun,* April 22, 1894, 1.

35. William G. Eidson, "Confusion, Controversy, and Quarantine: The Muncie Smallpox Epidemic of 1893," *Indiana Magazine of History* 56 (1990): 374–398.

36. "Anti-Vaccination Sentiment," *New York Daily Tribune,* April 15, 1894, 18.

37. Jewett, "Smallpox in Brooklyn"; "Vaccination in the Public Schools," *Brooklyn Medical Journal* 8 (1894): 294.

38. *Annual Report of the Board of Health of the City of Brooklyn for the Year 1894* (Brooklyn: 1895), 96.

39. "Modest Girls, Horrid Doctors," *New York Herald,* March 30, 1894, 8; "The Girls Fooled the Doctor," *Brooklyn Daily Eagle,* March 31, 1894, 1.

40. "Against Compulsory Vaccination," *New York Times,* April 22, 1894, 12; "Anti-Vaccinators Busy," *New York Herald,* April 28, 1894, 4.

41. Testimony of William H. Smith, *Smith v. Emery,* New York State Supreme Court Cases and Briefs, vol. 4269, Appellate Division, 1896–1911, 12–22.

42. *Annual Report of the Board of Health of the City of Brooklyn for the Year 1886* (Brooklyn, 1887), 39.

43. Testimony of William H. Smith, *Smith v. Emery,* New York State Supreme Court Cases and Briefs, 14–17.

44. Mortimer Smith, *William Jay Gaynor, Mayor of New York* (Chicago: Henry Regnery, 1951), 19–38. Gaynor was elected mayor of New York in 1910 and died in office in 1913.

45. "Judge Gaynor's Rulings," *New York Sun,* February 26, 1894, 6.

46. "Dangers of Smallpox," *Brooklyn Daily Eagle,* May 7, 1894, 5.

47. *In re Smith,* Ruling of William J. Gaynor, May 18, 1894, New York State Supreme Court Cases and Briefs, 35.

48. Testimony of Z. Taylor Emery, *Smith v. Emery,* New York State Supreme Court Cases and Briefs, 67.

49. "A Fight against Vaccination," *Brooklyn Daily Eagle,* May 5, 1894, 1; "Law as to Vaccination," *New York Times,* May 5, 1894, 9; "As to Compulsory Vaccination," *New York World,* May 5, 1894, 8; "Gaynor on the Health Board's Rights," *New York Daily Tribune,* May 5, 1894, 12.

50. "Smallpox Outbreak Feared," *Brooklyn Daily Eagle*, May 30, 1894, 1; "Refused to Be Vaccinated," *New York Times*, May 31, 1894, 9.

51. "Virus in an Italian Colony," *Brooklyn Daily Eagle*, May 7, 1894, 1. For an account of a similar sweep with police accompaniment in the Italian neighborhood of Red Hook, see "A Brooklyn Vaccinating Raid," *New York Sun*, April 19, 1894, 1.

52. "Slashed at the Doctors," *Brooklyn Daily Eagle*, May 8, 1894, 12.

53. "Want Emery Removed," *Brooklyn Daily Eagle*, May 29, 1894, 7.

54. "A Legal Contest over Vaccination," *New York Tribune*, July 13, 1894, 12; "Anti-Vaccination Test Cases," *New York Times*, July 13, 1894, 9.

55. "Vaccination and the Public Schools," *Brooklyn Medical Journal* 8 (1894): 637–639.

56. *Annual Report of the Board of Health of the City of Brooklyn for the Year 1894* (Brooklyn, 1895), 96. The number of house-to-house vaccinations was 164,306.

57. *In re Smith*, ruling of J. Dykman, February 14, 1895, Cases in the Court of Appeals, vol. 1442, New York Law Institute, 24.

58. *In re Smith*, 146 N.Y. 68 (1895).

59. *Smith v. Emery*, judgment of Charles F. Brown, December 16, 1895, New York State Supreme Court Cases and Briefs, 10.

60. *Smith v. Emery*, transcript, New York State Supreme Court Cases and Briefs, 43. The figure of 140 cases per day does not correspond to any health department data; it is probable that the judge here is speaking hyperbolically.

61. Ibid., 39–42 and passim.

62. See, e.g., *O'Brien v. Cunard Steamship Company*, 154 Mass. 272 (1891); "Vaccination Too Thorough," *New York Times*, January 22, 1903.

63. Randolph E. Bergstrom, *Courting Danger: Injury and Law in New York City, 1870–1910* (Ithaca, N.Y.: Cornell University Press, 1992), 19–21.

64. "$1,500 for Forced Vaccination," *New York Times*, November 16, 1895, 1.

65. "Death Followed the Vaccination," *New York Herald*, May 3, 1894, 11.

66. "Vaccine Suits in Brooklyn," *New York Times*, January 10, 1896, 9; "Light on that Vaccination," *New York Tribune*, January 11, 1896, 9.

67. "Burgraf vs. Emery," *Brooklyn Medical Journal* 19 (1896): 139–147. The spelling of the family name appears as "Burggraff" in most of the press accounts of the case.

68. "Lockjaw Germs Abound," *New York Times*, January 11, 1896, 14.

69. "The Burggraff Jury Discharged," *New York Times*, January 18, 1896, 9.

70. *Smith v. Emery*, 11 A.D. 10 (1896).

71. "Crowds Seek Vaccination," *New York Daily Tribune*, December 2, 1900, 6.

72. *Annual Report for the Board of Health of the Department of Health of the City of New York for the Year Ending December 31, 1901* (New York: Martin H. Brown, 1902), 13, 30.

73. Elizabeth Fee and Evelynn M. Hammonds, "Science, Politics and the Art of Persuasion: Promoting the New Scientific Medicine in New York City," in

David Rosner, ed., *Hives of Sickness: Public Health and Epidemics in New York City* (New Brunswick, N.J.: Rutgers University Press, 1995).

74. Hammonds, *Childhood's Deadly Scourge,* 169–173.

75. The distinction between treatment and prevention is not absolute. Antitoxin had limited immunizing powers against diphtheria, and vaccination, if performed very soon after exposure, could mitigate the effects of smallpox. But it was the curative power of antitoxin and the preventive properties of vaccination for which each was well known.

76. "Panic over Vaccination," *New York Daily Tribune,* April 28, 1902, 12.

77. *Annual Report for the Board of Health of the Department of Health of the City of New York for the Year Ending December 31, 1901* (New York: Martin H. Brown, 1902), 30. A total of 1,964 cases and 410 fatalities were recorded in 1901.

78. *Annual Report for the Board of Health of the Department of Health of the City of New York for the Year Ending December 31, 1902* (New York: Martin H. Brown, 1903), 8.

79. "Small-Pox in Suburbs Rouses City Health Board," *New York World,* January 19, 1902, 5.

80. Quoted in Charles E. Rosenberg, *Explaining Epidemics and Other Studies in the History of Medicine* (Cambridge: Cambridge University Press, 1992), 231.

81. "To Attack Disease in Lodging Houses," *New York Daily Tribune,* March 18, 1902, 5; "Vaccinated Six Thousand in a Night," ibid., March 20, 1902, 6.

82. "Information Wanted by the Committee on Vaccination," *New York State Journal of Medicine* 1 (1901): 138.

83. "Compulsory Vaccination," *New York Medical Journal* 75 (1902): 292; "To Make Vaccination Compulsory by Law," *New York World,* February 11, 1902, 4.

84. See, e.g., Hammonds, *Childhood's Deadly Scourge,* 11–12.

85. "Compulsory Vaccination," *Brooklyn Medical Journal* 16 (April 1902): 184.

86. "Vaccination under Indirect Compulsion," *New York Medical Journal* 75 (1902): 330.

87. Ibid., 331.

88. "The Amended Vaccination Act for New York State," *Medical Record* 61 (1902): 379.

89. J. N. McCormack, "The Value of State Control and Vaccination in the Management of Smallpox," *Journal of the American Medical Association* 38 (1902): 1434.

90. "Night Stations for Vaccination," *New York World,* February 9, 1902, 5.

91. "Compulsory Vaccination Law," *New York State Journal of Medicine* 2 (1902): 99.

92. Cyrus Edson, *A Plea for Compulsory Vaccination in Defence of Assembly Bill No. 474, Entitled "An Act Regulating Vaccination in the State of New York"* (New York: Trow's Printing and Bookbinding, 1889).

93. On Edson's aggressive use of police powers, see Howard Markel, *Quarantine! East European Jewish Immigrants and the New York City Epidemics of 1892* (Baltimore: John Hopkins University Press, 1997).

94. Michael R. Albert, Kristen G. Ostheimer, and Joel G. Breman, "The Last Smallpox Epidemic in Boston and the Vaccination Controversy, 1901–1903," *New England Journal of Medicine* 344, no. 5 (2001): 375–379.

95. The effort to repeal the Massachusetts law was ultimately unsuccessful (ibid.).

96. "Anti-Vaccination League," *New York Times*, January 6, 1901, 5.

97. *Annual Report for the Board of Health of the Department of Health of the City of New York for the Year Ending December 31, 1902*, 8.

98. James A. Tobey, *Public Health Law: A Manual for Sanitarians* (Baltimore: Williams & Wilkins, 1926), 89–98; William Fowler, "Smallpox Vaccination Laws, Regulations, and Court Decisions," *Public Health Reports,* suppl. 60 (1927): 1–21.

99. "The Cambridge Smallpox Epidemic," *Medical News* 80 (1902): 1231–1232; 1231.

100. Albert, Ostheimer, and Breman, "Last Smallpox Epidemic in Boston."

101. This biographical summary is drawn from "The Rev. Henning Jacobson," *New York Times*, October 15, 1930, 17; "Rev. Henning Jacobson," *Boston Herald*, October 15, 1930, 19; S. J. Sebelius, *My Church: An Illustrated Lutheran Manual* (Rock Island, Ill.: Augustana Book Concern, 1931); and *The Augustana Messenger* 1, no. 5 (1930), Archives of the Evangelical Lutheran Church in America.

102. *Transcript of Record, Supreme Court of the United States, Jacobson v. Massachusetts* (Washington, D.C.: Judd & Detweiler, 1903), 6.

103. Ibid., 7.

104. Ibid., 5.

105. *Commonwealth v. Pear, Commonwealth v. Jacobson,* 183 Mass. 242 (1903), 245.

106. Ibid., 246–247.

107. Ibid., 248.

108. "Final Appeal on Vaccination," *Boston Herald*, December 7, 1904, 16.

109. On Williams's life and career, see Gordon S. Wood, "The Massachusetts Mugwumps," *New England Quarterly* 33 (1960): 435–451; "Running for Governor," *New York Times*, October 20, 1895, 21; "The Bay State Democracy," *New York Times*, September 29, 1897, 3.

110. *Jacobson v. Massachusetts, Brief and Argument for Plaintiff in Error* (New York: Eastern Press, 1904), 23.

111. Ibid., 15.

112. *Jacobson v. Massachusetts, Brief and Argument for Defendant in Error* (New York: Eastern Press, 1904), 3.

113. *Jacobson v. Massachusetts,* 197 U.S. 11 (1905). The case has received surprisingly little analysis from historians or legal scholars. The best overview is Lawrence O. Gostin, *Public Health Law: Power, Duty, Restraint* (Berkeley: University of California Press, 2000), 66–69 and passim. A cogent analysis of

the case with respect to literal and metaphorical conceptions of bodily integrity is Alan Hyde, *Bodies of Law* (Princeton, N.J.: Princeton University Press, 1995), 241–252. See also Lynne Curry, *The Human Body on Trial* (Santa Barbara, Calif.: ABC-Clio, 2002), 51–54.

114. *Jacobson v. Massachusetts*, 25.

115. Ibid., 26.

116. Ibid., 27.

117. Ibid., 38–39.

118. Lawrence Gostin contends, "If there had been evidence that the vaccination would seriously impair Jacobson's health, he may have prevailed in this historic case." *Public Health Law*, 69. Alan Hyde, who believes *Jacobson* was correctly decided, nevertheless claims that the failure of the lower court to admit Jacobson's evidence that he was in physical danger from vaccination is "truly embarrassing ... to modern eyes." *Bodies of Law*, 244.

119. *Lochner v. New York*, 198 U.S. 45 (1905), 59.

120. Ibid., 70.

121. Ibid., 75.

122. *Boston Herald*, February 21, 1905, 6.

123. *New York Times*, February 22, 1905, 6.

2. SCIENCE IN A DEMOCRACY

1. James A. Loyster, *Vaccination Results in New York State in 1914* (Cazenovia, N.Y.: n.p., 1915).

2. Donald R. Hopkins, *Princes and Peasants: Smallpox in History* (Chicago: University of Chicago Press, 1983), 287–292.

3. Between 1908 and 1920, the number of deaths in New York state each year from smallpox never exceeded seven, and was sometimes zero, compared to deaths numbering in the hundreds or even thousands from conditions such as diphtheria, measles, and typhoid. Typescript, NYSDOH, series 13855, roll 28.

4. Dr. Hervey to deputy commissioner, December 27, 1926, NYSDOH, series 13855–84, reel 11.

5. See, e.g., correspondence in October 1917 between the Office of Hygienic Laboratory and the surgeon general regarding the National Vaccine and Antitoxin Institute, a manufacturer headquartered in Washington, D.C., which had its license suspended after samples were found to be contaminated with tetanus. NARA, RG 90, box 370, folder: Tetanus.

6. "Compulsory Vaccination," *New York State Journal of Medicine* 15 (1915): 3.

7. *Vaccination: What It Is, What It Does, What Its Claims Are on the People* (Albany, N.Y.: J. B. Lyon, 1908).

8. Jonathan Liebenau, *Medical Science and Medical Industry: The Formation of the American Pharmaceutical Industry* (Basingstoke: Macmillan, 1987); Louis Galambos with Jane Eliot Sewell, *Networks of Innovation: Vaccine Development at Merck, Sharp & Dohme, and Mulford, 1895–1995* (Cambridge: Cambridge University Press, 1995).

9. George W. McCoy to surgeon general, January 10, 1916, NARA, RG 90, box 368.

10. Plague vaccine, e.g., was used in outbreaks in San Francisco in 1900 and 1906. See Nayan Shah, *Contagious Divides: Epidemics and Race in San Francisco's Chinatown* (Berkeley: University of California Press, 2001).

11. Mazyck P. Ravenal, "The Control of Typhoid Fever by Vaccination," *Proceedings of the American Philosophical Society* 52 (1913): 226–233; Anne Hardy, "'Straight Back to Barbarism': Anti-Typhoid Inoculation and the Great War, 1914," *Bulletin of the History of Medicine* 74, no. 2 (2000): 265–90.

12. Selwyn D. Collins, "Frequency of Immunizing and Related Procedures in Nine Thousand Surveyed Families in Eighteen States," *Milbank Memorial Fund Quarterly* 15, no. 2 (1937): 150–172.

13. See, e.g., "Will Vaccine Be the Greatest Cure in Medical Science?" *New York Times,* August 21, 1910, V-12. See also Terra Ziporyn, *Disease in the Popular American Press: The Case of Diphtheria, Typhoid Fever, and Syphilis, 1870–1920* (New York: Greenwood Press, 1988); and Nancy Tomes, *The Gospel of Germs: Men, Women and the Microbe in American Life* (Cambridge, Mass.: Harvard University Press, 1998).

14. *Jacobson v. Massachusetts, Brief and Argument for Plaintiff in Error* (New York: Eastern Press, 1904), 29.

15. Christopher Lasch, *Haven in a Heartless World: The Family Besieged* (New York: Basic Books, 1977); see 12–21 for a discussion of "the appropriation of familial functions by agencies of socialized reproduction" (15). See also Andrew Polsky, *The Rise of the Therapeutic State* (Princeton, N.J.: Princeton University Press, 1991).

16. Angela Nugent, "Fit for Work: The Introduction of Physical Examinations in Industry," *Bulletin of the History of Medicine* 57 (1983): 578–595.

17. Audrey Davis, "Life Insurance and the Physical Examination: A Chapter in the Rise of American Medical Technology," *Bulletin of the History of Medicine* 55 (1981): 392–406.

18. S. S. Goldwater, "Wants Every New Yorker Physically Examined Yearly," *New York Times,* May 10, 1914, SM8.

19. H. B. Anderson, *State Medicine: A Menace to Democracy* (New York: Citizens Medical Reference Bureau, 1920), 23.

20. Theda Skocpol, *Protecting Soldiers and Mothers: The Political Origins of Social Policy in the United States* (Cambridge, Mass.: Belknap Press, 1992), 480–524; and Linda Gordon, *Pitied but Not Entitled: Single Mothers and the History of Welfare, 1890–1935* (New York: Free Press, 1994).

21. Stanley Joel Reiser, "The Emergence of the Concept of Screening for Disease," *Milbank Memorial Fund Quarterly* 56, no. 4 (1978): 403–425; Nadav Davidovitch, "Negotiating Dissent: Homeopathy and Anti-Vaccinationism at the Turn of the Twentieth Century," in Robert D. Johnston, ed., *The Politics of Healing: Histories of Alternative Medicine in Twentieth-Century North America* (New York: Routledge, 2004), 11–28.

22. Luther Halsey Gulick and Leonard P. Ayres, *Medical Inspection of Schools* (New York: Survey Associates, 1913).

23. Anderson, *State Medicine,* 23. See also 65–81 in the same book.

24. Cynthia Connolly, "Prevention through Detention: The Pediatric Tuberculosis Preventorium Movement in the United States, 1909–1951" (Ph.D. diss., University of Pennsylvania, 1999).

25. Ronald Numbers, *Almost Persuaded: American Physicians and Compulsory Health Insurance* (Baltimore: Johns Hopkins University Press, 1978).

26. On the Sheppard-Towner Act as the fruition of some of the most prominent Progressive Era ideals, see J. Stanley Lemons, "The Sheppard-Towner Act: Progressivism in the 1920s," *Journal of American History* 55, no. 4 (1969): 776–786.

27. Richard A. Meckel, *Save the Babies: American Public Health Reform and the Prevention of Infant Mortality 1850–1929* (Baltimore: Johns Hopkins University Press, 1990), 200–219; Skocpol, *Protecting Soldiers and Mothers*, 494–524.

28. Lynn Dumenil, "'The Insatiable Maw of Bureaucracy': Antistatism and Education Reform in the 1920s," *Journal of American History* 77, no. 2 (1990): 499–524.

29. Cited in Skocpol, *Protecting Soldiers and Mothers*, 500.

30. A 1912 publication of the Anti-Vaccination League of America listed regional directors in eight states.

31. On the relationship among Swedenborgianism, homeopathy, and antivaccinationism, see Davidovitch, "Negotiating Dissent," 315.

32. Richard R. Gladish, *John Pitcairn: Uncommon Entrepreneur* (Bryn Athyn, Pa.: Academy of the New Church, 1989), 330–335.

33. John Pitcairn, *Vaccination: An Address Delivered before the Committee on Public Health and Sanitation of the General Assembly of Pennsylvania at Harrisburg, March 5, 1907* (Philadelphia: Anti-Vaccination League of Pennsylvania, 1907), 1; emphasis in original.

34. Bernhard J. Stern, *Should We Be Vaccinated?* (New York: Harper & Brothers, 1927), 110.

35. "C. M. Higgins Dies; Ink Manufacturer" (obituary), *New York Times,* October 23, 1929, 27.

36. Anderson, *State Medicine*, 15.

37. The Pitcairn sons' commitment to the cause championed by their father recalls a similar legacy in Britain, where the work of one of the most prominent anti-vaccinationists of the nineteenth century, William Tebb, was carried on by his son, W. Scott Tebb. See W. Scott Tebb, *A Century of Vaccination and What It Teaches* (London: Swan Sonnenschein, 1899), which the younger Tebb dedicated to his father.

38. Norman Hapgood, ed., *Professional Patriots* (New York: Albert and Charles Boni, 1927), 170–172. On the Sentinels of the Republic, see also Walter I. Trattner, *Crusade for the Children: A History of the National Child Labor Committee and Child Labor Reform in America* (Chicago: Quadrangle Books, 1970), 166–167.

39. An excellent account of Little's life and career is provided in Robert D. Johnston, *The Radical Middle Class: Populist Democracy and the Question of Capitalism in Progressive Era Portland, Oregon* (Princeton, N.J.: Princeton University Press, 2003), 197–217, from which this biographical sketch is drawn.

40. In 1922, the letterhead of the American Medical Liberty League listed affiliates in thirty-six states and the District of Columbia.

41. Rennie B. Schoepflin, *Christian Science on Trial: Religious Healing in America* (Baltimore: Johns Hopkins University Press, 2003), 168–210 and app. 1.

42. Cited in Schoepflin, *Christian Science on Trial*, 179; see also Stephen Gottschalk, *The Emergence of Christian Science in American Religious Life* (Berkeley: University of California Press, 1973), 224–225.

43. Cited in Edwin Frander Dakin, *Mrs. Eddy: The Biography of a Virginal Mind* (New York: Charles Scribner's Sons, 1929), 369.

44. See, e.g., Julius Schiller to Edward S. Godfrey, January 13, 1924, NYSDOH, series 13855–84, reel 10; and "Deny School Clash," *New York Times*, June 27, 1929, 28.

45. See A. H. Flickwir to surgeon general, December 19, 1923, on the efforts of Christian Scientists to have the school vaccination requirement in Houston, Texas, repealed, NARA, RG 90, box 368; and Orwell Bradley Towne to Shirley W. Wynne, May 28, 1930, inquiring on behalf of the Christian Science Committee on Publication about the specifics of New York City's school entry law, NYCDOH, box 141356, folder: Vaccination.

46. See, e.g., "Public Defended as Schools Open," *Christian Science Monitor*, n.d. (August 1921), reporting on the efforts of Lora Little and the American Medical Liberty League to resist Chicago's compulsory school vaccination law. NARA, RG 90, box 366.

47. On physical culture and the life of Bernarr Macfadden, see William R. Hunt, *Body Love: The Amazing Career of Bernarr Macfadden* (Bowling Green, Ohio: Bowling Green State University Popular Press, 1989); Robert Ernst, "Macfadden, Bernarr," *American National Biography Online*, February 2000, www.anb.org/articles/16/16–02450.html (accessed December 16, 2002); and "Macfadden Dead; Health Cultist, 87" (obituary), *New York Times*, October 13, 1955, 31.

48. Felix Leopold Oswald, *Vaccination a Crime, with Comments on Other Sanitary Superstitions* (New York: Physical Culture Publishing, 1901).

49. Cited in Grace Perkins, *Chats with the Macfadden Family* (New York: Lewis Copeland, 1929), 81.

50. Hunt, *Body Love*, 105. Morris Fishbein, the editor of the *Journal of the American Medical Association* and Macfadden's most vituperative critic, charged that *Physical Culture* frequently published articles by bogus medical professionals. See Morris Fishbein, *The Medical Follies* (New York: Boni & Liveright, 1925), 177–178.

51. Stern, *Should We Be Vaccinated?* 107–108.

52. Bernarr Macfadden to "Dear Friend," February 8, 1930, NYCDOH, box 141356, folder: Vaccination.

53. Walter I. Wardwell, *Chiropractic: History and Evolution of a New Profession* (St. Louis: Mosby Year Book, 1992); see esp. 51–130.

54. On chiropractors' advocacy against vaccination, see Frederick R. Green to Hugh S. Cumming, April 5, 1920, NARA, RG 90, box 369; Ennion

G. Williams to Hugh S. Cumming, June 20, 1922, NARA, RG 90, box 367; Mosby G. Perrow to Hugh S. Cumming, October 31, 1923, NARA, RG 90, box 368; A. H. Flickwir to surgeon general, December 19, 1923, NARA, RG 90, box 368; "Offer to Risk Smallpox," *New York Times,* January 11, 1925, 2; "Vaccination Is Assailed," ibid., March 2, 1925, 21; "Opposes Vaccination of Daughter; Jailed," ibid., December 16, 1926, 49; and D. Pirie-Beyea to Shirley W. Wynne, December 12, 1929, NYCDOH, box 141353, folder: Vaccination.

55. Paul Starr, *The Social Transformation of American Medicine* (New York: Basic Books, 1982).

56. Eberhard Wolff, "Sectarian Identity and the Aim of Integration," *British Homeopathic Journal* 85 (1996): 95–114; Davidovitch, "Negotiating Dissent"; "Against Compulsory Vaccination," *New York Times,* April 22, 1894, 12; "Anti-Vaccinators Busy," *New York Herald,* April 28, 1894, 4.

57. On affinities between anti-vaccinationists and anti-vivisectionists in nineteenth-century England, see Richard D. French, *Antivivisection and Medical Science in Victorian Society* (Princeton, N.J.: Princeton University Press, 1975).

58. Susan Eyrich Lederer, "Hideyo Noguchi's Luetin Experiment and the Anti-Vivisectionists," *Isis* 76 (1985): 31–48; Susan E. Lederer, "Political Animals: The Shaping of Biomedical Research Literature in Twentieth-Century America," *Isis* 83 (1992): 61–79; Susan Lederer, "The Controversy over Animal Experimentation in America, 1880–1914," in Nicolaas Rupke, ed., *Vivisection in Historical Perspective* (London: Croom Helm, 1987).

59. On female Christian Scientists, see Schoepflin, *Christian Science on Trial,* 52–54; on female anti-vivisectionists, see Lederer, "Political Animals," 63.

60. Johnston's study of anti-vaccinationism in Portland, Oregon, finds strong middle-class roots in the movement ("a plebian alliance solidly anchored in the world of lower-level white collar work"); see *Radical Middle Class,* 216 and passim.

61. NARA, RG 90, box 364; spelling and punctuation as in original.

62. Higgins, *Vaccination and Lockjaw,* 11.

63. Anderson, *State Medicine,* 82.

64. See, e.g., the New York State health department publication *Vaccination: What It Is, What It Does, What Its Claims Are on the People* (Albany, N.Y.: J. B. Lyon, 1908).

65. Lora C. Little, *Crimes of the Cowpox Ring: Some Moving Pictures Thrown on the Dead Wall of Official Silence* (Minneapolis: Liberator Publishing, 1906), 6.

66. Manfred Waserman, "The Quest for a National Health Department in the Progressive Era," *Bulletin of the History of Medicine* 49 (1975): 353–380; Martin Kaufman, *Homeopathy in America: The Rise and Fall of a Medical Heresy* (Baltimore: Johns Hopkins University Press, 1971), 162–166.

67. For example, the American Medical Liberty League included copies of the newsletter of the Citizens Medical Reference Bureau in its mailings to legislators; see NARA, RG 90, box 367. The letterhead of the American Medical Liberty League identified the group as "endorsing the principles and aims of the

anti-vivisection societies." H. B. Anderson of the Citizens Medical Reference Bureau also spoke at anti-vivisection conferences. See "Foes of Vivisection Hold Annual Meeting," *New York Times*, May 18, 1927, 28. Activists who belonged to more than one organization included Diana Belais, the president of the New York Anti-Vivisection Society, and Nellie Williams, a member of the society, both of whom served as directors of the American Medical Liberty League; Williams was also a vice president of the Citizens Medical Reference Bureau. Jesse Mercer Gehman, a doctor of naturopathy who worked as an associate editor of Macfadden's *Physical Culture* magazine, became the secretary of the Citizen's Medical Reference Bureau in the 1930s and ultimately carried on the bureau's work after H. B. Anderson's death in 1953. See Donald R. McNeil, *The Fight for Fluoridation* (New York: Oxford University Press, 1957), 121; and Hunt, *Body Love*, 109.

68. Charles M. Higgins, *Unalienable Rights and Prohibition Wrongs* (Brooklyn: n.p., 1919), 5.

69. *The Medical Follies* attacked alternative healers such as chiropractors, homeopaths, and naturopaths, as well as popular fitness movements such as physical culture.

70. The group's honorary president was Charles W. Eliot, the former president of Harvard University, and its members included Yale University President James Rowland Angell, former New York governor and presidential candidate Charles Evans Hughes, and Edward Wigglesworth, the director of the Boston Museum of Natural History.

71. Benjamin C. Gruenberg, "Diphtheria Statistics," *New York Times*, September 21, 1927, 28.

72. American Association for Medical Progress, *Smallpox—A Preventable Disease* (New York: American Association for Medical Progress, 1924), 8–9.

73. Benjamin Gruenberg, "Science in a Democracy," in id. ed., *Modern Science and People's Health* (New York: Norton, 1926), 11–12.

74. "Friends of Medical Progress," *Journal of the American Medical Association* 81, no. 17 (1923): 1443–1444.

75. Lora Little to Hugh S. Cumming, June 5, 1922, NARA, RG 90, box 367. See also letters from Little to the health commissioners of Colorado, Virginia, South Carolina, Iowa, and New York in the same box.

76. Hugh S. Cumming to Edward S. Godfrey, June 21, 1922, NARA, RG 90, box 367.

77. Ennion G. Williams to Lora Little, June 20, 1922, NARA, RG 90, box 367.

78. John N. Force and James P. Leake, "Smallpox in Twenty States, 1915–1920," *Public Health Reports*, 1921: 1979–1989.

79. Ibid., 1989.

80. Raymond Pearl, *The Biology of Death* (Philadelphia: Lippincott, 1922); see 223–258 on the effects of public health efforts on mortality patterns.

81. Louis I. Dublin, "Does Health Work Pay?" reprint from *The Survey*, May 15, 1923, Louis I. Dublin papers, box 7, folder: Does Health Work Pay? 1923, National Library of Medicine.

82. "Child Toll of Smallpox," *New York Times*, August 13, 1922, II-14.

83. Stern, *Should We Be Vaccinated?* 109.

84. Samuel B. Woodward, "Legislative Aspects of Vaccination," *Boston Medical and Surgical Journal* 185, no. 11 (1921): 307–310.

85. C. C. Pierce, "Some Reasons for Compulsory Vaccination," *Boston Medical and Surgical Journal* 192, no. 15 (1925): 689–695; Force and Leake, "Smallpox in Twenty States," 1989.

86. Johnston, *Radical Middle Class*, 207–217.

87. Chester H. Rowell, "Medical and Anti-Medical Legislation in California," *American Journal of Public Health* 11 (1921): 128–132.

88. The vote on the anti-vaccination measure was 57 percent opposed and 43 percent in favor. "Defeat of Antivaccination and Antivivisection Measures on the Pacific Coast," *Public Health Reports* 35 (1920): 3040.

89. Charles M. Higgins, *Repeal of Compulsory Vaccination: Memorial to the Legislature and Governor of the State of New York* (n.p., 1909); "Renew War on Vaccination," *New York Times*, March 17, 1911, 3.

90. "Poll Gives Tie Vote in Fight on Barnes," *New York Times*, May 27, 1913, 2; "Keynote Address by Root," ibid., July 10, 1914, 4.

91. James A. Loyster, *Vaccination Results in New York State in 1914* (Cazenovia, N.Y.: n.p., 1915).

92. Louis K. Neff to Rupert Blue, February 1, 1915, NARA, RG 90, box 251, folder: 2796 (1915).

93. Abraham Jacobi, "Address in Opposition to the Jones-Tallett Amendment to the Public Health Law in Relation to Vaccination," *New York State Journal of Medicine* 15, no. 3 (1915): 90–92.

94. On Biggs's career, see C.-E. A. Winslow, *The Life of Hermann M. Biggs* (Philadelphia: Lea & Febiger, 1929); on Biggs's use of compulsion and the politics of such policies, see Daniel M. Fox, "Social Policy and City Politics: Tuberculosis Reporting in New York, 1889–1900," *Bulletin of the History of Medicine* 49, no. 2 (1975): 169–195.

95. Hermann M. Biggs, "Arguments in Favor of the Jones-Tallett Amendment to the Public Health Law in Relation to Vaccination," *New York State Journal of Medicine* 15, no. 3 (1915): 89–90.

96. Charles M. Higgins, *The Crime against the School Child* (Brooklyn: n.p., 1915), 5–9.

97. William Fowler, "Smallpox Vaccination Laws, Regulations, and Court Decisions," *Public Health Reports*, suppl. 60 (1927): 1–21.

98. The campaign against syphilis was also framed in this way. Allan Brandt, *No Magic Bullet: A Social History of Venereal Disease in the United States Since 1880* (New York: Oxford University Press, 1987), 52–121.

99. Circular Number 116 of the Public Health Service; see correspondence between the PHS and state and local health officers in NARA, RG 90, boxes 363 and 369.

100. See clippings and correspondence in NARA, RG 90, box 363.

101. President, Union Steel Products Company, to Rupert Blue, July 8, 1918, NARA, RG 90, box 369.

102. W. D. Heaton to medical officer in charge, July 29, 1918, NARA, RG 90, box 363.

103. On wartime labor unrest, see David Kennedy, *Over Here: The First World War and American Society* (New York: Oxford University Press, 1980), 258–270.

104. Fred C. Butler to surgeon general, July 10, 1918, NARA, RG 90, box 369.

105. Walker Hines to Rupert Blue, August 7, 1918, NARA, RG 90, box 369.

106. Nugent, "Fit for Work," 591.

107. W. O. Sweek to Rupert Blue, March 22, 1918; NARA, RG 90, box 363. See also Walter A. Scott to U.S. Public Health Service, NARA, RG 90, box 369; Rupert Blue to solicitor, Post Office Department, October 28, 1918, NARA, RG 90, box 364, folder: October 1918.

108. Johnston, *Radical Middle Class*, 210.

109. Matthias Nicoll, "Discussion," *American Journal of Public Health* 17 (1927): 206–207.

110. George Truman Palmer, Mahew Derryberry, and Philip Van Ingen, *Health Protection for the Preschool Child* (New York: Century, 1931), 50.

111. Ibid., 51.

112. Ibid., 7.

113. Selwyn D. Collins, "Frequency of Immunizing and Related Procedures in Nine Thousand Surveyed Families in Eighteen States," *Milbank Memorial Fund Quarterly* 15, no. 2 (1937): 150–172.

114. Palmer, Derryberry, and Van Ingen, *Health Protection for the Preschool Child*, 44, 111.

115. Ibid., 82–83, 112.

116. Matthias Nicoll, "The Age of Public Health," *New York State Journal of Medicine* 27 (1927): 114–116.

117. See, e.g., Edward Godfrey to Thomas E. Spaulding, August 19, 1924, and Paul Brooks to Thomas E. Spaulding, August 24, 1924, NYSDOH, series 13855–84, reel 11; and Dr. Brooks to Dr. Godfrey, March 19, 1927, NYSDOH, series 13855–84, reel 13.

118. Edward Godfrey to Dr. Sayer, March 26, 1927, NYSDOH, series 13855–84, reel 13.

119. Herman E. Hilleboe, "A Brief History of the New York State Department of Health and Its Activities," *New York State Journal of Medicine* 57 (1957): 533–542; 536.

120. Governor's Special Health Commission, *Public Health in New York State* (Albany: State of New York Department of Health, 1932), 38–39, 55–77.

121. Thomas E. Spaulding to H. F. Senftner, July 18, 1926, NYSDOH, series 13855–84, reel 11.

122. See, e.g., Dr. Hervey to deputy commissioner, October 27, 1926, NYSDOH, series 13855–84, reel 12.

123. Dr. Hervey to deputy commissioner, December 27, 1926, NYSDOH, series 13855–84, reel 11.

124. Lockport Board of Commerce to "Dear Employer," July 23, 1926, NYSDOH, series 13855–84, reel 11.

125. *Zucht v. King*, 260 U.S. 174 (1922).

126. Louis Brandeis to Felix Frankfurter, December 17, 1924, quoted in Melvin Urosky and David W. Levy, eds., *"Half Brother, Half Son": The Letters of Louis D. Brandeis to Felix Frankfurter* (Norman: University of Oklahoma Press, 1991).

127. Frank S. Swain to Matthias Nicoll, February 1, 1924, NYSDOH, series 13855–84, reel 9.

128. Dr. Conway to Dr. Brooks, February 6, 1924, NYSDOH, series 13855–84, reel 9.

129. Dr. Sayer to Dr. Brooks, April 26, 1928, NYSDOH, series 13855–84, reel 16.

130. Fowler, "Smallpox Vaccination Laws, Regulations, and Court Decisions."

131. *Jacobson v. Massachusetts*, 197 U.S. 11 (1905), 47.

132. H. B. Anderson to George J. Ryan, November 7, 1932, and William Snow to Shirley Wynne, November 26, 1932, NYCDOH, box 141354, folder: Vaccination.

133. "Seeks to Amend Law on Vaccinating Pupils," *New York Times*, November 13, 1932, 10; "Citizens Urge End of Vaccination Law," ibid., November 22, 1932, 10.

134. *Economic Security Act: Hearings before the Committee on Ways and Means, House of Representatives, Seventy-fourth Congress, First Session, on H.R. 4120* (Washington, D.C.: U.S. Government Printing Office, 1935), 652–653.

135. H. B. Anderson, *Public Health the American Way* (New York: Citizens Medical Reference Bureau, 1945).

136. See, e.g., H. B. Anderson to state and local departments of health, New York, Pennsylvania, New York City, Buffalo, and Philadelphia and vicinity, August 15, 1944, NYCDOH, box 141566, folder: Vaccination.

137. Starr, *Social Transformation of American Medicine*, 127.

138. The events described here are drawn from the following accounts: Israel Weinstein, "An Outbreak of Smallpox in New York City," *American Journal of Public Health* 37 (1947): 1376–1384; Berton Roueché, "A Man from Mexico," in *Eleven Blue Men* (Boston: Little, Brown, 1953), 100–120; Judith Walzer Leavitt, "'Be Safe. Be Sure.': New York City's Experience with Epidemic Smallpox," in David Rosner, ed., *Hives of Sickness: Public Health and Epidemics in New York City* (New Brunswick, N.J.: Rutgers University Press, 1995); and coverage in the *New York Times*, April 5–May 12, 1947.

139. "Report of Outbreak of Smallpox in New York City" (typescript, May 5, 1947), NYCDOH, box 141593, folder: Vaccination.

140. See letters in NYCDOH, box 141592, folder: Vaccination.

141. Teresa Scordino to William O'Dwyer, April 16, 1947, NYCDOH, box 141592, folder: Vaccination.

142. Karl Pretshold and Caroline C. Sulzer, "Speed, Action and Candor: The Public Relations Story of New York's Smallpox Emergency," *Channels* 25 (1947): 3–6; 3–4.

143. In the years following World War II, Leavitt contends, "The public retained something of an emergency mentality and easily followed government advice.... New Yorkers had already become accustomed to regulations that

affected the behavior of the whole population, from food rationing to blackout drills." Leavitt, "'Be Safe. Be Sure.,'" 102, 111.

144. H. B. Anderson to Paul L. Ross, April 24, 1947, NYCDOH, box 141592, folder: Vaccination.

145. Francis G. Velardi to health department, May 1, 1947, NYCDOH, box 141592, folder: Vaccination.

146. Pretshold and Sulzer, "Speed, Action and Candor," 6.

147. See letters in NYCDOH, box 141592, folder: Vaccination.

148. Weinstein, "Outbreak of Smallpox in New York City."

3. DIPHTHERIA IMMUNIZATION

1. "Children's Fete Aids Health Drive," *New York Times,* May 16, 1933, 19.

2. Evelynn Maxine Hammonds, *Childhood's Deadly Scourge: The Campaign to Control Diphtheria in New York City, 1880–1930* (Baltimore: Johns Hopkins University Press, 1999).

3. Abraham Zingher, "Diphtheria Preventive Work in the Public Schools of New York City," *Archives of Pediatrics* 38 (1921): 336–359. On the use of informed consent during this period, see Susan Eyrich Lederer, "Hideyo Noguchi's Leutin Experiment and the Antivivisectionists," *Isis* 76 (1985): 31–48.

4. Zingher, "Diphtheria Preventive Work," 338.

5. William H. Park, M. C. Schroder, and Abraham Zingher, "The Control of Diphtheria," *American Journal of Public Health* 13 (1923): 23–32.

6. H. B. Anderson, *Protest against Sending Nurses into Homes of School Children to Urge Medical Treatment, and against Using Public Schools to Promote the Schick Test, and Toxin-Antitoxin* (New York: Citizens Medical Reference Bureau, 1922).

7. F. W. Sears, "Can Diphtheria Be Eliminated?" *American Journal of Public Health* 15 (1925): 98–101; F. W. Sears, "Further Observations of the Schick and Toxin-Antitoxin Immunization against Diphtheria in the City of Auburn," *American Journal of Public Health* 15 (1925): 210–213.

8. George Sincerbeaux, "Auburn's Experience with Toxin-Antitoxin," *New York State Journal of Medicine* 26 (1926): 857–858.

9. Dr. Laidlaw to deputy commissioner, January 5, 1924, NYSDOH, series 13855–84, roll 9.

10. Dr. Laidlaw to deputy commissioner, February 23, 1924, NYSDOH, series 13855–84, roll 9.

11. Dr. Laidlaw to deputy commissioner, January 5, 1924, NYSDOH, series 13855–84, roll 9.

12. Ibid.

13. "A Plea to Physicians to Employ Active Immunization and So Prevent Deaths from Diphtheria," *Archives of Pediatrics* 38 (1921): 380–388.

14. "Communicable Disease Practice," *American Journal of Public Health* 16 (1926): 904–906.

15. See, e.g., Leslie Frank to U.S. surgeon general, October 29, 1919, NARA box 365; and T. F. Abercrombie to Hugh Cumming, August 25, 1921, NARA box 366.

16. Milton J. Rosenau, *Preventive Medicine and Hygiene,* 4th ed. (New York: D. Appleton, 1921), 200–201. The third edition, published in 1917, mentions that the curative use of antitoxin could produce a brief period of immunity, but there is no mention of active immunization through toxin-antitoxin. Milton J. Rosenau, *Preventive Medicine and Hygiene,* 3d ed. (New York: D. Appleton, 1917), 165–167.

17. William Osler, Thomas McCrae and Elmer H. Funk, eds., *Modern Medicine, Its Theory and Practice,* 3d ed. (Philadelphia: Lea & Febiger, 1925–1928), vol. 1, 727. The second edition, published in 1913, mentions the transient immunity produced by antitoxin and notes, "Active immunization is still in the experimental stage." William Osler and Thomas McCrae, eds., *Modern Medicine, Its Theory and Practice,* 2d ed. (Philadelphia: Lea & Febiger, 1913), 732.

18. Arnold Gesell, *The Pre-School Child from the Standpoint of Public Hygiene and Education* (Boston: Houghton Mifflin, 1923), 18.

19. "Preventive Diphtheria Work in the Public Schools of New York City," *Medical Record* 100 (1921): 34–35.

20. Park, Schroder, and Zingher, "Control of Diphtheria."

21. The trek was subsequently commemorated in the annual Iditarod dog sled race. Gay Salisbury and Laney Salisbury, *The Cruelest Miles: The Heroic Story of Dogs and Men in a Race against an Epidemic* (New York: Norton, 2003).

22. "Serum Foes Oppose a Statue for Balto," *New York Times,* March 29, 1925, 17.

23. "Deaths Following Toxin-Antitoxin," *Journal of the American Medical Association* 73 (1919): 1778.

24. "Health Officers' Exchange," *American Journal of Public Health* 14 (1924): 257–258.

25. John Duffy describes the early 1920s as "years of travail" for the New York City health department. John Duffy, *A History of Public Health in New York City, 1866–1966* (New York: Russell Sage Foundation, 1968), 343–374.

26. On public-private partnerships for child health during the first decades of the twentieth century, see Richard A. Meckel, *Save the Babies: American Public Health Reform and the Prevention of Infant Mortality, 1850–1929* (Baltimore: Johns Hopkins University Press, 1990), 124–158.

27. *Preventing Diphtheria in New York State* (New York: State Committee on Tuberculosis and Public Health and State Charities Aid Association, 1927), 3; "Aids Diphtheria Campaign," *New York Times,* January 12, 1928, 12.

28. On the use of short films to promote health issues, see Martin Pernick, "Thomas Edison's Tuberculosis Films: Mass Media and Health Propaganda," *Hastings Center Report* 8 (1978): 21–27.

29. Bruce V. Lewenstein, "Industrial Life Insurance, Public Health Campaigns, and Public Communication of Science, 1908–1951," *Public Understanding of Science* 1 (1992): 347–365; and William G. Rothstein, *Public Health and the Risk Factor: A History of an Uneven Medical Revolution* (Rochester, N.Y.: University of Rochester Press, 2003), 146–175.

30. Lee K. Frankel, "Insurance Companies and Public Health Activities," *American Journal of Public Health* 4 (1914): 1–10; 5.

31. Louis Dublin, "Child Health Protection or Neglect: The Ultimate Cost to the Community," presentation to the annual meeting, American Child Health Association, May 10, 1927, Dublin papers, box 10, folder: Child Welfare 1927.

32. Roland Marchand, *Creating the Corporate Soul: The Rise of Public Relations and Corporate Imagery in American Big Business* (Berkeley: University of California Press, 1998), 181–189.

33. On the health demonstrations, see Clyde V. Kiser, *The Milbank Memorial Fund: Its Leaders and Its Work, 1905–1974* (New York: Milbank Memorial Fund, 1975), 22–41.

34. Louis Dublin, "New York Health Demonstrations, Report of Technical Board to Board of Directors of the Milbank Memorial Fund" (typescript, March 19, 1925), Dublin papers, box 7, folder: Milbank Memorial Fund 1922–48.

35. "Annual Reports, 1926," *New York State Journal of Medicine* 27 (1927): 451–467.

36. *Preventing Diphtheria*, 7.

37. "War on Diphtheria From Air," *New York Times*, May 2, 1928, 19.

38. Louise Franklin Bache, *Health Education in an American City* (Garden City, N.Y.: Doubleday, Doran, 1934).

39. Evart G. Routzahn, "Education and Publicity," *American Journal of Public Health* 18 (1928): 518–519.

40. "Report of the Committee on Immunization of Children against Diphtheria," *New York State Journal of Medicine* 28 (1928): 604–607.

41. *City of New York Department of Health Annual Report 1929* (New York: F. Hubner, 1930), 20–32.

42. Niagara Falls, Syracuse, Yonkers, Rochester, Elmira, Schenectady, and Utica all had between 40 and 50 percent of their preschool children immunized. George Truman Palmer, Mahew Derryberry, and Philip Van Ingen, *Health Protection for the Preschool Child* (New York: Century, 1931), 113.

43. Ibid., 52, 113.

44. Ibid., 94.

45. Ibid., 60.

46. Ibid., 168–169.

47. Shirley W. Wynne to James J. Walker, December 14, 1931, NYCDOH, box 141372, folder: Diphtheria.

48. On the hookworm campaign, see John Ettling, *The Germ of Laziness: Rockefeller Philanthropy and Public Health in the New South* (Cambridge, Mass.: Harvard University Press, 1991), and William A. Link, "Privies, Progressivism, and Public Schools: Health Reform and Education in the Rural South, 1909–1920," *Journal of Southern History* 54, no. 4 (1988): 623–642; on yellow fever eradication, see Marcos Cueto, "Sanitation from Above: Yellow Fever and Foreign Intervention in Peru, 1919–1922," *Hispanic American Historical Review* 72 (1992): 1–22.

49. Hermann M. Biggs, "Arguments in Favor of the Jones-Tallett Amendment to the Public Health Law in Relation to Vaccination," *New York State Journal of Medicine* 15, no. 3 (1915): 89–90.

50. Elizabeth Toon, "Managing the Conduct of the Individual Life: Public Health Education and American Public Health, 1910 to 1940" (Ph.D. diss.,

University of Pennsylvania, 1998); Nancy Tomes, *The Gospel of Germs: Men, Women and the Microbe in American Life* (Cambridge, Mass.: Harvard University Press, 1998), 242–244; and John C. Burnham, *How Superstition Won and Science Lost* (New Brunswick, N.J.: Rutgers University Press, 1987), 56–62.

51. Toon, "Managing the Conduct of the Individual Life," 95.

52. Whether or not the "new public health" after the turn of the century represented a retreat from the reformist spirit of the profession's early days remains a matter of disagreement among historians. On this debate, see Judith Walzer Leavitt, "'Typhoid Mary' Strikes Back: Bacteriological Theory and Practice in Early Twentieth-Century Public Health," *Isis* 83 (1992): 608–629.

53. On health education aimed at reforming child health and maternal practices, see Meckel, *Save the Babies,* esp. 92–177.

54. Toon, "Managing the Conduct of the Individual Life," 70–80.

55. Gretchen A. Condran and Samuel H. Preston, "Child Mortality Differences, Personal Health Care Practices, and Medical Technology: The United States, 1900–1930," in Lincoln C. Chen, Arthur Kleinman and Norma C. Ware, eds., *Health and Social Change in International Perspective* (Boston: Department of Population and Family Health, Harvard School of Public Health, 1994).

56. William Leach, *Land of Desire: Merchants, Power and the Rise of a New American Culture* (New York: Vintage Books, 1993), and T. J. Jackson Lears, *Fables of Abundance: A Cultural History of Advertising in America* (New York: Basic Books, 1994).

57. Nancy Tomes, "Merchants of Health: Medicine and Consumer Culture in the United States, 1900–1940," *Journal of American History* 88, no. 2 (2001): 519–547; Rima Apple, *Vitamania: Vitamins in American Culture* (New Brunswick, N.J.: Rutgers University Press, 1996), 13–32.

58. Louis Galambos with Jane Eliot Sewell, *Networks of Innovation: Vaccine Development at Merck, Sharp & Dohme, and Mulford, 1895–1995* (Cambridge: Cambridge University Press, 1995), 19–20.

59. Dorothy Nelkin, *Selling Science: How the Press Covers Science and Technology* (New York: W. H. Freeman, 1987), 134.

60. Herman N. Bundesen, "Selling Health—A Vital Duty," *American Journal of Public Health* 18 (1928): 1451–1545; 1452.

61. *City of New York Department of Health Annual Report, 1928* (New York: F. Hubner, 1929), 23.

62. See, e.g., Edward A. Moree, "Public Health Publicity: The Art of Stimulating and Focusing Public Opinion," *American Journal of Public Health* 6 (1916): 97–108.

63. The term "pseudo-event" is from Daniel Boorstin: "It is not spontaneous, but comes about because someone has planned, planted or incited it.... It is planted primarily (not always exclusively) for the purpose of being reported or reproduced.... Its relation to the underlying reality of the situation is ambiguous. Its interest arises largely from this very ambiguity.... Usually it is intended to be a self-fulfilling prophecy." Daniel Boorstin, *The Image; or, What Happened to the American Dream* (New York: Atheneum, 1962), 11–12. On the career of Edward Bernays, see Leach, *Land of Desire,* 319–322.

64. Edward S. Godfrey, "Practical Uses of Diphtheria Immunization Records," *American Journal of Public Health* 23 (1933): 809–812; 810.

65. Iago Galdston, "Health Education and the Public Health of the Future," *Journal of the Michigan State Medical Society*, 1929: 32–35.

66. Charles Bolduan, "Health Education Today" (typescript, n.d. [1938?]), NYCMRL.

67. Elwin T. Nash and J. Graham Forbes, "Diphtheria Immunisation: Its Possibilities and Difficulties," *Public Health* 46 (1933): 245–271.

68. "The Supreme Court on Vaccination Laws," *American Journal of Public Health* 13 (1923): 120–121.

69. "The Evolution of Public Health Work," *New York State Journal of Medicine* 26 (1926): 614–616.

70. On the control of polio during the Progressive Era, which involved both quarantine and "Swat the Fly" education campaigns, see Naomi Rogers, *Dirt and Disease: Polio before FDR* (New Brunswick, N.J.: Rutgers University Press, 1992).

71. Brandt, *No Magic Bullet*.

72. Judith Walzer Leavitt, *Typhoid Mary: Captive to the Public's Health* (Boston: Beacon Press, 1996). Mallon remained on North Brother Island until her death in 1938.

73. On rhetoric of parental blame, see Hammonds, *Childhood's Deadly Scourge*, 200–207.

74. *Little Boy Blue* (pamphlet, Orleans County Committee on Tuberculosis and Public Health, n.d.), NYCDOH box 141380, folder: Diphtheria.

75. Cited in "Diphtheria Is Called Conquered Disease," *New York Times*, September 3, 1926, 14.

76. Apple, *Vitamania*, 13–32.

77. In one successful prosecution, a judge fined a Newark father $50 and sentenced him to one month in jail for refusing to have his son immunized against diphtheria; the father relented rather than go to jail. "Faces Jail for Refusing Son Immunization," *New York Sun*, January 28, 1936; "9 Children Are So Healthy, She Fights Immunization," *New York World-Telegram*, January 29, 1936, 36; "Allows Schick Test," *New York Sun*, January 29, 1936, 10.

78. Mrs. E. C. Schoeler to Shirley Wynne, June 7, 1933, NYCDOH, box 141421, folder: Diphtheria. Punctuation as in original.

79. On tensions between the professions of public health and medicine, see Allan M. Brandt and Martha Gardner, "Antagonism and Accommodation: Interpreting the Relationship Between Public Health and Medicine in the United States during the 20th Century," *American Journal of Public Health* 90 (2000): 707–715; John Duffy, "The American Medical Profession and Public Health: From Support to Ambivalence," *Bulletin of the History of Medicine* 53 (1979): 1–15; and Paul Starr, *The Social Transformation of American Medicine* (New York: Basic Books, 1982), 180–197.

80. Sydney A. Halpern, *American Pediatrics: The Social Dynamics of Professionalism, 1880–1980* (Berkeley: University of California Press, 1988), 90–98; and Charles R. King, *Children's Health in America: A History* (New York: Twayne, 1993), 124–142.

81. Matthias Nicoll, "The Past, Present and Future of Preventive Medicine," *New York State Journal of Medicine* 26 (1926): 883–886.

82. Ibid., 886.

83. Howard Gilmartin, "The Medical Society's Share in Protecting the Children of Schenectady against Diphtheria," *New York State Journal of Medicine* 28 (1928): 1097–1100.

84. "The Tri-State Conference," *New York State Journal of Medicine* 27 (1927): 733–736.

85. C.-E. A. Winslow, *A City Set on a Hill* (Garden City, N.Y.: Doubleday, Doran, 1934), 123.

86. "Public Health vs. Private Practice," *New York Medical Week* 9 (January 18, 1930): 6.

87. On the alleged abuse of medical charity services by the middle class, see Halpern, *American Pediatrics*, 98–102.

88. Morris Myers to Shirley Wynne, June 15, 1932, NYCDOH box 141380, folder: Diphtheria.

89. Shirley Wynne to Morris Myers, June 18, 1932, NYCDOH, box 141380, folder: Diphtheria.

90. Morris Fishbein, "Present-Day Trends of Private Practice in the United States," *Journal of the American Medical Association* 98 (1933): 2039–2045; 2044.

91. Assistant sanitary superintendent, Queens, to commissioner, August 25, 1933, NYCDOH, box 141421, folder: Diphtheria.

92. "Prevent Diphtheria," *New York Medical Week* 12 (May 20, 1933): 3–4.

93. Michael Katz, *In the Shadow of the Poorhouse: A Social History of Welfare in America* (New York: Basic Books, 1996).

94. "State Medicine," *New York State Journal of Medicine* 27 (1927): 723.

95. See Shirley W. Wynne, "Diphtheria Must Go," in Edward Fisher Brown, ed., *How to Protect Children from Diphtheria* (New York: Department of Health, n.d. [1929]), 7.

96. "Dear Doctor" letter, May 17, 1929, NARA box 425, folder: New York Cities & Counties 0115–0425. See also "Wynne Acts to Widen Immunization Drive," *New York Times*, May 27, 1929, 20.

97. Shirley Wynne to Hugh Cumming, June 19, 1930, NARA box 425, folder: New York Cities & Counties 0875–1658.

98. "More Immunization Needed," *New York City Department of Health Weekly Report* 21 (July 2, 1932): 204–205.

99. Shirley W. Wynne to Homer Folks, January 8, 1932, NYCDOH, box 141380, folder: Diphtheria.

100. John Rice to Henry Vaughan, October 19, 1934, NYCDOH, box 141406, folder: Diphtheria.

101. "Torture of the Innocents," *Chiropractic News*, January 31, 1929, NYCDOH box 141349, folder: Bellevue-Yorkville Health Demonstration.

102. Edgar H. Bauman to Shirley Wynne, February 23, 1932; *Beware the Schick Test* (New York Anti-Vivisection Society leaflet, n.d.), NYCDOH, box 141359, folder: Diphtheria.

103. "Ready to Immunize 1,000,000 Children," *New York Times,* July 6, 1930, II-3.

104. Fred L. Mickert to Shirley Wynne, June 26, 1933, NYCDOH, box 141421, folder: Diphtheria.

105. Miss Casey to Shirley Wynne, [n.d., June 1932], NYCDOH, box 141380, folder: Diphtheria.

106. See, e.g., Anna Robinson to Shirley Wynne, January 23, 1932, and Katherine F. Blake to Shirley W. Wynne, February 8, 1932, NYCDOH, box 141380, folder: Diphtheria.

107. Acting director, Bureau of Nursing, to commissioner, June 27, 1930, NYCDOH, box 141359, folder: Diphtheria.

108. Mrs. M. Messner to John Rice, January 2, 1934, NYCDOH, box 141410, folder: Vaccination.

109. Max Bernstein to New York City Health Department, May 28, 1934, NYCDOH, box 141406, folder: Diphtheria.

110. Frances B. Morley to Shirley Wynne, February 5, 1932, NYCDOH, box 141380, folder: Diphtheria.

111. Acting director, Bureau of Nursing, to commissioner, June 27, 1930, NYCDOH, box 141359, folder: Diphtheria.

112. William Rost to Shirley Wynne, July 3, 1930, NYCDOH, box 141356, folder: Vaccination.

113. Shirley Wynne to Homer Folks, January 8, 1932, NYCDOH, 141380, folder: Diphtheria.

114. Gretchen A. Condran and Ellen A. Kamarow, "Child Mortality among Jewish Immigrants to the United States," *Journal of Interdisciplinary History* 22 (1991): 223–254; Alice Goldstein, Susan Cotts Watkins and Ann Rosen Spector, "Childhood Health-Care Practices among Italians and Jews in the United States, 1910–1940," *Health Transition Review* 4 (1994): 45–61.

115. "Warns of Diphtheria," *New York Times,* June 28, 1930, 14; "Diphtheria Rate Studied," ibid., May 25, 1931, 3; Hammonds, *Childhood's Deadly Scourge,* 199.

116. Acting director, Bureau of Nursing, to commissioner, June 27, 1930, NYCDOH, box 141359, folder: Diphtheria.

117. Shirley Wynne to Ernst Boas, February 5, 1931, NYCDOH, box 141372, folder: Diphtheria.

118. Shirley Wynne to James C. Quinn, May 12, 1932, NYCDOH, box 141380, folder: Diphtheria.

119. Robert A. Strong, "The Newer Conception of Diphtheria Immunization," *Archives of Pediatrics* 49 (1932): 614–620.

120. H. A. Reisman to Shirley Wynne, October 12, 1933, NYCDOH, box 141421, folder: Diphtheria.

121. John L. Rice to Charles Weymuller, February 1, 1935, NYCDOH, box 141436, folder: Diphtheria; see also attached "Diphtheria Warning!" card.

122. Herman N. Bundesen to John L. Rice, March 22, 1938, NYCDOH, box 141488, folder: Diphtheria.

123. Lewis I. Coriell, "Recommendation and Schedules for Immunization," *Archives of Environmental Health* 15 (1967): 521–527.

124. Harry M. Marks, *The Progress of Experiment: Science and Therapeutic Reform in the United States, 1900–1990* (Cambridge: Cambridge University Press, 1997).

125. Samuel Frant, "Survey of Diphtheria New York City 1937" (typescript, February 1938), NYCMRL.

126. "Diphtheria Mortality in Large Cities in the United States in 1930," *Journal of the American Medical Association* 96 (1930): 1768–1771; 1771.

127. Donald B. Armstrong to Shirley Wynne, March 21, 1933, NYCDOH, box 141421, folder: Diphtheria.

128. John L. Rice to Herman N. Bundesen, April 30, 1936, NYCDOH, box 141451, folder: Diphtheria.

129. Committee on Neighborhood Health Development, *Statistical Reference Data, Five-Year Period, 1929–1933* (New York: Department of Health, 1935).

130. "Diphtheria War Is Begun," *New York Times,* March 21, 1937, II-7; director, Bureau of School Hygiene, to John L. Rice, March 26, 1937, NYCDOH, box 141527, folder: Diphtheria.

131. Deputy commissioner to the commissioner, April 8, 1933, NYCDOH, box 141392, folder: Diphtheria.

132. "Preventive Diphtheria Work in the Public Schools of New York City," *Medical Record* 11 (1921): 34–35.

133. For example, a joint committee of the Bronx County Tuberculosis and Health Committee and the Bronx County Medical Society made such a recommendation in 1931, and the following year, the Bronx County Medical Society passed a formal resolution in support of a school entry law.

134. Ernst Boas to Shirley Wynne, February 2, 1931; and Shirley Wynne to Ernst Boas, February 5, 1931, NYCDOH, box 141372, folder: Diphtheria.

135. Shirley W. Wynne to I. J. Landsman, June 7, 1932, NYCDOH, box 141380, folder: Diphtheria; see also Shirley Wynne to H. F. Dana, January 25, 1933, NYCDOH, box 141421, folder: Diphtheria.

136. The most frequent age to administer toxin-antitoxin was between one and two; the most frequent age to vaccinate against smallpox was between five and six. *Health Protection for the Preschool Child,* 59, 62.

137. Assistant sanitary superintendent to commissioner, July 6, 1932, NYCDOH, box 141380, folder: Diphtheria.

138. Thomas J. Duffield to Ernest Stebbins, March 10, 1943, NYCDOH, box 141549, folder: Diphtheria; Thomas J. Duffield to Ernest Stebbins, November 6, 1943, NYCDOH, box 141549, folder: Diphtheria.

139. Kansas, New Jersey, West Virginia, and the territory of Alaska required immunization for school entry; Illinois, Kentucky, West Virginia, and New York had miscellaneous provisions (New York required the procedure for children entering the state reconstruction home at Haverstraw). William Fowler, "State Diphtheria Immunization Requirements," *Public Health Reports* 57 (1942): 325–328.

140. Leona Baumgartner, "Attitude of the Nation toward Immunization Procedures," *American Journal of Public Health* 33 (1943): 256–260. The survey respondents were all white, and the article did not specify their ethnic background.

141. Oliver E. Byrd, ed. *Health Instruction Yearbook 1943* (London: Oxford University Press, 1943), 106–107.

142. Joseph H. Lapin, "Combined Immunization of Infants against Diphtheria, Tetanus and Whooping Cough," *American Journal of Diseases of Children* 63 (1942): 225–237.

143. "Pertussis Vaccines Omitted from N.N.R.," *Journal of the American Medical Association* 96, no. 8 (1931): 613.

144. R. S. Lepsotta to health commissioner, December 17, 1934, NYCDOH, box 141410, folder: Whooping Cough.

145. John L. Rice to Dr. Oleson, December 19, 1934, NYCDOH, box 141410, folder: Whooping Cough.

146. Baker, "Immunization and the American Way."

147. Josephine H. Kenyon, "Immunize Your Child against Whooping Cough," *Good Housekeeping,* March 1935, 95.

148. See NYCDOH, box 141432, folder: Whooping Cough.

149. John L. Rice to Donald Armstrong, January 13, 1941, NYCDOH, box 141525, folder: Whooping Cough.

150. Donald B. Armstrong to John L. Rice, January 14, 1942, NYCDOH, box 141525, folder: Whooping Cough.

151. Harriet M. Felton and Cecilia Y. Willard, "Current Status of Prophylaxis by Hemophilus Pertussis Vaccine," *Journal of the American Medical Association* 126 (1944): 294–299.

152. Paul de Kruif, "We Can Wipe Out Whooping Cough," *Reader's Digest,* January 1943, 124–126.

153. Catherine Mackenzie, "Diphtheria Cases Termed Unnecessary; New City Booklet Tells of Immunization," *New York Times,* October 12, 1944, 30.

154. Benjamin Spock, *The Common Sense Book of Baby and Child Care* (New York: Duell, Sloan & Pearce, 1946), 187–192.

4. HARD CORES AND SOFT SPOTS

1. A. D. Langmuir, "Epidemiologic Considerations," *Journal of the American Medical Association* 175 (1962): 840–843; 840.

2. Naomi Rogers, *Dirt and Disease: Polio before FDR* (New Brunswick, N.J.: Rutgers University Press, 1992).

3. Neal Nathanson and John R. Martin, "The Epidemiology of Poliomyelitis: Enigmas Surrounding Its Appearance, Epidemicity, and Disappearance," *American Journal of Epidemiology* 110 (1979): 672–692.

4. Amy L. Fairchild, "The Polio Narratives: Dialogs with FDR," *Bulletin of the History of Medicine* 75 (2001): 488–534.

5. Jane S. Smith, *Patenting the Sun: Polio and the Salk Vaccine* (New York: Doubleday, 1990), 64–68 and passim.

6. John R. Paul, *History of Poliomyelitis* (New Haven, Conn.: Yale University Press, 1971), 233–239.

7. Saul Benison, "The History of Polio Research in the United States: Appraisal and Lessons," in Gerald Holton, ed., *The Twentieth Century Sciences: Studies in the Biography of Ideas* (New York: Norton, 1972). Enders and

his colleagues Frederick Robbins and Thomas Weller received the Nobel Prize in medicine in 1954 for their work.

8. Paul, *History of Poliomyelitis.*

9. Paul Starr, *The Social Transformation of American Medicine* (New York: Basic Books, 1982), 343. On the rise of biomedical research in the public and private sectors during and after World War II, see also Harry M. Marks, *The Progress of Experiment: Science and Therapeutic Reform in the United States, 1900–1990* (Cambridge: Cambridge University Press, 1997), 98–128.

10. See, e.g., Stephen B. Withey, "Public Opinion about Science and Scientists," *Public Opinion Quarterly* 23 (1959): 382–388. Based on public opinion polls this article concluded that "for the public the caduceus of medicine sits proudly at the top of the totem pole of science" (388).

11. The details of the Salk vaccine trials have been described extensively in the scientific and popular literature and will not be recounted here. See the official report on the trials by the University of Michigan evaluation center: Tom Rivers, *Evaluation of the 1954 Field Trial of Poliomyelitis Vaccine* (Ann Arbor, Mich.: Poliomyelitis Evaluation Center, 1957). For subsequent scholarly evaluations, see Paul, *History of Poliomyelitis,* 426–440; Arnold S. Monto, "Francis Field Trial of Inactivated Poliomyelitis Vaccine: Background and Lessons for Today," *Epidemiological Reviews* 21 (1999): 7–22; Jeffrey P. Baker, "Immunization and the American Way: 4 Childhood Vaccines," *American Journal of Public Health* 90 (2000): 199–207. For more journalistic accounts, see Smith, *Patenting the Sun;* John Rowan Wilson, *Margin of Safety* (Garden City, N.Y.: Doubleday, 1963), 79–99; Richard Carter, *Breakthrough: The Saga of Jonas Salk* (New York: Trident Press, 1966), 207–267; Aaron Klein, *Trial by Fury: The Polio Vaccine Controversy* (New York: Charles Scribner's Sons, 1972), 66–126.

12. Hazel Gaudet Erskine, "The Polls: Exposure to Domestic Information," *Public Opinion Quarterly* 27 (1963): 491–500; 498. See also National Association of Science Writers, *Science, the News, and the Public: Who Gets What Science News, Where They Get It, and What They Think About It* (New York: New York University Press, 1958), 31–33.

13. Carter, *Breakthrough,* 301–302.

14. On Baumgartner's life and career, see Farnsworth Fowle, "Wagner Names 2 Women to Cabinet," *New York Times,* January 1, 1954, 1; "Her Vigil: City's Health," *New York Times,* March 7, 1957, 14; and "Dr. Leona Baumgartner, 88, Dies; Led New York Health Department," *New York Times,* January 17, 1991, B10.

15. Carter, *Breakthrough,* 303–304.

16. Leona Baumgartner to Paul R. Hays, May 12, 1955, NYCDOH, box 141647, folder: Polio January–June.

17. Leona Baumgartner to Robert F. Wagner, May 23, 1955, NYCDOH, box 141647, folder: Polio January–June.

18. B. J. Cutler, "Jail for Vaccine Black Marketers; Adults Got Shots, City for Rationing," *New York Herald-Tribune,* April 30, 1955, 1.

19. Alexander D. Langmuir, Neal Nathanson and William Jackson Hall, "Surveillance of Poliomyelitis in the United States in 1955," *American Journal of Public Health* 46 (1956): 75–88; Neal Nathanson and Alexander D. Langmuir,

"The Cutter Incident: Poliomyelitis Following Formaldehyde-Inactivated Poliovirus Vaccination in the United States during the Spring of 1955," *American Journal of Hygiene* 78 (1963): 16–28. For a historical and ethical analysis of the Cutter incident, see Allan M. Brandt, "Polio, Politics, Publicity, and Duplicity: Ethical Aspects in the Development of the Salk Vaccine," *Connecticut Medicine* 43 (1979): 581–590.

20. "Physician Suspended by Society, 3 Reprimanded for Adult Shots," *New York Herald-Tribune*, May 5, 1955, 1.

21. Morris Kaplan, "Vaccine Misuse Laid to 5 Doctors," *New York Times*, May 1, 1955, 57.

22. Smith, *Patenting the Sun*, 368; Brandt, "Polio, Politics, Publicity, and Duplicity."

23. Benison, "Polio Research in the United States," 330.

24. Herman Hilleboe to "Dear Doctor," May 27, 1955, NYCDOH, box 141647, folder: Polio July–December.

25. B. J. Cutler, "Few Parents Canceling Salk-Shots Permission," *New York Herald-Tribune*, May 6, 1955, 1.

26. Leona Baumgartner to "Dear Parents," March 1955, NYCDOH, box 141647, folder: Polio January–June.

27. New York State Advisory Committee on Polio Vaccine, minutes, May 3, 1955, NYCDOH, box 141647, folder: Polio January–June.

28. "Sidewalk Interviews," *Amsterdam News*, June 4, 1955, 55.

29. James Osborne to all state reps in Region IV, July 14, 1955, MOD, series 3, file: Vaccine Promotion and Education 1955.

30. Smith, *Patenting the Sun*, 65, 81.

31. James Osborne to all state reps in Region IV, July 14, 1955, MOD, series 3, file: Vaccine Promotion and Education 1955.

32. George P. Voss to Basil O'Connor, MOD, series 3, file: Vaccine Promotion and Education 1955.

33. Robert F. Wagner Jr. to President Dwight Eisenhower, April 13, 1955, NYCDOH, box 141647, folder: Polio January–June.

34. "U.S. Vaccine Rule Urged by Parents," *New York Post*, June 12, 1955, 4; Abel Silver, "Call Rally to Demand U.S. Vaccine Controls," ibid., June 21, 1955, 2; "Civic Club Asks Effective Salk Vaccine Control Plan," *New York Amsterdam News*, July 2, 1955, 24.

35. Smith, *Patenting the Sun*.

36. James L. Sundquist, *Politics and Policy: The Eisenhower, Kennedy, and Johnson Years* (Washington, D.C.: Brookings Institution, 1968), 290–293.

37. *Poliomyelitis Vaccine*, 116.

38. Ibid., 115.

39. William M. Blair, "Mrs. Hobby Terms Free Vaccine Idea a Socialistic Step," *New York Times*, June 15, 1955, 1.

40. "Mrs. Hobby Says Responsibility for Vaccine Plan is Dr. Scheele's," *New York Times*, June 21, 1955, 1.

41. *Extension of Poliomyelitis Vaccination Assistance Act, Hearing before a Subcommittee of the Committee on Interstate and Foreign Commerce, House of Representatives, Eighty-fourth Congress, Second Session, January 24, 1956* (Washington, D.C.: Government Printing Office, 1956), 4.

42. "Report on Poliomyelitis Vaccine Situation" (typescript, July 15, 1955), NYCDOH, box 141647, folder: Polio July–December.

43. See, e.g., Leona Baumgartner to Ruth Shatz, March 17, 1955; Shirley Lacy (Tompkins Parents Association) to Leona Baumgartner, June 8, 1955; Jessie Futerman (Parents Association of P.S. 28) to Robert F. Wagner, June 15, 1955; New York State Advisory Committee on Polio Vaccine, minutes, May 3, 1955, NYCDOH, box 141647, folder: Polio January–June; and Sylvia LeVine to Leona Baumgartner, November 26, 1956, NYCDOH, box 141657, folder: Polio July–December.

44. Mildred Hochman to Leona Baumgartner, March 26, 1956, NYCDOH, box 141657, folder: Polio January–June.

45. Leona Baumgartner to Leon Greenspan, April 5, 1956, NYCDOH, box 141657, folder: Polio January–June.

46. New York State Advisory Committee on Polio Vaccine, minutes, September 26, 1955, NYCDOH, box 141647, folder: Polio July–December. On this issue, see also Roscoe P. Kandle to Hollis Ingraham, November 9, 1955, NYCDOH, box 141647, folder: Polio July–December; Leon Greenspan to Leona Baumgartner, April 5, 1956, NYCDOH, box 141657, folder: Polio January–June.

47. Brooklyn Academy of Pediatrics, "Resolution re Salk Poliomyelitis Vaccine" (typescript, January 25, 1956), NYCDOH, box 141657, folder: Polio January–June.

48. Leona Baumgartner to Adolph Emerson, February 1, 1956, NYCDOH, box 141657, folder: Polio January–June.

49. Morris Greenberg to Leona Baumgartner, February 23, 1956, NYCDOH, box 141657, folder: Polio January–June.

50. Dorothy Ducas to Members of Vaccine Education Committee, February 2, 1956, MOD, series 3, file: Vaccine Promotion and Education 1956.

51. "17 States Return Share of Vaccine," New York Times, July 25, 1956, 27.

52. Judd Marmor, Viola W. Bernard, and Perry Ottenberg, "Psychodynamics of Group Opposition to Health Programs," American Journal of Orthopsychiatry 30 (1960): 330–345.

53. On the battles against fluoridation, see Gretchen Ann Reilly, "'Not a So-Called Democracy': Anti-Fluoridationists and the Fight Over Drinking Water," in Robert D. Johnston, ed., The Politics of Healing: Histories of Alternative Medicine in Twentieth-Century North America (New York: Routledge, 2004); Donald R. McNeil, The Fight for Fluoridation (New York: Oxford University Press, 1957); Brian Martin, Scientific Knowledge in Controversy: The Social Dynamics of the Fluoridation Debate (Albany: State University of New York Press, 1991).

54. Fluoridation of Water, Hearings before the Committee on Interstate and Foreign Commerce, House of Representatives, Eighty-third Congress, Second Session (Washington, D.C.: Government Printing Office, 1954), 239.

55. Flora Rheta Schreiber, "The Fear Campaign against the Polio Vaccine," Redbook, April 1956.

56. Polio Prevention Inc., flyer, March 25, 1955, NYCDOH, box 141647, folder: Polio January–June; emphases in original.

57. Leona Baumgartner to Albert H. Douglas, October 12, 1956, NYCDOH, box 141657, folder: Polio July–December.

58. Karl Pretshold to Leona Baumgartner, October 3, 1956, NYCDOH, box 141657, folder: Polio July–December.

59. Wilber Crawford to Headquarters List # 1, September 28, 1956, MOD, series 3, file: Vaccine Promotion and Education.

60. Vaccine Education Committee Meeting minutes, May 2, 1957, MOD, series 3, file: Vaccine Promotions and Education 1957.

61. "Elvis Shielded from Mob of Teeners on Broadway," *New York Tribune*, October 29, 1956; "Presley Receives a City Polio Shot," *New York Times*, October 29, 1956. The idea for vaccinating Presley had originated within the NFIP's public relations department in the summer of 1956 as part of its response to the sluggish demand for the vaccine. See Dorothy Ducas to Raymond H. Barrows, August 28, 1956, MOD, series 3, file: Vaccine Promotion and Education.

62. Ruth Migdal to Leona Baumgartner, February 8, 1957, NYCDOH, box 141667, folder: Poliomyelitis.

63. Dorothy Ducas to regional public relations representatives, March 11, 1957, MOD, series 3, file: Vaccine Promotion and Education 1957.

64. See, e.g., Leona Baumgartner to Frank LaGattuta, October 5, 1956, NYCDOH, box 141657, folder: Polio July–December. Baumgartner believed the disease was "a dead subject" as far as the major newspapers were concerned.

65. "National Foundation Report of Youth Conference on Polio Vaccination" (typescript, August 28, 1957), MOD, series 3, file: Youth Conference on Polio Vaccination 1957.

66. "Medical Group's Protests Stop Polio Shot Project in Brooklyn," *New York Times*, September 12, 1956, 39; "Salk 'Clinics' Dropped," ibid., September 19, 1956, 39.

67. Aaron Kottler to "Dear Doctor," September 13, 1956, NYCDOH, box 141657, folder: Polio July–December.

68. Karl Pretshold to Leona Baumgartner, January 18, 1957, NYCDOH, box 141657, folder: Polio July–December.

69. Michael Antell to Roscoe P. Kandle, November 14, 1956, NYCDOH, box 141657, folder: Polio July–December.

70. "Dear Doctor" letter, December 5, 1956, NYCDOH, box 141657, folder: Polio July–December.

71. Abe A. Brown to Public Health Educators, December 10, 1956, NYCDOH, box 141657, folder: Polio July–December.

72. Vaccine Education Committee Meeting, minutes, February 6, 1957, MOD, series 3, file: Vaccine Promotion and Education 1957.

73. George P. Voss to state representatives, January 13, 1958, MOD, series 3, file: Vaccine Promotion and Education 1958.

74. Sundquist, *Politics and Policy,* 296–321.

75. American Medical Association, *Polio Inoculation Clinic* (brochure, n.d. [1958]), NYCDOH, box 141677, folder: Poliomyelitis.

76. Summary of Discussion, Second Meeting of the Governor's Committee to End Polio by Vaccination, June 26, 1958, NYCDOH, box 141677, folder: Poliomyelitis.

77. "Summary of Question and Answer Session with the Honorable Arthur S. Flemming, Secretary, Department of Health, Education and Welfare" (typescript, n.d. [1958]), ASTHO Archives, box 8, folder: Proceedings, 1958 Annual Conference, Surgeon General, Children's Bureau, State and Territorial Health Officers.

78. Melvin A. Glasser, "A Study of the Public's Acceptance of the Salk Vaccine Program," *American Journal of Public Health* 48 (1958): 141–146.

79. John A. Clausen, M. A. Seidenfeld, and Leila Calhoun Deasy, "Parent Attitudes toward Participation of Their Children in Polio Vaccine Trials," *American Journal of Public Health* 44 (1954): 1526–1536; Leila Calhoun Deasy, "Socio-economic Status and Participation in the Poliomyelitis Vaccine Trial," *American Sociological Review* 21 (1956): 185–191.

80. John C. Belcher, "Acceptance of the Salk Polio Vaccine," *Rural Sociology* 23 (1958): 158–170; Malcolm H. Merrill, Arthur C. Hollister, Stephen F. Gibbs, et al., "Attitudes of Californians toward Poliomyelitis Vaccination," *American Journal of Public Health* 48 (1958): 146–152; David L. Sills and Rafael E. Gill, "Young Adults' Use of the Salk Vaccine," *Social Problems* 6 (1958–59): 246–252; Warren Winklestein Jr. and Saxon Graham, "Factors in Participation in the 1954 Poliomyelitis Vaccine Field Trials, Erie County, New York," *American Journal of Public Health* 49 (1959): 1454–1466; Irwin M. Rosenstock, Mayhew Derryberry, and Barbara K. Carriger, "Why People Fail to Seek Poliomyelitis Vaccination," *Public Health Reports* 74 (1959): 98–103; Walter E. Boek, Lewis E. Patrie, and Violet M. Huntley, "Poliomyelitis Vaccine Injection Levels and Sources," *New York State Journal of Medicine* 59 (1959): 1783–1785; Francis A. Ianni, Robert M. Albrecht, Walter E. Boek, et al., "Age, Social, and Demographic Factors in Acceptance of Polio Vaccination," *Public Health Reports* 75 (1960): 545–556; Monroe G. Sirkin and Berthold Brenner, *Population Characteristics and Participation in the Poliomyelitis Vaccination Program*, Public Health Monograph No. 61 (Washington, D.C.: Government Printing Office, 1960); Constantine A. Yeracaris, "The Acceptance of Polio Vaccine: An Hypothesis," *American Catholic Sociological Review* 224 (1961): 299–305; id., "Social Factors Associated with the Acceptance of Medical Innovations: A Pilot Study," *Journal of Health and Human Behavior* 3 (1962): 193–198; Albert L. Johnson, C. David Jenkins, Ralph Patrick, et al., *Epidemiology of Polio Vaccine Acceptance: A Social and Psychological Analysis*, Florida State Board of Health Monograph No. 3 (Jacksonville, Fla.: Florida State Board of Health, 1962); Robert E. Serfling and Ida L. Sherman, "Survey Evaluation of Three Poliomyelitis Immunization Campaigns," *Public Health Reports* 78 (1963): 413–418; Carol N. D'Onofrio, *Reaching Our "Hard to Reach"—The Unvaccinated* (Berkeley: California Department of Health Services, 1966).

81. On the growth in survey research during this period, see, inter alia, Jean M. Converse, *Survey Research in the United States: Roots and Emergence 1890–1960* (Berkeley: University of California Press, 1987); Seymour Sudman and Norman M. Bradburn, "The Organizational Growth of Public Opinion Research in the United States," *Public Opinion Quarterly* 51 (1987): S67–S78; and William H. Sewell, "Some Reflections on the Golden Age of Interdisciplinary Social Psychology," *Social Psychology Quarterly* 52 (1989): 88–97.

82. "Surveillance of Poliomyelitis in the United States, 1958–61," *Public Health Reports* 77 (1962): 1011–1020.

83. Neal Nathanson, Lauri D. Thrup, Wm. Jackson Hall, et al., "Epidemic Poliomyelitis during 1956 in Chicago and Cook County, Illinois," *American Journal of Hygiene* 70 (1959): 107–168.

84. Alexander D. Langmuir, "Progress in Conquest of Paralytic Poliomyelitis," *Journal of the American Medical Association* 171 (1959): 271–273.

85. Roscoe P. Kandle to Barry L. McCarthy, February 3, 1959, NYCDOH, box 141690, folder: Poliomyelitis.

86. E. Russell Alexander, "The Extent of the Poliomyelitis Problem," *Journal of the American Medical Association* 175 (1961): 837–840.

87. Robert E. Serfling, R. G. Cornell, and Ida L. Sherman, "The CDC Quota Sampling Technic with Results of 1959 Poliomyelitis Vaccination Surveys," *American Journal of Public Health* 50 (1960): 1847–1857.

88. Selwyn D. Collins, "Frequency of Immunizing and Related Procedures in Nine Thousand Surveyed Families in Eighteen States," *Milbank Memorial Fund Quarterly* 15, no. 2 (1937): 150–172.

89. Carl M. Brauer, "Kennedy, Johnson, and the War on Poverty," *Journal of American History* 69 (1982): 98–119.

90. John Kenneth Galbraith, *The Affluent Society* (Boston: Houghton Mifflin, 1958). See pp. 325–327 for Galbraith's discussion of "insular" poverty—entire communities in which "everyone or nearly everyone is poor"—as distinct from "case poverty," an individual or family that is poor because of some misfortune or personal shortcoming.

91. Roscoe Kandle to Leona Baumgartner, December 8, 1958, NYCDOH, box 141677, folder: Poliomyelitis. Emphasis in original.

92. S. M. Wishik to Leona Baumgartner, April 5, 1961, NYCDOH, box 141907, folder: Poliomyelitis.

93. Al Burns to Dorothy Ducas, December 20, 1957, MOD, series 3, file: Vaccine Promotion and Education 1957.

94. Harold R. Moskovit to Leona Baumgartner, March 24, 1959, NYCDOH, box 141690, folder: Poliomyelitis.

95. Leona Baumgartner to Harold R. Moskovit, March 31, 1959 (draft), NYCDOH, box 141690, folder: Poliomyelitis.

96. The Board of Health first urged fluoridation of the city's water supply in 1954, with Baumgartner as one of the proposal's leading proponents, but after years of often vociferous public protest, the effort remained stalled. Fluoride was not added to the city's water until 1965.

97. Leona Baumgartner to Harold R. Moskovit, April 6, 1959, NYCDOH, box 141690, folder: Poliomyelitis.

98. William A. Allen and Michael J. Burke, "Poliomyelitis Immunization House to House," *Public Health Reports* 75 (1960): 245–250.

99. Karl Presthold to Leona Baumgartner, June 1, 1960, NYCDOH, box 141703, folder: Poliomyelitis.

100. "City Health Head Gives Polio Shots in Sunday School," *New York Times,* June 6, 1960, 33.

101. Leona Baumgartner to Robert E. Condon, August 21, 1959, NYCDOH, box 141690, folder: Poliomyelitis.

102. Simon Podair to Abe A. Brown, July 5, 1961, NYCDOH, box 141907, folder: Poliomyelitis.

103. Leroy E. Burney, "Poliomyelitis Vaccination," *Public Health Reports* 74 (1959): 95–96; 96.

104. Thomas M. Rivers to selected chapters, April 24, 1959, MOD, series 3, file: Vaccine Prevention and Education 1959.

105. The cities were Indianapolis, Indiana; Louisville, Kentucky; Minneapolis, Minnesota; St. Louis, Missouri; Kansas City, Missouri; and Oklahoma City, Oklahoma. Gabriel Stickle to Hubert E. White, July 27, 1959, MOD, series 3, file: Vaccine Promotion and Education 1959. On the progress of the "soft spots" program, see also memos dated June 15 and June 29 in the same folder.

106. Surgeon General's Committee on Poliomyelitis Control, *Babies and Breadwinners, Proposal for a 1961 Neighborhood Polio Vaccination Campaign* (Washington, D.C.: Government Printing Office, 1961), 4, 5.

107. Ibid., 13; emphases in original.

108. Alexander, "Extent of the Poliomyelitis Problem."

109. John R. Paul, "Status of Vaccination against Poliomyelitis, with Particular Reference to Oral Vaccination," *New England Journal of Medicine* 264 (1961): 651–658.

110. Alexander Langmuir told the American Medical Association in 1960 that the "basic miscalculation" of those who hoped for complete control of polio in 1955 was overestimating popular acceptance of the killed vaccine. Langmuir, "Epidemiologic Considerations," 840.

111. "3 Polio Shots Ruled Enough by Experts," *New York Times*, March 21, 1958, 8; Damon Stetson, "Vaccination Held Major Polio Need," ibid., January 7, 1959, 66.

112. Harold Jacobziner to Leona Baumgartner, August 25, 1959, NYCDOH, box 141690, folder: Poliomyelitis.

113. Wilson, *Margin of Safety*, 217.

114. Sumner Berkovich, Jack E. Pickering, and Sidney Kibrick, "Paralytic Poliomyelitis in a Well Vaccinated Population," *New England Journal of Medicine* 264 (1961): 1323–1329.

115. Rowan, *Margin of Safety*; Paul, *History of Poliomyelitis*, 452.

116. In addition to Albert Sabin's preparation, the other leading contenders to develop a live attenuated virus were Herald Cox of Lederle Laboratories and Hilary Koprowski of the Wistar Institute. Wilson, *Margin of Safety*, 168–190.

117. Saul Benison, "International Medical Cooperation: Dr. Albert Sabin, Live Poliovirus Vaccine and the Soviets," *Bulletin of the History of Medicine* 56 (1982): 460–483; Dorothy M. Horstmann, "The Sabin Live Poliovirus Trials in the USSR, 1959," *Yale Journal of Biology and Medicine* 64 (1991): 499–512. Field trials of live attenuated vaccine developed by Sabin as well as other researchers were conducted in several other countries during the second half of the 1950s; Paul, *History of Poliomyelitis*, 454.

118. Cases of polio per 100,000 population had averaged 14.6 for the period 1950–1965, while the case rate for the years 1957–1961 averaged 1.8, a

decline of 88 percent. "Oral Poliomyelitis Vaccines," *Journal of the American Medical Association* 190 (1964): 49–51.

119. The vaccine itself was slightly more expensive than the Salk inactivated vaccine, but because no hypodermic needles were required, overall costs of administering it were less. Harold T. Fuerst to Leona Baumgartner, April 5, 1962, NYCDOH, box 141921, folder: Poliomyelitis.

120. Domenic G. Iezzoni to Leona Baumgartner, January 31, 1961, NYCDOH, box 141907, folder: Poliomyelitis.

121. A senior manager at the foundation noted in 1962 that "the decision was made to soft-peddle Sabin's name … for fear that to do otherwise would dilute Salk's name." George P. Voss to Jack Major, August 30, 1962, MOD, series 3, file: Vaccine Promotion and Education 1957–1962.

122. *Polio Vaccines, Hearings before a Subcommittee of the Committee on Interstate and Foreign Commerce, House of Representatives, Eighty-seventh Congress, First Session, March 16 and 17, 1961* (Washington, D.C.: Government Printing Office, 1961).

123. Albert B. Sabin, Richard H. Michaels, Ilya Spigland, et al., "Community-Wide Use of Oral Poliovirus Vaccine," *American Journal of Diseases of Children* 101 (1961): 38–59; John R. Paul, "The 1961 Middletown Oral Poliovirus Vaccine Program," *Yale Journal of Biology and Medicine* 34 (1962): 439–446.

124. "Recommendation on Oral Poliomyelitis Vaccine," *Public Health Reports* 78 (1963): 273–274.

125. "Many Polio Inoculation Drives to Continue Despite Advice to Bar Type III Oral Vaccine," *Wall Street Journal*, September 17, 1962, 4.

126. See, e.g., Donald Day, "Enlisting Community Support of a Polio Vaccine Program," *Public Health Reports* 80 (1965): 737–740.

127. "Oral Poliomyelitis Vaccines," *Journal of the American Medical Association* 190 (1964): 49–51.

128. U.S. Department of Health, Education and Welfare, *Immunization Activities Statistical Report* (Atlanta: Communicable Disease Center, 1965), 9.

129. "Immunization Campaign, Communicable Disease Activities—FY 1962" (typescript, n.d. [1961]), NARA, RG 442, box 105229, folder: Associations, Committees etc., 1961.

130. James L. Goddard, "Smallpox, Diphtheria, Tetanus, Pertussis, and Poliomyelitis Immunization," *Journal of the American Medical Association* 187 (1964): 1009–1012; 1012. Emphasis in original.

131. Theodore J. Bauer to Luther Terry, August 2, 1961, NARA, RG 442, box 105229, folder: Associations, Committees etc., 1961.

132. "Immunization against Polio and Other Diseases, Summary of Previous Report" (typescript [draft], April 24, 1961), NARA, RG 442, box 105229, folder: Associations, Committees etc., 1961.

133. Elizabeth W. Etheridge, *Sentinel for Health: A History of the Centers for Disease Control* (Berkeley: University of California Press, 1992), 143. On the Kennedy administration's health care policy, see Starr, *Social Transformation of American Medicine*, 363–369.

134. "Kennedy Calls for 'Mass Immunization' against Diseases; No Details Supplied," *Wall Street Journal*, January 12, 1962, 2.

135. John D. Morris, "Kennedy Presses Congress to Pass Bill on Aged Care," *New York Times,* February 28, 1962, 1.

136. U.S. Department of Health, Education and Welfare, *Fact Book Relating to the Vaccination Assistance Act of 1962,* NYCDOH, box 141997.

137. Herman Hilleboe to David Sencer, March 13, 1962, NYCDOH, box 141921, folder: Poliomyelitis.

138. *Intensive Immunization Programs,* 25.

139. Clarence H. Webb to James L. Goddard, February 1, 1963, NARA, RG 442, box 108381, folder: Immunization Activities 1963.

140. F. Robert Freckleton, "Federal Government Programs in Immunization," *Archives of Environmental Health* 15 (1967): 512–514; 513.

141. On this point, see Patrick M. Vivier, "National Policies for Childhood Immunization in the United States: A Historical Perspective" (Ph.D. diss., Johns Hopkins University, 1996), 66–105.

142. Dorothy Ducas to Basil O'Connor, January 20, 1956, MOD, series 3, file: Vaccine Promotion and Education 1956.

143. "Draft Statement Pertaining to Responsibilities of the Advisory Committee on Immunization Practice" (typescript, n.d. [July 1964]), NARA, RG 90, box 334062, folder: Advisory Committee on Immunization Practice.

144. *Reports and Recommendations of the National Immunization Work Groups, March 15, 1977* (McLean, Va.: JRB Associates, 1977), table 2 (n.p.).

145. "Recommendation on Oral Poliomyelitis Vaccine," *Public Health Reports* 78 (1963): 273–274.

5. ERADICATIONISM AND ITS DISCONTENTS

1. J. L. Conrad, Robert Wallace, John J. Witte, "The Epidemiologic Rationale for the Failure to Eradicate Measels in the United States," *American Journal of Public Health* 61 (1971): 2304–2310.

2. James D. Cherry, Ralph D. Feigin, Louis A. Lobes Jr., et al., "Urban Measles in the Vaccine Era: A Clinical, Epidemiologic, and Serologic Study," *Journal of Pediatrics* 81 (1972): 217–230.

3. Peter M. Strebel, Mark J. Papania, and Neal A. Halsey, "Measles Vaccine," in Stanley A. Plotkin and Walter A. Orenstein, eds., *Vaccines,* 4th ed. (Philadelphia: Elsevier, 2004).

4. Ibid.

5. Vincent A. Fulginiti, Jerry J. Eller, Allan W. Downie, et al., "Altered Reactivity to Measles Virus," *Journal of the American Medical Association* 202 (1967): 101–106. Between 600,000 and 900,000 children were estimated to have received the killed measles vaccine before it was taken off the market. Strebel, Papania, and Halsey, "Measles Vaccine."

6. John J. Goldman, "New Measles Vaccines Fail to Curb Incidence of Disease This Year," *Wall Street Journal,* June 25, 1964, 1.

7. William E. Mosher, "Statement for the New York State Senate Committee on Public Health," March 10, 1965, NYSDOH, series 13307–82, box 42, folder: Measles 1963–1970; "Twelve Million Children Immunized against Measles; Cases Drop Sharply," *Journal of the American Medical Association*

196 (1966): 29–30, 38–39; George James, "Testimony before the New York State Senate Committee on Public Health," March 10, 1965, NYSDOH, series 13307–82, box 42, folder: Measles 1963–1970.

8. Louis Galambos with Jane Eliot Sewell, *Networks of Innovation: Vaccine Development at Merck, Sharp & Dohme, and Mulford, 1895–1995* (Cambridge: Cambridge University Press, 1995), 115.

9. *Public Health Grants and Construction of Health Research Facilities, Hearing before the Subcommittee on Health of the Committee on Labor and Public Welfare, United States Senate, Eighty-ninth Congress, First Session, January 27, 1965* (Washington, D.C.: Government Printing Office, 1965), 114.

10. Warren A. Rasmussen, "Maintenance Immunization Programs," in U.S. Department of Health, Education and Welfare, *1st Immunization Conference Proceedings* (Atlanta: Communicable Disease Center, 1965), 56.

11. "Statement on the Status of Measles Vaccine by the Ad Hoc Advisory Committee on Measles Control (March 21, 1963) as Revised by the Advisory Committee on Immunization Practice May 25, 1964," NARA, RG 90, box 334062, folder: Advisory Committee on Immunization Practices.

12. Advisory Committee on Immunization Practices, minutes, Meeting No. 4, June 11, 1965, NARA, RG 90, box 334062, folder: Advisory Committee on Immunization Practices.

13. Milton D. Stewart to guest witnesses, March 1, 1965, NYSDOH, series 13307–82, box 42, folder: Measles 1963–1970.

14. "A Crash Program to Combat Measles Debated in Albany," *New York Times*, March 11, 1965, 38.

15. James L. Goddard, "Information on Measles Vaccination for Public Hearing of the New York State Senate Committee on Public Health" (March 10, 1965), NYSDOH, series 13307–82, box 42, folder: Measles 1963–1970.

16. George James, "Testimony before the New York State Senate Committee on Public Health" (March 10, 1965), NYSDOH, series 13307–82, box 42, folder: Measles 1963–1970.

17. George James, "Health Challenges Today," *American Review of Respiratory Diseases* 90 (1964): 349–358; 351. Emphases in original.

18. Fred L. Soper, "Rehabilitation of the Eradication Concept in Prevention of Communicable Diseases," *Public Health Reports* 80 (1965): 855–869.

19. Donald A. Henderson, "The History of Smallpox Eradication," *Henry E. Sigerist Supplements to the Bulletin of the History of Medicine* 4 (1980): 99–108.

20. F. Fenner, A. J. Hall, and W. R. Dowdle, "What Is Eradication?" in W. R. Dowdle and D. R. Hopkins, eds., *The Eradication of Infectious Diseases* (New York: John Wiley & Sons, 1998), 9.

21. Fred L. Soper, "Problems to Be Solved if the Eradication of Tuberculosis Is to Be Realized," *American Journal of Public Health* 52 (1962): 734–739.

22. Justin M. Andrews and Alexander D. Langmuir, "The Philosophy of Disease Eradication," *American Journal of Public Health* 53 (1963): 1–6.

23. James, "Health Challenges Today."

24. Amy Fairchild, James Colgrove, and Ronald Bayer, "The Myth of Exceptionalism: The History of Venereal Disease Reporting in the Twentieth Century," *Journal of Law, Medicine and Ethics* 31 (2003): 624–637.

25. T. Aidan Cockburn, "Eradication of Infectious Diseases," *Science* 133 (1961): 1050–1058; 1058.

26. *Report of the Department of Health of the City of New York for the Years 1961–1962* (New York: Department of Health, 1963), 9.

27. René Dubos, *Man Adapting* (New Haven, Conn.: Yale University Press, 1965), 378.

28. Ibid., 346.

29. On the influence of social science on government programs in the 1960s, see Daniel P. Moynihan, *Maximum Feasible Misunderstanding: Community Action in the War on Poverty* (New York: Free Press, 1969); Carl M. Brauer, "Kennedy, Johnson, and the War on Poverty," *Journal of American History* 69 (1982): 98–119; and Byron G. Lander, "Group Theory and Individuals: The Origin of Poverty as a Political Issue in 1964," *Western Political Quarterly* 24 (1971): 514–526.

30. Ira Katznelson, "Was the Great Society a Lost Opportunity?" in Steve Fraser and Gary Gerstle, eds., *The Rise and Fall of the New Deal Order, 1930–1980* (Princeton, N.J.: Princeton University Press, 1989).

31. Anne-Marie Foltz, *An Ounce of Prevention: Child Health Politics under Medicaid* (Cambridge, Mass.: MIT Press, 1982).

32. "Twelve Million Children Immunized against Measles; Cases Drop Sharply," *Journal of the American Medical Association* 196 (1966): 29–30, 38–39.

33. Richard G. Lennon, Craig D. Turnbull, and William R. Elsea, "Measles Immunization in a Northeastern Metropolitan County," *Journal of the American Medical Association* 200 (1967): 815–819.

34. Lawrence Bergner and Alonzo S. Yerby, "Low Income and Barriers to Use of Health Services," *New England Journal of Medicine* 278 (1968): 541–546. See also New York City Department of Health, "Health Services General Project Grant" (typescript, September 10, 1968), NYCDOH, box 142241, folder: Preventable Disease.

35. Charlotte Muller, "Income and the Receipt of Medical Care," *American Journal of Public Health* 55 (1965): 510–521.

36. Alexander D. Langmuir, "Medical Importance of Measles," *American Journal of Diseases of Children* 103 (1962): 224–226, at 224; "2 Measles Vaccines Licensed; U.S. Sees End of Disease in 1965," *New York Times*, March 22, 1963, 1.

37. James L. Goddard, "Future Goals of Immunization Activities," in U.S. Department of Health, Education and Welfare, *2nd Immunization Conference Proceedings* (Atlanta: Communicable Disease Center, 1965), 9.

38. "Statement of Executive Committee of Conference of State and Territorial Epidemiologists on Measles—September 1966," ASTHO archives, box 3, folder: Conference of State and Territorial Epidemiologists.

39. Earl B. Byrne, Beryl J. Rosenstein, Alexander A. Jaworski, et al., "A Statewide Mass Measles Immunization Program," *Journal of the American Medical Association* 199 (1967): 619–623; and James E. Bowes, "Rhode Island's End Measles Campaign," *Public Health Reports* 82 (1967): 409–415.

40. On this point, see Patrick M. Vivier, "National Policies for Childhood Immunization in the United States: A Historical Perspective" (Ph.D. diss., Johns Hopkins University, 1996).

41. Robert E. Serfling, "Historical Review of Epidemic Theory," *Human Biology* 24 (1952): 145–166.

42. W. C. Tapley and G. S. Wilson, "The Spread of Bacterial Infection: The Problem of Herd Immunity," *Journal of Hygiene* 21 (1923): 243–249. The "herd" in question were mice used in laboratory experiments on the spread of bacterial infections. See Paul E. M. Fine, "Community Immunity," in Plotkin and Orenstein, eds., *Vaccines*, 1443–1462.

43. Major Greenwood, *Epidemics and Crowd-Diseases: An Introduction to the Study of Epidemiology* (New York: Macmillan, 1935), 68–77.

44. Edward S. Godfrey, "Practical Uses of Diphtheria Immunization Records," *American Journal of Public Health* 23 (1933): 809–812; 811.

45. F. Robert Freckleton, "Preschool Diphtheria Immunization Status of a New York State Community," *American Journal of Public Health* 39 (1949): 1439–1440.

46. William J. Meyer, "Determination of Immunization Status of School Children in New York State," *New York State Journal of Medicine* 60 (1960): 2869–2873; 2869.

47. A. W. Hedrich, "The Corrected Average Attack Rate from Measles among City Children," *American Journal of Hygiene* 11 (1930): 576–600.

48. David J. Sencer, H. Bruce Dull, and Alexander D. Langmuir, "Epidemiologic Basis for Eradication of Measles in 1967," *Public Health Reports* 82 (1967): 253–256.

49. "U.S. Plans Drive to End Measles," *New York Times*, March 7, 1967, 43.

50. New York City Health Services Administration, Public Service Announcement, May 1, 1967, NYCDOH, box 142024, folder: Measles.

51. Helen S. Stone to Edward O'Rourke, May 8, 1967; Helen S. Stone to Edward O'Rourke, May 22, 1967, NYCDOH, box 142024, folder: Measles.

52. "Measles Trends in New York City 1968" (typescript), NYCDOH, box 142241, folder: Preventable Disease.

53. "Immunization Activities Project: First City-Wide Mailing of Birth Certificates Follow-up Program," *Bulletin to Professors of Preventive Medicine*, February 1967, 2; "City Plans Drive for Immunization," *New York Times*, March 2, 1967, 37; Department of Health, "Health Services General Project Grant" (typescript), September 10, 1968, NYCDOH, box 142241, folder: Preventable Disease.

54. U.S. Department of Health, Education and Welfare, *3rd Immunization Conference Proceedings* (Atlanta: Communicable Disease Center, 1966), passim.

55. The sociologist Frank Riessman popularized the term "indigenous nonprofessional" in studies conducted under the aegis of the National Institute of Labor Education on community mental health services. See Frank Riessman, *Mental Health for the Poor* (New York: Free Press of Glencoe, 1964), and Arthur Pearl and Frank Riessman, *New Careers for the Poor: The Nonprofessional in Human Service* (New York: Free Press, 1965). On the influence of Riessman's

work on immunization programs, see Russell H. Richardson, "Getting Community Response," in U.S. Department of Health, Education and Welfare, *3rd Immunization Conference Proceedings*.

56. See, e.g., Herbert Domke, Gladys Coffey, "The Neighborhood-Based Public Health Worker: Additional Manpower for Community Heath Services," *American Journal of Public Health* 56 (1966): 603–608; Jane Luckham and David W. Swift, "Community Health Aides in the Ghetto: The Contra Costa Project," *Medical Care* 7 (1969): 332–339; James C. Stewart and William R. Hood, "Using Workers from 'Hard-Core' Areas to Increase Immunization Levels," *Public Health Reports* 85 (1970): 177–185; Theodore J. Colombo, Donald K. Freeborn, John P. Mullooly, and Vicky R. Burnham, "The Effect of Outreach Workers' Educational Efforts on Disadvantaged Preschool Children's Use of Preventive Services," *American Journal of Public Health* 69 (1979): 465–468.

57. Joel G. Bremen and Isao Arita, "The Confirmation and Maintenance of Smallpox Eradication," *New England Journal of Medicine* 303 (1980): 1263–1273.

58. George Horne, "Idlewild Inspectors Keep Close Watch for Smallpox," *New York Times*, October 20, 1963, 86.

59. James L. Goddard, "Smallpox, Diphtheria, Tetanus, Pertussis, and Poliomyelitis Immunization," *Journal of the American Medical Association* 187 (1964): 1009–1012; John C. Devlin, "Smallpox Alert Is Sounded Here," *New York Times*, August 20, 1962, 17; Lawrence O'Kane, "Broad Search on in Smallpox Case," ibid., August 21, 1962, 21; "Smallpox Danger Is Over, City Health Chief Says," ibid., August 29, 1962, 20.

60. Richard R. Leger, "Doctors See Danger in Low Level of U.S. Immunity to Disease," *Wall Street Journal*, December 18, 1963, 1.

61. Morris Greenberg, "Complications of Vaccination against Smallpox," *American Journal of Diseases of Children* 76 (1948): 492–502.

62. G. W. McCoy to S. W. Wynne, October 13, 1930, NYCDOH, box 141375, folder: Vaccination. Four months later Wynne reported to McCoy that after consultation with all of his bureau chiefs, "not a single case has come to the attention of this Department since your communication was received." S. W. Wynne to G. W. McCoy, February 10, 1931, NYCDOH, box 141375, folder: Vaccination.

63. Stimson cautioned, however, that this information "could hardly be made public and should only be given out to health officials in confidence," a stance that underscores the paternalism that underlay medical ethics in that era. A. M. Stimson to Dr. Williams (n.d. [December 1930]), NARA, box 425, folder: New York Cities & Counties—Niagara Falls—Seneca Lake.

64. C. Henry Kempe, "Studies on Smallpox and Complications of Smallpox Vaccination," *Pediatrics* 26 (1960): 176–189.

65. John M. Neff, Michael Lane, James H. Pert, et al., "Complications of Smallpox Vaccination. I. National Survey in the United States, 1963," *New England Journal of Medicine* 276 (1967): 125–132.

66. "Recommendation of the Public Health Service Advisory Committee on Immunization Practices," *Morbidity and Mortality Weekly Report* 15 (1966): 404–407; 405.

67. Lewis L. Coriell, "Smallpox Vaccination: When and Whom to Vaccinate," *Pediatrics* 37 (1966): 493–496; C. Henry Kempe, Abram S. Benenson, "Smallpox Immunization in the United States," *Journal of the American Medical Association* 194 (1965): 141–146.

68. J. Michael Lane, Frederick L. Ruben, John M. Neff, et al., "Complications of Smallpox Vaccination, 1968," *New England Journal of Medicine* 281 (1969): 1201–1207; J. Michael Lane, Frederick L. Ruben, John M. Neff, et al., "Complications of Smallpox Vaccination, 1968: Results of Ten Statewide Surveys," *Journal of Infectious Diseases* 122 (1970): 303–309; J. Michael Lane, Frederick L. Ruben, Elias Abrutyn, et al., "Deaths Attributable to Smallpox Vaccination, 1959 to 1966, and 1968," *Journal of the American Medical Association* 212 (1970): 441–444.

69. Saul Krugman and Samuel L. Katz, "Smallpox Vaccination," *New England Journal of Medicine* 281 (1969): 1241–1242; George J. Galasso, "Projected Studies on Immunization against Smallpox," *Journal of Infectious Diseases* 121 (1970): 575–577.

70. George Dick, "Smallpox: A Reconsideration of Public Health Policies," *Progress in Medical Virology* 8 (1966): 1–29.

71. Thomas M. Mack, "Smallpox in Europe, 1950–1971," *Journal of Infectious Diseases* 125 (1972): 161–169; 168.

72. John M. Neff, "The Case for Abolishing Routine Childhood Smallpox Vaccination in the United States," *American Journal of Epidemiology* 93 (1971): 245–247.

73. "Recommendations of the Public Health Service Advisory Committee on Immunization Practices," *Morbidity and Mortality Weekly Report*, suppl. 18 (1969): 23–25.

74. J. Michael Lane and J. D. Millar, "Routine Childhood Vaccination against Smallpox Reconsidered," *New England Journal of Medicine* 281 (1969): 1220–1224.

75. Center for Disease Control, "Public Health Service Recommendation on Smallpox Vaccination," *Morbidity and Mortality Weekly Report* 20 (1971): 339–345; 339.

76. "Revised Recommendations of the Committee on Infectious Disease of the American Academy of Pediatrics, October 17, 1971, for Infants and Children in the United States," *Clinical Pediatrics* 11 (1972): 3.

77. Alan R. Hinman to William H. Wisely, January 7, 1972, NYSDOH, series 13855, roll 4.

78. "Smallpox-Vaccination Laws May Be Revoked by States, Cities in Line with Federal Advice," *Wall Street Journal*, October 8, 1971, 24.

79. Lawrence K. Altman, "All States Drop Smallpox Vaccinations," *New York Times*, January 29, 1976, 30; "Smallpox Vaccination No Longer Required for Entrance to School" (memorandum, State Education Department, April 1972), NYSDOH, series 13855, reel 4.

80. Alan R. Hinman, A. David Brandling-Bennett, and P. I. Nieburg, "The Opportunity and Obligation to Eliminate Measles from the United States," *Journal of the American Medical Association* 242 (1979): 1157–1162.

81. *Report and Recommendations of the National Immunization Work Groups March 15, 1977* (McLean, Va.: JRB Associates, 1977), n.p.

82. George E. Hardy, Ira Kassanoff, Hyman G. Orbach, et al., "The Failure of a School Immunization Campaign to Terminate an Urban Epidemic of Measles," *American Journal of Epidemiology* 91 (1970): 286–293; 290–291.

83. "South Bronx Children to Get Measles-Immunization Shots," *New York Times,* February 10, 1969, 35.

84. "Outbreak of Measles in City Is Now Termed an Epidemic," *New York Times,* April 8, 1969, 93; Jane E. Brody, "Measles Outbreak Prompts City to Press Vaccination Campaign," ibid., April 11, 1969, 30.

85. D. Harris to Vincent Guinee, October 8, 1969, NYCDOH, box 142261, folder: Bureau of Infectious Disease.

86. Conrad, Wallace, and Witte, "Epidemiologic Rationale."

87. Jonathan Spivak, "Measles Resurgence Sparks New Campaign to Immunize Children," *Wall Street Journal,* February 20, 1970, 1.

88. "Measles Eradication at a Stand-Still," *Journal of the American Medical Association* 209 (1969): 191–192.

89. "Report of Proceedings, Conference on 'Measles Eradication 1967' and School Health Programs" (typescript, August 18, 1967), NARA, RG 90, box 334062, folder: Measles Eradication 1967.

90. John P. Fox, Lila Elveback, William Scott, et al., "Herd Immunity: Basic Concept and Relevance to Public Health Immunization Practices," *American Journal of Epidemiology* 94 (1971): 179–189.

91. Conrad, Wallace, and Witte, "Epidemiologic Rationale," 2309–2310.

92. Hinman, Brandling-Bennett, and Nieburg, "Opportunity and Obligation to Eliminate Measles."

93. Michael Harrington, *The Other America* (New York: Macmillan, 1962); see pp. 15 and 169 for discussions of the relationship between poverty and health.

94. John A. Ross, "Social Class and Medical Care," *Journal of Health and Human Behavior* 3 (1962): 35–40.

95. Edward A. Suchman, "Sociomedical Variations among Ethnic Groups," *American Journal of Sociology* 70 (1964): 319–331; 323.

96. James A. Kent, C. Harvey Smith, "Involving the Urban Poor in Health Services through Accommodation—The Employment of Neighborhood Representatives," *American Journal of Public Health* 57 (1967): 997–1003; 997.

97. John Sibley, "Measles Up 300% Here, but Peak Is Believed Passed," *New York Times,* July 31, 1971, 25.

98. William Schaffner, "Measles Eradication: The Impossible Dream? Or the New Heresy of an 'Old Boy'," in U.S. Department of Health, Education and Welfare, *8th Immunization Conference Proceedings* (Atlanta: Communicable Disease Center, 1971), 16; emphases in original.

99. Alexander D. Langmuir, "Changing Concepts of Airborne Infection of Acute Contagious Diseases: A Reconsideration of Classic Epidemiologic Theories," *Annals of the New York Academy of Sciences* 353 (1980): 35–44; 38.

100. Wilbur Hoff, "Why Health Programs Are Not Reaching the Unresponsive in Our Communities," *Public Health Reports* 81 (1966): 654–658; 656.

101. James C. Stewart, "Analysis of the Diphtheria Outbreak in Austin, Texas, 1967–69," *Public Health Reports* 85 (1970): 949–954.

102. Bernard Guyer, Steven J. Baird, Robert H. Hutcheson, et al., "Failure to Vaccinate Children against Measles during the Second Year of Life," *Public Health Reports* 91 (1976): 133–137; 136.

103. Herbert A. Schreier, "On the Failure to Eradicate Measles," *New England Journal of Medicine* 290 (1974): 803–804; 804.

104. Health Policy Advisory Center, *The American Health Empire: Power, Profits, and Politics* (New York: Random House, 1970).

105. Schreier, "On the Failure to Eradicate Measles"; William J. Dougherty, "Community Organization for Immunization Programs," *Medical Clinics of North America* 51 (1967): 837–842.

106. Edward M. Kennedy to William H. Stewart, July 7, 1967; and John Bagby to Edward M. Kennedy, July 27, 1967, NARA, RG 442, box 43434, folder: Information 1967–68.

107. F. Robert Freckleton, "Status Report by CDC," in U.S. Department of Health, Education and Welfare, *4th Immunization Conference Proceedings* (Atlanta: Communicable Disease Center, 1967).

108. Kay A. Johnson, Alice Sardell, Barbara Richards, "Federal Immunization Policy and Funding: A History of Responding to Crisis," *American Journal of Preventive Medicine* 19 (2000): 99–112.

109. Vivier, "National Policies for Childhood Immunization in the United States," 110–131.

110. Ibid., 160; Elizabeth W. Etheridge, *Sentinel for Health: A History of the Centers for Disease Control* (Berkeley: University of California Press, 1992), 174–177.

111. John J. Witte, "Recent Advances in Public Health. Immunization," *American Journal of Public Health* 64 (1974): 939–944.

112. Johnson, Sardell, and Richards, "Federal Immunization Policy and Funding."

113. Vivier, "National Policies for Childhood Immunization in the United States."

114. Tom Rivers, the foundation's medical director, who had served on the New York City Board of Health for many years, was skeptical about the constitutionality of compulsory laws; he claimed that "health boards keep the laws on the books by keeping them out of court where they would be declared invalid." Wilber Crawford to Elaine Whitelaw, February 27, 1959, MOD, series 3, file: Vaccine Promotion and Education 1959.

115. The commissioner and members of his staff testified against a proposal to make polio immunization mandatory on the grounds that it would detract from efforts to get parents to immunize their children in infancy. A. L. Marshall Jr. and Andrew C. Offutt, "A Noncompulsory Immunization Law for Indiana School Children," *Public Health Reports* 75 (1960): 967–969.

116. "Compulsory Inoculation," *Journal of the South Carolina Medical Association* 57 (1961): 171.

117. William J. Dougherty, Adele C. Shepard, and Curtis F. Culp, "New Jersey's Action Program to Prevent Poliomyelitis," *Public Health Reports* 75 (1960): 659–664.

118. "An Act to amend the public health law, in relation to requiring the vaccination of school children against poliomyelitis" (February 10, 1965), NYCDOH, box 141983, folder: Poliomyelitis.

119. George James to Alexander Chananau, June 8, 1965, NYCDOH, box 141983, folder: Poliomyelitis.

120. By 1963, only eight states had enacted laws requiring polio vaccination for students: California, Kansas, Kentucky, Michigan, Missouri, New Hampshire, North Carolina, and Ohio. Adelaide M. Hunter, Robert Ortiz, Joe Martinez, "Compulsory and Voluntary School Immunization Programs in the United States," *Journal of School Health* 33 (1963): 98–102. See also *Intensive Immunization Programs*, 14. Requirements for vaccination before school entry were also adopted at the local level as well; many states had laws that allowed localities to enact such regulations, although the number of cities that did so is unknown.

121. "Status Report by CDC," 4.

122. The foundation was established in 1946 and named in honor of one of Joseph Kennedy Sr.'s sons who had been killed in World War II. It funded scientific research into the causes and treatment of mental retardation and sponsored the annual "Special Olympics." John Clinton, ed., *National Guide to Foundation Funding in Health* (New York: Foundation Center, 1988). On the research funded by the foundation, see George A. Jervis, ed., *Mental Retardation: A Symposium from the Joseph P. Kennedy, Jr. Foundation* (Springfield, Ill.: C. C. Thomas, 1967).

123. Harold T. Fuerst to Arthur Bushel, May 26, 1966, NYCDOH, box 142007, folder: Preventable Diseases.

124. See, e.g., Eunice Kennedy Shriver to John A. Volpe, January 22, 1968, NARA, RG 442, box 43435, folder: Programs & Projects 1967–68.

125. Nicholas Fiumara to Fred Bledsoe, February 2, 1968, NARA, RG 442, box 43435, folder: Programs & Projects 1967–68. On James Bowes's involvement in the work of the Kennedy Foundation, see "Status Report on Measles Programs" (memo, June 7, 1967), Joseph P. Kennedy Jr. Foundation, NARA, RG 442, box 43434, folder: Information 1967–68.

126. Hollis Ingraham to Jacob Javits, February 16, 1968, NYSDOH, series 13307–82, box 42, folder: Measles 1963–1970.

127. *Journal of the Senate of the State of New York, 189th Session*, vol. 1 (Albany, N.Y.: Williams Press, 1966), 454; *Journal of the Senate of the State of New York, 191st Session*, vol. 1 (Albany, N.Y.: Williams Press, 1966), 794–795.

128. New York State Department of Health, news release, April 11, 1970, NYSDOH, series 13307–82, box 42, folder: Measles 1963–70. It is unclear whether or not Rockefeller ever saw the Kennedy Foundation's letter or was persuaded by the foundation's efforts.

129. Philip J. Landrigan, "Epidemic Measles in a Divided City," *Journal of the American Medical Association* 221 (1972): 567–570.

130. "Measles—United States," *Morbidity and Mortality Weekly Report* 26 (1977): 109–111.

131. Hinman, Brandling-Bennett, and Nieburg, "Opportunity and Obligation to Eliminate Measles."

132. Charles A. Jackson, "State Laws on Compulsory Immunization in the United States," *Public Health Reports* 84 (1969): 787–795.

133. Jeanette L. Hale, "School Laws Update," in *16th Immunization Conference Proceedings* (Atlanta: Centers for Disease Control, 1981).

134. Alan Hinman, "Position Paper," *Pediatric Research* 13 (1979): 689–696; 695.

135. Samuel L. Katz, "The Case for Continuing 'Routine' Childhood Smallpox Vaccination in the United States," *American Journal of Epidemiology* 93 (1971): 241–244; 243.

136. Opinion Research Corporation, *Public Attitudes toward Immunization: August 1977 and February 1978* (Princeton, N.J.: Opinion Research Corporation, 1978), 84–85.

137. Department of Health, Education and Welfare, memo, June 22, 1970, NYSDOH, series 13307–82, box 41, folder: Legislation—State—1970.

138. John Enders, "Rubella Vaccination," *New England Journal of Medicine* 283 (1970): 261–263.

139. Matthew L. Wald, "Rubella Debate Divides Doctors and Lawmakers," *New York Times*, March 26, 1978, xxiii-1.

140. Vincent A. Fulginiti, "Controversies in Current Immunization Policy and Practices: One Physician's Viewpoint," *Current Problems in Pediatrics* 6 (1976): 3–35; 17.

141. Lawrence E. Klock and Gary S. Rachelefsky, "Failure of Rubella Herd Immunity during an Epidemic," *New England Journal of Medicine* 288 (1973): 69–72; 71.

142. Louis Weinstein and Te-Wen Chang, "Rubella Immunization," *New England Journal of Medicine* 288 (1973): 100–101.

143. "Measles and Rubella Immunization: Statement of the Committee on Infectious Diseases, American Academy of Pediatrics," *Postgraduate Medicine* 61 (1977): 269–272.

144. Rita Swan, "On Statutes Depriving a Class of Children of Rights to Medical Care: Can This Discrimination be Litigated?" *Quinnipiac Health Law Journal* 2 (1988–1999): 73–95; William J. Curran, "Smallpox Vaccination and Organized Religion," *American Journal of Public Health* 61 (1971): 2127–2128; and Rennie B. Schoepflin, *Christian Science on Trial: Religious Healing in America* (Baltimore: Johns Hopkins University Press, 2003), 196–199.

145. C. Ross Cunningham to Charles Rubano, January 20, 1967, NYCDOH, box 142023, folder: Legislation. The only two votes in the legislature against the bill had come from members who opposed the exemption. Sydney H. Schanberg, "Assembly Votes Polio Shots Bill," *New York Times*, June 21, 1966, 26.

146. *McCartney v. Austin*, 293 N.Y.S. 2d 188 (1968).

147. *In re Elwell*, 284 N.Y.S. 2d 924 (1967), 930.

148. Stephen R. Redmond, "Immunization and School Records," *Journal of the New York State School Nurse Teachers Association* 6 (1974): 11–16.

149. Richard J. McDonald to Hollis Ingraham, October 31, 1967, NYSDOH, series 13307-82, box 41, folder: Legislation—New York State—1967–1970.

150. Ibid.

151. Norman S. Moore to Hollis Ingraham, January 17, 1968, NYSDOH, series 13307-82, box 41, folder: Legislation—New York State—1967–1970.

152. *Maier v. Good*, 325 F. Supp. 1268 (1971), 1270.

153. *Maier v. Besser*, 73 Misc. 2d. 241 (1972).

154. *Dalli v. Board of Education*, 358 Mass. 753 (1971).

155. *Avard v. Dupuis*, 376 F. Supp. 479 (1974).

156. Ibid., 483.

157. *Kleid v. Board of Education*, 406 F. Supp. 902 (1976).

158. "Follow-Up on Poliomyelitis," *Morbidity and Mortality Weekly Report* 21 (1972): 365–366.

159. Stanley W. Ferguson, "Mandatory Immunization," *New England Journal of Medicine* 288 (1973): 800.

160. *Prince v. Massachusetts*, 321 U.S. 158 (1944), 170.

161. Ibid., 166–167.

162. On this point, see James G. Hodge and Lawrence O. Gostin, "School Vaccination Requirements: Historical, Social, and Legal Perspectives," *Kentucky Law Journal* 90 (2001–2002): 831–890; 860.

6. CONSENT, COMPULSION, AND COMPENSATION

1. David T. Karzon, "Immunization on Public Trial," *New England Journal of Medicine* 297 (1977): 275–276; 275.

2. Elena O. Nightingale, "Recommendation for a National Policy on Poliomyelitis Vaccination," *New England Journal of Medicine* 297 (1977): 249–253.

3. *Gottsdanker v. Cutter*, 182 Cal. App. 2d 602 (1960).

4. Paul A. Offit, *The Cutter Incident: How America's First Polio Vaccine Led to the Growing Vaccine Crisis* (New Haven: Yale University Press, 2005).

5. See, e.g., Albert B. Sabin, "Vaccine-Associated Poliomyelitis Cases," *Bulletin of the World Health Organization* 40 (1969): 947–949.

6. *Davis v. Wyeth*, 399 F.2d 121 (1968).

7. *Reyes v. Wyeth*, 498 F.2d. 1264 (1974).

8. William J. Curran, "Public Warnings of the Risk in Oral Polio Vaccine," *American Journal of Public Health* 65 (1975): 501–502.

9. *Reyes v. Wyeth*, 1294.

10. "Discussion on the Implications of Litigation Regarding Vaccine-Associated Injury" (typescript, February 25, 1975), ASTHO archives, box 23, folder: Immunization Programs 1975–76.

11. "Report and Recommendations, National Immunization Work Group on Liability," in *Reports and Recommendations of the National Immunization Work Groups, March 15, 1977* (McLean, Va.: JRB Associates, 1977), 20.

12. William J. Curran, "Drug-Company Liability in Immunization Programs," *New England Journal of Medicine* 281 (1969): 1057–1058; 1057, emphasis in original.

13. Louis Galambos with Jane Eliot Sewell, *Networks of Innovation: Vaccine Development at Merck, Sharp & Dohme, and Mulford, 1895–1995* (Cambridge: Cambridge University Press, 1995), 213–214.

14. *Reports and Recommendations of the National Immunization Work Groups*, 2.

15. Nightingale, "Recommendation for a National Policy on Poliomyelitis Vaccination." See also the committee's full report: Institute of Medicine, *Evaluation of Poliomyelitis Vaccines: Report of the Committee for the Study of Poliomyelitis Vaccines* (Washington, D.C.: National Academy of Sciences, 1977).

16. §402 A of the Restatement (Second) of Torts, 1965, increased the ability of consumers who were injured by defective products to recover damages from manufacturers. The Restatement considered vaccines to belong to a class of products that were "unavoidably unsafe"; therefore their manufacturers were not to be held to the same standards of strict liability that applied to other products, provided that proper warnings were given to recipients. The courts in both the *Davis* and *Wyeth* cases held that the warnings that had been given did not fulfill the duty imposed under §402 A. Bonnie L. Siber, "Apportioning Liability in Mass Inoculations: A Comparison of Two Views and a Look at the Future," *Review of Law and Social Change* 6 (1977): 239–262; Andrea Peterson Woolley, "Informed Consent to Immunization: The Risks and Benefits of Individual Autonomy," *California Law Review* 65 (1977): 1286–1314; Thomas E. Baynes Jr., "Liability for Vaccine-Related Injuries: Public Health Considerations and Some Reflections on the Swine Flu Experience," *Legal Medicine Annual* (1978): 195–224; Fay F. Spence, "Alternatives to Manufacturer Liability for Injuries Caused by the Sabin-Type Oral Polio Vaccines," *William and Mary Law Review* 28 (1987): 711–742.

17. David J. Rothman, *Strangers at the Bedside* (New York: Basic Books, 1991), 101–147.

18. See, e.g., Allan Mazur, "Public Confidence in Science," *Social Studies of Science* 7 (1977): 123–125, which concluded that the percentage of the public expressing great confidence in medicine declined from almost three-quarters to about one-half between 1966 and 1975. Confidence in other institutions such as the military, the education system, and religion underwent similar declines. On this phenomenon, see Paul Starr, *The Social Transformation of American Medicine* (New York: Basic Books, 1982), 379–393.

19. Sarah H. Newman, "Consumer Perspective: Position Paper," *Pediatric Research* 13 (1979): 705–706; 706.

20. Ruth R. Faden and Tom Beauchamp, *A History and Theory of Informed Consent* (New York: Oxford University Press, 1986).

21. On informed consent for children, see American Academy of Pediatrics Committee on Bioethics, "Informed Consent, Parental Permission, and Assent in Pediatric Practice," *Pediatrics* 95 (1995): 314–317.

22. LeRoy B. Walters, "Response," *Pediatric Research* 13 (1979): 700.

23. Alan R. Hinman, "Information Forms," in U.S. Department of Health, Education and Welfare, *13th Immunization Conference Proceedings* (Atlanta: Center for Disease Control, 1978), 17.

24. Advisory Committee on Immunization Practices, minutes, Meeting No. 4, June 11, 1965, NARA, RG 90, box 334062, folder: Advisory Committee on Immunization Practices.

25. Richard D. Krugman, "Immunization 'Dyspractice': The Need for 'No Fault' Insurance," *Pediatrics* 56 (1975): 159–160; 160.

26. Nightingale, "Recommendation for a National Policy on Poliomyelitis Vaccination."

27. Geoffrey Evans, "Vaccine Injury Compensation Programs Worldwide," *Vaccine* 17 (1999): S25–S35.

28. Richard E. Neustadt and Harvey V. Fineberg, *The Epidemic That Never Was: Policy-Making and the Swine Flu Affair* (New York: Vintage Books, 1982).

29. Diana B. Dutton, "Medical Risks, Disclosure, and Liability: Slouching Toward Informed Consent," *Science, Technology & Human Values* 12 (1987): 48–59.

30. Pascal James Imperato, "The United States Swine Flu Influenza Immunization Program: A New York City Perspective," *Bulletin of the New York Academy of Medicine* 55 (1979): 285–302.

31. Neustadt and Fineberg, *Epidemic That Never Was;* Cyril Wecht, "The Swine Flu Immunization Program: Scientific Venture or Political Folly?" *American Journal of Law & Medicine* 3 (1978): 425–445.

32. Elizabeth W. Etheridge, *Sentinel for Health: A History of the Centers for Disease Control* (Berkeley: University of California Press, 1992), 274–275.

33. New York State Department of Health, "Annual Report, Immunization Program, April 1976–March 1977," NYSDOH, series 13307–82, box 8, folder: Immunizations (1977–78).

34. Harold M. Schmeck, "Califano to Outline a Major Drive to Immunize More U.S. Children," *New York Times*, April 6, 1977, 1.

35. Opinion Research Corporation, *Public Attitudes toward Immunization: August 1977 and February 1978* (Princeton, N.J.: Opinion Research Corporation, 1978), v.

36. Neustadt and Fineberg, *Epidemic That Never Was*, 105–108.

37. "Report and Recommendations, National Immunization Work Group on Consent," in *Reports and Recommendations*, 17.

38. Ibid., 5–6.

39. Ibid., 4.

40. The dissenting group comprised Robert Veatch, Ruth Faden, Barbara Katz, and Lois Schiffer. Ibid., C-2.

41. Ibid., C-8.

42. The dissent was by Joanne E. Finley, health commissioner of New Jersey. Ibid., C-3.

43. Institute of Medicine, *Evaluation of Poliomyelitis Vaccines.*

44. Hinman, "Information Forms," in U.S. Department of Health, Education and Welfare, *13th Immunization Conference Proceedings*, 17.

45. Donald O. Lyman to Alan R. Hinman, February 3, 1978, NYSDOH, series 13855, roll 4.

46. Nicholas J. Fiumara to Joseph A. Califano, November 8, 1977, ASTHO Archives, box 23, folder: Immunization Programs 1977–78.

47. Hans H. Neumann, "For a Federal Immunization Insurance Corporation," *Connecticut Medicine* 41 (1977): 118–119; 119. Punctuation in original.

48. Patrick M. Vivier, "National Policies for Childhood Immunization in the United States: A Historical Perspective" (Ph.D. diss., Johns Hopkins University, 1996), 166–169.

49. Ibid., 169–170.

50. Alan R. Hinman, "Opening Statement," in U.S. Department of Health, Education and Welfare, *13th Immunization Conference Proceedings* (Atlanta: Center for Disease Control, 1978).

51. George S. Lovejoy, James W. Giandelia, and Mildred Hicks, "Successful Enforcement of an Immunization Law," *Public Health Reports* 89 (1974): 456–458.

52. James E. Donoho, "Missouri Vaccine Delivery Program—'The Force that Achieved Our Means,'" in U.S. Department of Health, Education and Welfare, *13th Immunization Conference Proceedings* (Atlanta: Center for Disease Control, 1978).

53. Donald O. Lyman to Richard J. Jackson, undated memo (Fall 1976), NYSDOH, series 13855, reel 10.

54. Donald O. Lyman to Saul Smoller, December 30, 1976, NYSDOH, series 13855, reel 10.

55. Donald Lyman to Robert Whalen, March 13, 1978, NYSDOH, series 13307–82, box 8, folder: Immunizations (1977–78).

56. Donald Lyman to Robert Whalen, March 13, 1978, NYSDOH, series 13307–82, box 8, folder: Immunizations (1977–78); Michael Alexander, "Measles Order Bars 90 Pupils in Oceanside," *Newsday*, March 11, 1978.

57. In the Matter of Robert D. Whalen, May 5, 1978, NYSDOH, series 13307–82, box 8, folder: Immunizations (1977–78).

58. Alan Hinman, "Immunization, Equity, and Human Rights," in U.S. Department of Health and Human Services, *36th National Immunization Conference Proceedings* (Atlanta: Centers for Disease Control, 2002).

59. Olive E. Pitkin to Margaret Grossi, April 7, 1978; and Lloyd Novick to Reinaldo Ferrer, April 10, 1978, NYCDOH, box 142299, folder: School Health.

60. Barry Ensminger, "Political Commitment to Immunization Programs at the Local Level," in U.S. Department of Health, Education and Welfare, *15th Immunization Conference Proceedings* (Atlanta: Centers for Disease Control, 1980); Joseph B. Treaster, "School Inoculation Data Missing; Director of City Program Ousted," *New York Times*, November 19, 1978, 47.

61. Bernard Bihari to Edward I. Koch, December 27, 1979, NYCDOH, box 142361, folder: School Health.

62. Reinaldo Ferrer to Robert F. Wagner Jr., January 29, 1981, NYCDOH, box 142304, folder: Ferrer's Personal File.

63. Frank Macchiarola to Reinaldo Ferrer, December 21, 1979, NYCDOH, box 142361, folder: School Health.

64. Wilfredo Lopez to Irwin Davison, March 5, 1980, NYCDOH, box 142361, folder: School Health.

65. Josh Barbanel, "Students Given a Month's Reprieve on Inoculations," *New York Times,* September 28, 1980, 32.

66. Dr. Grossi to Dr. Ferrer, October 31, 1980; and Reinaldo Ferrer to Jack Kirby, November 21, 1980, NYCDOH, box 142304, folder: Ferrer's personal file.

67. Mona Solomon to Reinaldo Ferrer, September 25, 1980, NYCDOH, box 142304, folder: Ferrer's personal file; Ari L. Goldman, "Pupils Lacking Inoculations Face High School Ban Today," *New York Times,* November 3, 1980, B1.

68. William G. Blair, "11 School Principals Accused of Violating Immunization Statute," *New York Times,* June 2, 1981, B2.

69. Sydney H. Schanberg, "Why Punish the Kids?" *New York Times,* October 17, 1981, 23.

70. Pascal James Imperato, "The High Cost of Attempting to Rid America of Measles," *New York Times,* October 28, 1981, 26.

71. Louis Z. Cooper, Anne E. Gershon, and James G. Lione, "The Worth of New York City's Child Immunization Program," *New York Times,* December 15, 1981, 30.

72. Dennis G. Olsen to Burton Lincoln, April 25, 1978, NYCDOH, box 142299, folder: School Health; Nicholas Anthony, Mary Reed, Arnold M. Leff, et al., "Immunization: Public Health Programming through Law Enforcement," *American Journal of Public Health* 67 (1977): 763–764; "Detroit Turns Away Unvaccinated Pupils," *New York Times,* October 25, 1977, 18.

73. *Brown v. Stone,* 378 So. 2d 218 (1979).

74. *Davis v. Maryland,* 294 Md. 370 (1982).

75. *Hanzel v. Arter,* 625 F. Supp. 1259 (1985).

76. *Sherr v. Northport-East Northport Union Free School District,* 672 F. Supp. 81 (1987); 89.

77. Ross D. Silverman, "No More Kidding Around: Restructuring Childhood Immunization Exemptions to Ensure Public Health Protection," *Annals of Health Law* 12 (2003): 277–294.

78. *Sherr v. Northport-East Northport Union Free School District,* 95–96.

79. Ibid., 97.

80. Kenneth B. Robbins, A. David Brandling-Bennett, and Alan R. Hinman, "Low Measles Incidence: Association with Enforcement of School Immunization Laws," *American Journal of Public Health* 71 (1981): 270–274.

81. Joanne E. Finley, commissioner of health for New Jersey, to Lyman J. Olsen, president of the Association of State and Territorial Health Officials, February 24, 1978, ASTHO Archives, box 23, folder: Immunization Programs 1977–78.

82. Martin H. Smith, "American Academy of Pediatrics' Proposal for a Vaccine Compensation System," in U.S. Department of Health and Human Services, *18th Immunization Conference Proceedings* (Atlanta: Centers for Disease Control, 1983), 69–70.

83. Office of Technology Assessment, *Compensation for Vaccine-Related Injuries: A Technical Memorandum* (Washington, D.C.: OTA, 1980).

84. Ibid.

85. Neustadt and Fineberg, *Epidemic That Never Was.*

86. Office of Technology Assessment, *Compensation for Vaccine-Related Injuries.*

87. Matthew Brody and Ralph G. Sorley, "Neurologic Complications following the Administration of Pertussis Vaccine," *New York State Journal of Medicine* 47 (1947): 1016–1017.

88. Curran, "Drug-Company Liability in Immunization Programs"; Baynes, "Liability for Vaccine-Related Injuries."

89. M. Kulenkampff, J. S. Schwartzman, and J. Wilson, "Neurologic Complications of Pertussis Inoculation," *Archives of Disease in Childhood* 49 (1974): 46–49.

90. James D. Cherry, "The Epidemiology of Pertussis and Pertussis Immunization in the United Kingdom and the United States: A Comparative Study," *Current Problems in Pediatrics* 14 (1978): 1–78.

91. Gordon T. Stewart, "Vaccination against Whooping Cough: Efficacy versus Risks," *Lancet* no. 8005 (1977): 243–237.

92. E. J. Gangarosa, A. M. Galazka, C. R. Wolfe, et al., "Impact of Anti-Vaccine Movements on Pertussis Control: The Untold Story," *Lancet* 351 (1998): 356–361.

93. D. L. Miller, R. Alderslade, and E. M. Ross, "Whooping Cough and Whooping Cough Vaccine: The Risks and Benefits Debate," *Epidemiologic Reviews* 4 (1982): 1–24.

94. Jeffrey P. Koplan, Stephen C. Schoenbaum, Milton C. Weinstein, et al., "Pertussis Vaccine—An Analysis of Risks, Benefits, and Costs," *New England Journal of Medicine* 301 (1979): 906–911.

95. Harrison C. Stetler, "Adverse Events—Current Trends in Surveillance," in U.S. Department of Health and Human Services, *18th Immunization Conference Proceedings* (Atlanta: Centers for Disease Control, 1983).

96. John R. Mullen and Harrison C. Stetler, "Implementation of Revisions in the Monitoring System for Adverse Events following Immunization," in U.S. Department of Health and Human Services, *19th Immunization Conference Proceedings* (Atlanta: Centers for Disease Control, 1984).

97. Richard H. Bruce, "Update on Vaccine Litigation: The Vaccine Litigation Monitoring System (VLMS)," in *18th Immunization Conference Proceedings* (Atlanta: Centers for Disease Control, 1983).

98. Elizabeth Rasche González, "TV Report on DTP Galvanizes U.S. Pediatricians," *Journal of the American Medical Association* 248 (1982): 12–22.

99. Ibid.

100. *Immunization and Preventive Medicine, 1982, Hearing before the Subcommittee on Investigations and General Oversight of the Committee on Labor and Human Resources, United States Senate, Ninety-seventh Congress, Second Session* (Washington, D.C.: Government Printing Office, 1982), 79.

101. A good summary of the formation of DPT and its early political battles over a federal compensation program is Robert D. Johnston, "Contemporary Anti-Vaccination Movements in Historical Perspective," in id., ed., *The Politics of Healing: Histories of Alternative Medicine in Twentieth-Century North America* (New York: Routledge, 2004).

102. *Immunization and Preventive Medicine, 1982*, 3.

103. Alan R. Hinman, "The National Vaccine Program and the National Childhood Vaccine Injury Compensation Act," in U.S. Department of Health and Human Services, *23rd Immunization Conference Proceedings* (Atlanta: Centers for Disease Control, 1989).

104. Gary L. Freed, Samuel L. Katz, and Sarah J. Clark, "Safety of Vaccinations: Miss America, the Media, and Public Health," *Journal of the American Medical Association* 276 (1996): 1869–1872.

105. *Childhood Immunizations: A Report Prepared by the Subcommittee on Health and the Environment of the Committee on Energy and Commerce, U.S. House of Representatives* (Washington, D.C.: Government Printing Office, 1986), 61.

106. *Vaccine Injury Compensation, Hearing before the Subcommittee on Health and the Environment of the Committee on Energy and Commerce, House of Representatives, Ninety-ninth Congress, Second Session, July 25, 1986* (Washington, D.C.: Government Printing Office, 1987), 189.

107. *Childhood Immunizations: A Report*, 68–70.

108. "The Cost of Ignoring Vaccine Victims," *New York Times*, A18.

109. Harris L. Coulter and Barbara Loe Fisher, *DPT: A Shot in the Dark* (New York: Harcourt Brace Jovanovich, 1985).

110. For skeptical reviews of the book, see, e.g., Harry Schwartz, "Shots or Not?" *New York Times*, February 3, 1985, BR 19; and Ezekiel J. Emanuel, "Politicizing Whooping Cough," *Wall Street Journal*, March 7, 1985, 30.

111. *Vaccine Injury Compensation, Hearing before the Subcommittee on Health and the Environment of the Committee on Energy and Commerce, House of Representatives, Ninety-eighth Congress, Second Session, September 10 and December 19, 1984* (Washington, D.C.: Government Printing Office, 1985), 92.

112. Marsha F. Goldsmith, "AMA Offers Recommendations for Vaccine Injury Compensation," *Journal of the American Medical Association* 252 (1984): 2937–2943.

113. Leah R. Young, "Reagan Inks Vaccine Bill," *Journal of Commerce*, November 17, 1986, 12A.

114. Robert Pear, "U.S. Plan to Curb Damage Claims Aims to Avert Vaccine Shortages," *New York Times*, April 7, 1985, 1.

115. *Vaccine Injury Compensation, September 10 and December 19, 1984*, 261.

116. *Vaccine Injury Compensation, July 25*, 189–190.

117. Ibid., 2.

118. Spencer Rich, "Vaccine Injury Measure Signed by President," *Washington Post*, November 15, 1986, A8; Robert Pear, "Reagan Signs Bill on Drug Exports and Payment for Vaccine Injuries," *New York Times*, November 15, 1986, 1.

119. Geoffrey Evans, Deborah Harris, and Emily Marcus Levine, "Legal Issues," in Stanley A. Plotkin and Walter A. Orenstein, eds., *Vaccines*, 4th ed. (Philadelphia: Elsevier, 2004).

120. Wendy K. Mariner, "Legislative Report: The National Vaccine Injury Compensation Program," *Health Affairs* 11 (1992): 255–265; Evans, Harris and Levine, "Legal Issues."

121. Evans, Harris and Levine, "Legal Issues."

122. Institute of Medicine, *Adverse Effects of Pertussis and Rubella Vaccines* (Washington, D.C.: National Academies Press, 1991).

123. Institute of Medicine, *Adverse Events Associated with Childhood Vaccines: Evidence Bearing on Causality* (Washington, D.C.: National Academies Press, 1994), 16–17.

7. EXPANSION AND BACKLASH

1. *Vaccines—Finding the Balance between Public Safety and Personal Choice, Hearing before the Committee on Government Reform, House of Representatives, One Hundred Sixth Congress, First Session, August 3, 1999* (Washington, D.C.: Government Printing Office, 2000), 4.

2. Chris Feudtner and Edgar K. Marcuse, "Ethics and Immunization Policy: Promoting Dialogue to Sustain Consensus," *Pediatrics* 107 (2001): 1158–1164.

3. Elizabeth Zell, Vance Dietz, John Stevenson, et al., "Low Vaccination Levels of US Preschool and School-Children," *Journal of the American Medical Association* 271 (1994): 833–839.

4. Kay A. Johnson, Alice Sardell, and Barbara Richards, "Federal Immunization Policy and Funding: A History of Responding to Crisis," *American Journal of Preventive Medicine* 19 (2000): 99–112; Robert Pear, "Proposal Would Tie Welfare to Vaccinations of Children," *New York Times*, November 29, 1990, A1.

5. Deirdre Carmody, "State Agency Acts to Put Welfare Mothers to Work," *New York Times*, September 23, 1971, 57.

6. "Points Lost," *New York Times*, November 7, 1971, E5; Eveline M. Burns, "Incentive Plan for Welfare Clients," ibid., October 29, 1971, 40.

7. Larry C. Kerpelman, David B. Connell, and Walter J. Gunn, "Effect of a Monetary Sanction on Immunization Rates of Aid to Families with Dependent Children," *Journal of the American Medical Association* 284 (2000): 53–59; 59.

8. National Vaccine Advisory Committee, "The Measles Epidemic: The Problems, Barriers, and Recommendations," *Journal of the American Medical Association* 266 (1991): 1547–1552.

9. Felicity T. Cutts, Walter A. Orenstein, and Roger H. Bernier, "Causes of Low Preschool Immunization Coverage in the United States," *Annual Review of Public Health* 13 (1992): 385–398; 395.

10. Gary L. Freed, W. Clayton Bordley, Gordon H. DeFriese, "Childhood Immunization Programs: An Analysis of Policy Issues," *Milbank Memorial Fund Quarterly* 71 (1993): 65–96.

11. Edgar K. Marcuse, "Obstacles to Immunization in the Private Sector," in U.S. Department of Health and Human Services, *25th National Immunization Conference Proceedings* (Atlanta: Centers for Disease Control, 1991).

12. Daniel Yankelovich, "The Debate That Wasn't: The Public and the Clinton Plan," *Health Affairs* 14 (1995): 7–22.

13. Theda Skocpol, *Boomerang: Clinton's Health Security Effort and the Turn against Government in U.S. Politics* (New York: Norton, 1996).

14. Walter A. Orenstein, "Building the Immunization Superhighway: Childhood Immunization Initiative as the Framework," in U.S. Department of Health

and Human Services, *28th National Immunization Conference Proceedings* (Atlanta: Centers for Disease Control, 1994).

15. *Comprehensive Child Immunization Act of 1993, Joint Hearing before the Committee on Labor and Human Resources, United States Senate and the Subcommittee on Health and the Environment of the Committee on Energy and Commerce, House of Representatives, One Hundred Third Congress, First Session, April 21, 1993* (Washington, D.C.: Government Printing Office, 1993), 4.

16. Ibid., 46.

17. National Vaccine Information Center web site, www.909shot.com/ Issues/ICA.htm (accessed September 13, 2003).

18. The group that opposed the Clinton purchase plan was DPT SHOT (Determined Parents to Stop Hurting Our Tots). *Comprehensive Child Immunization Act of 1993*, 192.

19. Ibid., 30.

20. "Reported Vaccine-Preventable Diseases—United States, 1993, and the Childhood Immunization Initiative," *Morbidity and Mortality Weekly Report* 43 (1994): 57–60.

21. Walter A. Orenstein, Lance Rodewald, and Alan R. Hinman, "Immunization in the United States," in Stanley A. Plotkin and Walter A. Orenstein, eds., *Vaccines*, 4th ed. (Philadelphia: Elsevier, 2004).

22. Gary L. Freed and Samuel L. Katz, "The Comprehensive Childhood Immunization Act of 1993: Toward a More Rational Approach," *New England Journal of Medicine* 329 (1993): 1957–1960; 1959.

23. Orenstein, "Building the Immunization Superhighway."

24. James L. Goddard, "Future Goals of Immunization Programs," in U.S. Department of Health, Education and Welfare, *2nd Immunization Conference Proceedings* (Atlanta: Communicable Disease Center, 1965).

25. Gordon H. DeFriese, Kathleen M. Faherty, Victoria A. Freeman, et al., "Developing Child Immunization Registries," in Stephen L. Isaacs and James R. Knickman, eds., *To Improve Health and Health Care, 1997* (Princeton, N.J.: Robert Wood Johnson Foundation, 1997).

26. Kay Johnson, "Proposal for a National Vaccination Registry," in U.S. Department of Health and Human Services, *25th National Immunization Conference Proceedings* (Atlanta: Centers for Disease Control, 1991).

27. William C. Watson, Kristin Nicholson Sarlaas, Ruby Hearn, et al., "The All Kids Count National Program: A Robert Wood Johnson Foundation Initiative to Develop Immunization Registries," *American Journal of Preventive Medicine* 13 (1997): 3–6.

28. See, e.g., the testimony of Ed Thompson, interim health officer of Mississippi, and Michael Moen, director of disease prevention for the Minnesota Health Department, in congressional hearings on the bill. *Comprehensive Child Immunization Act of 1993*, 80, 86 and passim.

29. Victoria A. Freeman and Gordon H. DeFriese, "The Challenge and Potential of Childhood Immunization Registries," *Annual Review of Public Health* 24 (2003): 227–246.

30. Lawrence O. Gostin and Zita Lazzarini, "Childhood Immunization Registries: A National Review of Public Health Information Systems and the Protection of Privacy," *Journal of the American Medical Association* 274 (1995): 1793–1799.

31. Philip R. Horne, Kristin N. Sarlaas, and Alan R. Hinman, "Costs of Immunization Registries: Experiences from the All Kids Count II Projects," *American Journal of Preventive Medicine* 19 (2000): 94–98.

32. David Wood, Kristin N. Sarlaas, Moira Inkelas, et al., "Immunization Registries in the United States: Implications for the Practice of Public Health in a Changing Health Care System," *Annual Review of Public Health* 20 (1999): 231–255.

33. Lawrence O. Gostin, James G. Hodge, and Ronald O. Valdiserri, "Informational Privacy and the Public's Health: The Model State Public Health Privacy Act," *American Journal of Public Health* 91 (2001): 1388–1392.

34. Wood, Sarlaas, Inkelas, et al., "Immunization Registries in the United States."

35. Centers for Disease Control and Prevention, "Findings of Focus Group Research on Immunization Registries," National Immunization Program web site, www.cdc.gov/nip/registry/fg/fg01.pdf (accessed January 12, 2004).

36. Wood, Sarlaas, Inkelas, et al., "Immunization Registries in the United States."

37. Barbara Loe Fisher, "Statement, Immunization Registries Workgroup on Privacy and Confidentiality," National Vaccine Information Center web site, www.909shot.com/Loe_Fisher/blf51498tracking.html (accessed September 17, 2003).

38. Caroline Breese Hall, Harold Margolis, "Hepatitis B Immunization: Premonitions and Perceptions of Pediatricians," *Pediatrics* 91 (1993): 841–843.

39. K. A. Woodin, L. E. Rodewald, S. G. Humiston, et al., "Physicians and Parent Opinions: Are Children Becoming Pincushions from Immunizations?" *Archives of Pediatric and Adolescent Medicine* 149 (1995): 845–849.

40. Jon S. Abramson, "The Immunization Schedule: Friend or Foe," in U.S. Department of Health and Human Services, *34th National Immunization Conference Proceedings* (Atlanta: Centers for Disease Control, 2000).

41. Neal A. Halsey, "Safety of Combination Vaccines: Perception versus Reality," *Pediatric Infectious Disease Journal* 20 (2001): S40–S44.

42. Paul A. Offit, Jessica Quarles, Michael A. Gerber, et al., "Addressing Parents' Concerns: Do Multiple Vaccines Overwhelm or Weaken the Infant's Immune System?" *Pediatrics* 109 (2002): 124–128.

43. Robert T. Chen, Robert L. Davis, and Kristine M. Sheedy, "Safety of Immunizations," in Plotkin and Orenstein, eds., *Vaccines,* 4th ed.

44. This phenomenon has inspired a voluminous literature. For a good summary, see Cass Sunstein, *Risk and Reason: Safety, Law and the Environment* (Cambridge: Cambridge University Press, 2002). See also Michael Fitzpatrick, "MMR: Risk, Choice, Chance," *British Medical Bulletin* 69 (2004): 143–153; and J. A. Muir Gray, "Postmodern Medicine," *Lancet* 354 (1999): 1550–1553.

45. Leslie Ball, John Glasser, Sharon Humiston, et al., "How Do You Know, and How Do You Let Your Patients Know, that Vaccines are Safe?" in U.S. Department of Health and Human Services, *30th National Immunization Conference Proceedings* (Atlanta: Centers for Disease Control, 1996); Ann Bostrom, "Vaccine Risk Communication: Lessons from Risk Perception, Decision Making and Environmental Risk Communication Research," *Risk: Health, Safety, and the Environment* 8 (1997): 183–200; Leslie K. Ball, Geoffrey Evans, and Ann Bostrom, "Risky Business: Challenges in Vaccine Risk Communication," *Pediatrics* 101 (1998): 453–458; C.J. Clements, G. Evans, S. Dittman, and A.V. Reeler, "Vaccine Safety Concerns Everyone," *Vaccine* 17 (1999): S90–S94.

46. Institute of Medicine, *Risk Communication and Vaccination: Workshop Summary* (Washington, D.C.: National Academies Press, 1997).

47. A.J. Wakefield, S.H. Murch, A. Anthony, et al., "Ileal-Lymphoid-Nodular Hyperplasia, Non-Specific Colitis, and Pervasive Developmental Disorder in Children," *Lancet* 351 (1998): 637–641.

48. Jeremy Laurance, "Doctors Warn of a New Child Vaccine Danger," *Independent* (London), February 27, 1998, 5.

49. Sarah Boseley, "Fear of Needles," *Guardian* (London), June 3, 1999, 4.

50. Robert T. Chen and Frank DeStefano, "Vaccine Adverse Events: Causal or Coincidental?" *Lancet* 351 (1998): 611–612.

51. James Colgrove and Ronald Bayer, "Could It Happen Here? Vaccine Risk Controversies and the Specter of Derailment," *Health Affairs* 24 (2005): 729–739.

52. Thomas H. Maugh, "State Study Finds Sharp Rise in Autism Rate," *Los Angeles Times,* April 16, 1999, 1.

53. See, e.g., Eric Fombonne, "Is There an Epidemic of Autism?" *Pediatrics* 107 (2001): 411–413; and Marie McCormick, "The Autism 'Epidemic': Impressions from the Perspective of Immunization Safety," *Ambulatory Pediatrics* 3 (2003): 119–120.

54. Steven Lee Myers, "U.S. Armed Forces to Be Vaccinated against Anthrax," *New York Times,* December 16, 1997, 1.

55. Ruth K. Miller, "Informed Consent in the Military: Fighting a Losing Battle against the Anthrax Vaccine," *American Journal of Law and Medicine* 28 (2002): 325–343.

56. Otto Kreisher, "Despite Furor, Anthrax Shots Continue; House Panel's Sharp Criticism Fails to Sway the Pentagon," *San Diego Union-Tribune,* February 18, 2000, A1.

57. Philippe Monteyne, Francis E. Andre, "Is There a Causal Link Between Hepatitis B Vaccination and Multiple Sclerosis?" *Vaccine* 18 (2000): 1994–2001.

58. Cited in Charles Marwick and Mike Mitka, "Debate Revived on Hepatitis B Vaccine Value," *Journal of the American Medical Association* 281 (1999): 15–17; 16.

59. *Hepatitis B Vaccine: Helping or Hurting Public Health, Hearing before the Subcommittee on Criminal Justice, Drug Policy and Human Resources of the Committee on Government Reform, House of Representatives, One Hundred Sixth Congress, First Session, May 18, 1999* (Washington, D.C.: Government Printing Office, 2000), 87.

60. The EPA maximum was the most conservative of threshold levels that were set by three different U.S. government agencies, which differed because of variations in the types of data each agency used to formulate them, their methods of calculation, and the safety factors they adopted. While the amount of mercury in childhood vaccines exceeded the EPA threshold, the most conservative of the three, it was under the limit set by the Food and Drug Administration and Agency for Toxic Substances and Disease Registry. Leslie K. Ball, Robert Ball, and R. Douglas Pratt, "Assessment of Thimerosal Use in Childhood Vaccines," *Pediatrics* 107 (2001): 1147–1154.

61. Gary L. Freed, Margie C. Andreae, Anne E. Cowan, et al., "The Process of Public Policy Formulation: The Case of Thimerosal in Vaccines," *Pediatrics* 109 (2002): 1153–1159; 1159.

62. "Thimerosal in Vaccines: A Joint Statement of the American Academy of Pediatrics and the Public Health Service," *Morbidity and Mortality Weekly Report* 48, no. 26 (1999): 563–565.

63. Paul A. Offitt, "Preventing Harm from Thimerosal in Vaccines," *Journal of the American Medical Association* 283 (2000): 2104; Stanley A. Plotkin, "Preventing Harm from Thimerosal in Vaccines," *Journal of the American Medical Association* 283 (2000): 2104–2105; and John B. Seal and Robert S. Daum, "What Happened to *Primum Non Nocere?*" *Pediatrics* 107 (2001): 1177–1178.

64. "Impact of the 1999 AAP/USPHS Joint Statement on Thimerosal in Vaccines on Infant Hepatitis B Vaccination Practices," *Morbidity and Mortality Weekly Report* 50 (2001): 94–97.

65. American Academy of Pediatrics, "Thimerosal in Vaccines—An Interim Report to Clinicians," *Pediatrics* 104 (1999): 570–574.

66. H. Fred Clark, Paul A. Offit, Roger I. Glass, et al., "Rotavirus Vaccines," in Plotkin and Orenstein, eds., *Vaccines*, 4th ed.

67. M. Carolina Danovaro-Holliday, Allison L. Wood, and Charles W. LeBaron, "Rotavirus Vaccine and the News Media, 1987–2001," *Journal of the American Medical Association* 287 (2002): 1455–1462.

68. Margaret B. Rennels, "The Rotavirus Vaccine Story: A Clinical Investigator's View," *Pediatrics* 106 (2000): 123–125.

69. Heather McPhillips and Edgar K. Marcuse, "Vaccine Safety," *Current Problems in Pediatrics* 31 (2001): 95–121.

70. Jon S. Abramson and Larry K. Pickering, "US Immunization Policy," *Journal of the American Medical Association* 287 (2002): 505–509.

71. Institute of Medicine, *Immunization Safety Review: Measles-Mumps-Rubella Vaccine and Autism* (Washington, D.C.: National Academies Press, 2001); id., *Immunization Safety Review: Thimerosal-Containing Vaccines and Neurodevelopmental Disorders* (Washington, D.C.: National Academies Press, 2001); id., *Immunization Safety Review: Multiple Immunizations and Immune Dysfunction* (Washington, D.C.: National Academies Press, 2002); id., *Immunization Safety Review: Hepatitis B Vaccine and Demyelinating Neurological Complications* (Washington, D.C.: National Academies Press, 2002); id., *Immunization Safety Review: Vaccinations and Sudden Unexpected Death in Infancy* (Washington, D.C.: National Academies Press, 2003); id., *Immunization*

Safety Review: SV40 Contamination of Polio Vaccine and Cancer (Washington, D.C.: National Academies Press, 2003).

72. Institute of Medicine, *Measles-Mumps-Rubella Vaccine and Autism*, 6.

73. *Autism—Why the Increased Rates? A One-Year Update. Hearings before the Committee on Government Reform, House of Representatives, One Hundred Seventh Congress, First Session, April 25 and 26, 2001* (Washington, D.C.: Government Printing Office, 2001), 214–215.

74. Institute of Medicine, *Immunization Safety Review: Multiple Immunizations and Immune Dysfunction*.

75. Phil Brown, "Popular Epidemiology: Community Response to Toxic Waste-Induced Disease in Woburn, Massachusetts," *Science, Technology, and Human Values* 12 (1987): 78–85.

76. Steven G. Epstein, *Impure Science: AIDS, Activism, and the Politics of Knowledge* (Berkeley: University of California Press, 1996).

77. For profiles of some of the scientists who questioned the orthodox view of vaccination, see National Vaccine Information Center, *Third International Public Conference on Vaccination 2002, Program*, National Vaccine Information Center web site, www.909shot.com (accessed January 13, 2004).

78. Barbara Loe Fisher, "Anti-Science Activists Label Pro-Vaccine Safety Advocates 'Anti-Vaccine' in June 26 JAMA Article," National Vaccine Information Center web site, www.909shot.com (accessed October 2, 2003). The sociologist Phil Brown, who has termed lay activism around disease "popular epidemiology," argues that "it is not antiscience. Rather, it has a different concept of what science is, whom it should serve, and who should control it." Brown, "Popular Epidemiology," 83.

79. National Vaccine Information Center, *Third International Public Conference on Vaccination 2002, Program*, National Vaccine Information Center web site, www.909shot.com (accessed January 13, 2004).

80. *The Status of Research Into Vaccine Safety and Autism, Hearing before the Committee on Government Reform, House of Representatives, One Hundred Seventh Congress, Second Session, June 19, 2002* (Washington, D.C.: Government Printing Office, 2002), 2.

81. See, e.g., Sandy Mintz, "Contemporary Legends—How to Lie With Statistics," Vaccination News web site, www.vaccinationnews.com/Scandals/Aug_9_02/Scandal28.htm (accessed February 1, 2004).

82. Robert M. Wolfe, Lisa K. Sharpe, and Martin S. Lipsky, "Content and Design Attributes of Antivaccination Web Sites," *Journal of the American Medical Association* 287 (2002): 3245–3248; P. Davies, S. Chapman, and J. Leask, "Antivaccination Activists on the World Wide Web," *Archives of Diseases of Childhood* 87 (2002): 22–25.

83. "Vaccines. An Issue of Trust," *Consumer Reports* 66 (2001): 17–24.

84. Jeffrey P. Baker, "The Pertussis Vaccine Controversy in Great Britain, 1974–1986," *Vaccine* 21 (2003): 4003–4010.

85. Katherine Seligman, "Vaccination Backlash," *San Francisco Chronicle*, May 25, 2003.

86. Arthur Allen, "Bucking the Herd," *Atlantic* 290 (September 2002).

87. F. Colley and M. Haas, "Attitudes on Immunization: A Survey of American Chiropractors," *Journal of Manipulative and Physiological Therapy* 17 (1994): 584–590. On the diversity of views among chiropractors, see also Joel Alcantara, "Vaccination Issues: A Chiropractor's Perspective," www.chiroweb.com/archives/17/03/13.html (accessed February 19, 2000).

88. E. Ernst, "Rise in Popularity of Complementary and Alternative Medicine: Reasons and Consequences for Vaccination," *Vaccine* 20 (2000): S90–S93.

89. James B. Campbell, Jason W. Busse, and H. Stephen Injeyan, "Chiropractors and Vaccination: A Historical Perspective," *Pediatrics* 105 (2000): e43.

90. Phyllis Schlafly, "Compulsory Medical Treatment is Un-American," *Copley News Service,* October 12, 1998.

91. "Doctors' Group Votes to Oppose Vaccine Mandates," news release, November 2, 2000, American Association of Physicians and Surgeons web site, www.aapsonline.org/press/nrvacres.html (accessed January 8, 2004).

92. National Vaccine Information Center web site, www.909shot.com (accessed September 13, 2003).

93. Vaccination Liberation web site, www.vaclib.org/index.htm (accessed January 14, 2004).

94. Jennifer S. Rota, Daniel A. Salmon, Lance E. Rodewald, et al., "Processes for Obtaining Nonmedical Exemptions to State Immunization Laws," *American Journal of Public Health* 91 (2001): 645–648.

95. Daniel A. Salmon, Jason W. Sapsin, Stephen Teret, et al., "Public Health and the Politics of School Immunization Requirements," *American Journal of Public Health* 95 (2005): 778–783.

96. James G. Hodge and Lawrence O. Gostin, "School Vaccination Requirements: Historical, Social, and Legal Perspectives," *Kentucky Law Journal* 90 (2001–2002): 831–890.

97. Rota, Salmon, Rodewald, et al., "Processes for Obtaining Nonmedical Exemptions."

98. Edgar K. Marcuse, "Life, Liberty, and the Pursuit of Public Health: Reflections on Mandates and Exemptions," in U.S. Department of Health and Human Services, *36th National Immunization Conference Proceedings* (Atlanta: Centers for Disease Control, 2002).

99. Daniel A. Salmon, Saad B. Omer, Lawrence H. Moulton, et al., "Exemptions to School Immunization Requirements: The Role of School-Level Requirements, Policies, and Procedures," *American Journal of Public Health* 95 (2005): 436–440.

100. Marcuse, "Life, Liberty, and the Pursuit of Public Health."

101. Natalie J. Smith, "Vaccine Safety: A View from the Front Lines," in U.S. Department of Health and Human Services, *33rd National Immunization Conference Proceedings* (Atlanta: Centers for Disease Control, 1999).

102. Bruce G. Gellin, Edward W. Maibach, and Edgar K. Marcuse, "Do Parents Understand Immunizations? A National Telephone Survey," *Pediatrics* 106 (2000): 1097–1102.

103. Pamela Fitch and Andrew Racine, "Parental Beliefs about Vaccination among an Ethnically Diverse Inner-City Population," *Journal of the National Medical Association* 96 (2004): 1047–1050.

104. Gary L. Freed et al., "Parental Vaccine Safety Concerns: The Experiences of Pediatricians and Family Physicians," *American Journal of Preventive Medicine* 26 (2004): 11–14.

105. Shannon Brownlee, "Clear and Present Danger," *Washington Post*, October 28, 2001, W8.

106. Tara O'Toole, Michael Mair, and Thomas V. Inglesby, "Shining Light on 'Dark Winter,'" *Clinical Infectious Diseases* 34 (2002): 972–983.

107. Ronald Bayer and James Colgrove, "Rights and Dangers: Bioterrorism and the Ideologies of Public Health," in Jonathan Moreno, ed., *In the Wake of Terror: Medicine and Morality in a Time of Crisis* (Boston: MIT Press, 2003).

108. Center for Law and the Public's Health, *The Model State Emergency Health Powers Act, October 23, 2001* (Washington, D.C.: Center for Law and the Public's Health, 2001).

109. George J. Annas, "Bioterrorism, Public Health, and Civil Liberties," *New England Journal of Medicine* 346 (2002): 1337–1342; 1340.

110. Lawrence O. Gostin, Jason W. Sapsin, Stephen P. Teret, et al., "The Model State Emergency Health Powers Act: Planning for and Response to Bioterrorism and Naturally Occurring Infectious Diseases," *Journal of the American Medical Association* 288 (2002): 622–628.

111. Center for Law and the Public's Health, *The Model State Emergency Health Powers Act, December 21, 2001* (Washington, D.C.: Center for Law and the Public's Health, 2001).

112. Judith Miller, Sheryl Gay Stolberg, "Sept. 11 Attacks Led to Push for More Smallpox Vaccine," *New York Times*, October 22, 2001, 1.

113. Justin Gillis and Ceci Connolly, "U.S. Details Response to Smallpox," *Washington Post*, November 27, 2001, A1.

114. Alex R. Kemper, Matthew M. Davis, and Gary L. Freed, "Expected Adverse Events in a Mass Smallpox Vaccination Campaign," *Effective Clinical Practice* 5 (2002): 84–90.

115. William J. Bicknell, "The Case for Voluntary Smallpox Vaccination," *New England Journal of Medicine* 346 (2002): 1323–1325; 1323.

116. Veronique de Rugy and Charles V. Peña, *Responding to the Threat of Smallpox Bioterrorism: An Ounce of Prevention is Best Approach*, Cato Policy Analysis No. 434, April 18, 2002, www.cato.org/pubs/pas/pa-434es.html (accessed January 8, 2004); Association of American Physicians and Surgeons, "AAPS: Feds' Smallpox Plans Fatally Flawed," news release, September 25, 2002, www.aapsonline.org/press/nrsmallpox.html (accessed January 8, 2004).

117. Association of American Physicians and Surgeons, "Clarification on the AAPS Position on Vaccines," September 27, 2002, www.aapsonline.org/testimony/explainvc.html (accessed January 8, 2004). Emphasis in original.

118. The figure could vary according to the density and mixing patterns of the population affected. Roy M. Anderson and Robert M. May, "Immunisation and Herd Immunity," *Lancet* 335 (1990): 641–645.

119. Martin Enserink, "How Devastating Would a Smallpox Attack Really Be?" *Science* 296 (2002): 1592–1594.

120. Martin I. Meltzer, Inger Damon, James W. LeDuc, et al., "Modeling Potential Responses to Smallpox as a Bioterrorist Weapon," *Emerging Infectious Diseases* 7

(2001): 959–969; Edward H. Kaplan, David L. Craft, and Lawrence M. Wein, "Emergency Response to a Smallpox Attack: The Case for Mass Vaccination," *Proceedings of the National Academy of Sciences* 99 (2002): 10935–10940.

121. David Brown, "Panel Alters Advice on Smallpox Shots; Wider Use for Health Workers Backed," *Washington Post*, October 17, 2002, A3; David Brown, "Panel Leery of Mass Smallpox Doses; Major Risks Outweigh Benefits of Immunizing the General Public, Experts Say," *Washington Post*, October 18, 2002, A2.

122. Robert J. Blendon, Catherine M. DesRoches, John M. Benson, et al., "The Public and the Smallpox Threat," *New England Journal of Medicine* 348 (2003): 426–432.

123. Ceci Connolly and Dana Milbank, "U.S. Revives Smallpox Shot; Bush Says He Will Receive Vaccine With Military, Emergency Workers," *Washington Post*, December 14, 2002, A1.

124. "Protection against Smallpox," *New York Times*, December 14, 2002, A28.

125. Lawrence K. Altman, "Limited Vaccination Plan Is Applauded," *New York Times*, December 14, 2002, A13.

126. Richard W. Stevenson and Sheryl Gay Stolberg, "Bush Lays Out Plan on Smallpox Shots; Military Is First," *New York Times*, December 14, 2002, A1.

127. William Foege, "Can Smallpox Be as Simple as 1–2–3?" *Washington Post*, December 29, 2002, B5.

128. Linda Rosenstock, "Smallpox Vaccine Policy Is Bad Science," *Los Angeles Times*, December 29, 2002.

129. Ceci Connolly, "Bush Smallpox Inoculation Plan Near Standstill," *Washington Post*, February 24, 2003, A6; "Smallpox Vaccination, United States, 2003: An Interim Report Card," in U.S. Department of Health and Human Services, *37th National Immunization Conference Proceedings* (Atlanta: Centers for Disease Control, 2003).

130. Gerald Markowitz and David Rosner, *Emergency Preparedness, Bioterrorism and the States: The First Two Years after September 11th* (New York: Milbank Memorial Fund, 2004); Daniel J. Kuhles and David M. Ackman, "The Federal Smallpox Vaccination Program: Where Do We Go from Here?" *Health Affairs* web exclusive, October 22, 2003, content.healthaffairs.org/cgi/reprint/hlthaff.w3.503v1.pdf (accessed February 1, 2004).

131. "Smallpox Vaccination Program Status by State," www.cdc.gov/od/oc/media/spvaccin.htm (accessed January 7, 2004).

132. Anita Manning, "Smallpox Vaccination Plan 'Ceased,'" *USA Today*, October 16, 2003, 1A.

133. "National, State, and Urban Area Vaccination Coverage among Children Aged 19–35 Months—United States, 2004," *Morbidity and Mortality Weekly Report* 54 (2005): 717–721.

134. Susan Y. Chu, Lawrence E. Barker, and Phillip J. Smith, "Racial/Ethnic Disparities in Preschool Immunizations: United States, 1996–2001," *American Journal of Public Health* 94 (2004): 973–977.

135. "National, State, and Urban Area Vaccination Coverage among Children Aged 19–35 Months—United States, 2003," *Morbidity and Mortality Weekly Report* 53 (July 30, 2004): 658–661.

136. James Colgrove and Ronald Bayer, "Could It Happen Here? Vaccine Safety Controversies and the Specter of Derailment," *Health Affairs* 24 (2005): 729–739.

137. Institute of Medicine, *Vaccine Safety Research, Data Access, and Public Trust* (Washington, D.C.: National Academies Press, 2004).

138. Anahad O'Connor and Gardiner Harris, "Health Agency Splits Program amid Vaccination Dispute," *New York Times*, February 25, 2005, 18.

139. Institute of Medicine, *Immunization Safety Review: Vaccines and Autism* (Washington, D.C.: National Academies Press, 2004).

140. Ibid.

141. "SafeMinds Analysis of IOM Report: The Failures, the Flaws and the Conflicts of Interest," news release, SafeMinds, Wednesday, May 19, 2004.

142. "A Statement by the Editors of The Lancet," February 23, 2004, The Lancet online, image.thelancet.com/extras/statement20Feb2004web.pdf (accessed March 4, 2004).

143. Anahad O'Connor, "Researchers Retract a Study Linking Autism to Vaccination," *New York Times*, March 4, 2004, A15.

144. *McCarthy v. Boozman*, 212 F. Supp. 2d 945; 948.

145. Salmon, Sapsin, Teret, et al., "Public Health and the Politics of School Immunization Requirements."

146. Institute of Medicine, *Financing Vaccines in the Twenty-First Century: Assuring Access and Availability* (Washington, D.C.: National Academies Press, 2004).

147. Robert Griffin, Kathleen Stratton, and Rosemary Chalk, "Childhood Vaccine Finance and Safety Issues," *Health Affairs* 23 (2004): 98–111; 106.

Archival Sources

Archives of the Evangelical Lutheran Church in America

Association of State and Territorial Health Officers Archives, History of Medicine Division, National Library of Medicine (ASTHO Archives, NLM)

Chicago Foreign Language Press Archive, Chicago Public Library

Herman Hilleboe Papers, Hammer Health Sciences Library Manuscripts and Special Collections, Columbia University

Louis I. Dublin Papers, History of Medicine Division, National Library of Medicine (Dublin Papers, NLM)

March of Dimes Archives, Series 3, Salk and Sabin Polio Vaccines (MOD)

Records of the Brooklyn Department of Health, Medical Research Library of Brooklyn, State University of New York

Records of the Centers for Disease Control and Prevention, National Archives and Records Administration, Record Group 442 (NARA, RG 442)

Records of the New York City Department of Health, New York City Municipal Archives (NYCDOH)

Records of the New York State Department of Health, New York State Archives (NYSDOH)

Records of the U.S. Public Health Service, National Archives and Records Administration, Record Group 90 (NARA, RG 90)

Index

317